Urinary Tract Infections: Pathogenesis and Clinical Management

Urinary Tract Infections: Pathogenesis and Clinical Management

Editor: Jameson Lopez

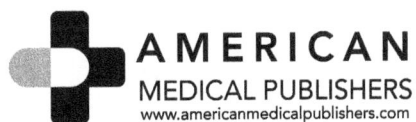

AMERICAN
MEDICAL PUBLISHERS
www.americanmedicalpublishers.com

AMERICAN
MEDICAL PUBLISHERS
www.americanmedicalpublishers.com

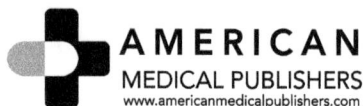

Cataloging-in-Publication Data

Urinary tract infections : pathogenesis and clinical management / edited by Jameson Lopez.
  p. cm.
Includes bibliographical references and index.
ISBN 978-1-63927-516-8
1. Urinary tract infections. 2. Urinary tract infections--Treatment.
3. Urinary organs--Diseases--Pathogenesis. I. Lopez, Jameson.
RC901.8 .U75 2022

616.6--dc23

American Medical Publishers,
41 Flatbush Avenue,
1st Floor, New York,
NY 11217, USA

ISBN 978-1-63927-516-8 (Hardback)

Contents

Preface IX

Chapter 1   The impact of trimethoprim-sulfamethoxazole as *Pneumocystis jiroveci*
pneumonia prophylaxis on the occurrence of asymptomatic bacteriuria and
urinary tract infections among renal allograft recipients 1
Ramandeep Singh, Frederike J. Bemelman, Caspar J. Hodiamont, Mirza M. Idu,
Ineke J. M. ten Berge and Suzanne E. Geerlings

Chapter 2   Carbapenem resistance, inappropriate empiric treatment and outcomes
among patients hospitalized with Enterobacteriaceae urinary tract infection,
pneumonia and sepsis 11
Marya D. Zilberberg, Brian H. Nathanson, Kate Sulham, Weihong Fan and
Andrew F. Shorr

Chapter 3   A single center observational study on emergency department clinician
non-adherence to clinical practice guidelines for treatment of uncomplicated
urinary tract infections 24
Catherine Zatorski, Mark Zocchi, Sara E. Cosgrove, Cynthia Rand, Gillian Brooks
and Larissa May

Chapter 4   Extended spectrum beta lactamase producing organisms causing urinary tract
infections in Sri Lanka and their antibiotic susceptibility pattern.................. 33
M. M. P. S. C. Fernando, W. A. N. V. Luke, J. K. N. D. Miththinda,
R. D. S. S. Wickramasinghe, B. S. Sebastiampillai, M. P. M. L. Gunathilake,
F. H. D. S. Silva and R. Premaratna

Chapter 5   Effect of prior receipt of antibiotics on the pathogen distribution and
antibiotic resistance profile of key Gram-negative pathogens among patients
with hospital-onset urinary tract infections 39
Monique R. Bidell, Melissa Palchak Opraseuth, Min Yoon, John Mohr and
Thomas P. Lodise

Chapter 6   Use of antimicrobial resistance information and prescribing guidance for
management of urinary tract infections: survey of general practitioners
in the West Midlands... 46
Dean Ironmonger, Obaghe Edeghere, Savita Gossain and Peter M. Hawkey

Chapter 7   Detection of CTX-M-15 beta-lactamases in Enterobacteriaceae causing
hospital- and community-acquired urinary tract infections as early as 2004,
in Dar es Salaam, Tanzania... 52
Joel Manyahi, Sabrina J. Moyo, Marit Gjerde Tellevik, Faustine Ndugulile,
Willy Urassa, Bjørn Blomberg and Nina Langeland

Chapter 8   Urinary tract infection among fistula patients admitted at Hamlin fistula
hospital, Addis Ababa, Ethiopia... 58
Matifan Dereje, Yimtubezinesh Woldeamanuel, Daneil Asrat and
Fekade Ayenachew

Chapter 9   **Cost-effectiveness of ceftolozane/tazobactam compared with piperacillin/tazobactam as empiric therapy based on the in-vitro surveillance of bacterial isolates in the United States for the treatment of complicated urinary tract infections** 66
Teresa L Kauf, Vimalanand S. Prabhu, Goran Medic, Rebekah H. Borse, Benjamin Miller, Jennifer Gaultney, Shuvayu S. Sen and Anirban Basu

Chapter 10   **Outcomes of high-dose levofloxacin therapy remain bound to the levofloxacin minimum inhibitory concentration in complicated urinary tract infections** 76
Eliana S. Armstrong, Janelle A. Mikulca, Daniel J. Cloutier, Caleb A. Bliss and Judith N. Steenbergen

Chapter 11   **Management of febrile urinary tract infection among spinal cord injured patients** 82
Aurélien Dinh, Adnène Toumi, Constance Blanc, Alexis Descatha, Frédérique Bouchand, Jérôme Salomon, Thomas Hanslik, Benjamin Bernuz, Pierre Denys and Louis Bernard

Chapter 12   **The influence of antibiotic prophylaxis on bacterial resistance in urinary tract infections in children with spina bifida** 88
Sebastiaan Hermanus Johannes Zegers, Jeanne Dieleman, Tjomme van der Bruggen, Jan Kimpen and Catharine de Jong-de Vos van Steenwijk

Chapter 13   **Characteristics of gram-negative urinary tract infections caused by extended spectrum beta lactamases: pivmecillinam as a treatment option within South Dublin, Ireland** 97
Fardod O'Kelly, Siobhan Kavanagh, Rustom Manecksha, John Thornhill and Jérôme P. Fennell

Chapter 14   **Antimicrobial susceptibilities of aerobic and facultative gram-negative bacilli isolated from Chinese patients with urinary tract infections between 2010 and 2014** 104
Qiwen Yang, Hui Zhang, Yao Wang, Zhipeng Xu, Ge Zhang, Xinxin Chen, Yingchun Xu, Bin Cao, Haishen Kong, Yuxing Ni, Yunsong Yu, Ziyong Sun, Bijie Hu, Wenxiang Huang, Yong Wang, Anhua Wu, Xianju Feng, Kang Liao, Yanping Luo, Zhidong Hu, Yunzhuo Chu, Juan Lu, Jianrong Su, Bingdong Gui, Qiong Duan, Shufang Zhang, Haifeng Shao and Robert E. Badal

Chapter 15   **Oral fosfomycin for treatment of urinary tract infection** 113
Philippa C. Matthews, Lucinda K. Barrett, Stephanie Warren, Nicole Stoesser, Mel Snelling, Matthew Scarborough and Nicola Jones

Chapter 16   **Randomized controlled trial of piperacillin-tazobactam, cefepime and ertapenem for the treatment of urinary tract infection caused by extended-spectrum beta-lactamase-producing *Escherichia coli*** 124
Yu Bin Seo, Jacob Lee, Young Keun Kim, Seung Soon Lee, Jeong-a Lee, Hyo Youl Kim, Young Uh, Han-Sung Kim and Wonkeun Song

Chapter 17   **Restriction of in vivo infection by antifouling coating on urinary catheter with controllable and sustained silver release** 133
Kedar Diwakar Mandakhalikar, Rong Wang, Juwita N. Rahmat, Edmund Chiong, Koon Gee Neoh and Paul A. Tambyah

Chapter 18   **Species distribution and antibiotic susceptibility profile of bacterial uropathogens among patients complaining urinary tract infections** 142
Adane Bitew, Tamirat Molalign and Meseret Chanie

Chapter 19   **The impact of cathelicidin, the human antimicrobial peptide LL-37 in urinary tract infections** 150
Ibrahim H. Babikir, Elsir A. Abugroun, Naser Eldin Bilal, Abdullah Ali Alghasham, Elmuataz Elmansi Abdalla and Ishag Adam

Chapter 20   **Empiric antibiotic therapy in urinary tract infection in patients with risk factors for antibiotic resistance in a German emergency department** 158
Sebastian Bischoff, Thomas Walter, Marlis Gerigk, Matthias Ebert and Roger Vogelmann

Chapter 21   **Hospitalization for community-acquired febrile urinary tract infection: validation and impact assessment of a clinical prediction rule** 165
Janneke E. Stalenhoef, Willize E. van der Starre, Albert M. Vollaard, Ewout W. Steyerberg, Nathalie M. Delfos, Eliane M.S. Leyten, Ted Koster, Hans C. Ablij, Jan W. van't Wout, Jaap T. van Dissel and Cees van Nieuwkoop

Chapter 22   **Carbapenem susceptibilities of Gram-negative pathogens in intra-abdominal and urinary tract infections: updated report of SMART 2015 in China** 174
Hui Zhang, Haishen Kong, Yunsong Yu, Anhua Wu, Qiong Duan, Xiaofeng Jiang, Shufang Zhang, Ziyong Sun, Yuxing Ni, Weiping Wang, Yong Wang, Kang Liao, Huayin Li, Chunxia Yang, Wenxiang Huang, Bingdong Gui, Bin Shan, Robert Badal, Qiwen Yang and Yingchun Xu

Chapter 23   **Prevalence and antibiotic susceptibility of Uropathogens from cases of urinary tract infections (UTI) in Shashemene referral hospital, Ethiopia** 182
Wubalem Desta Seifu and Alemayehu Desalegn Gebissa

Chapter 24   **Distribution of virulence genes and their association with antimicrobial resistance among uropathogenic *Escherichia coli* isolates from Iranian patients** 191
Yalda Malekzadegan, Reza Khashei, Hadi Sedigh Ebrahim-Saraie and Zahra Jahanabadi

Chapter 25   **Prevalence of antimicrobial resistant *Escherichia coli* from patients with suspected urinary tract infection in primary care, Denmark** 200
Gloria Córdoba, Anne Holm, Frank Hansen, Anette M. Hammerum and Lars Bjerrum

Permissions

List of Contributors

Index

Preface

It is often said that books are a boon to mankind. They document every progress and pass on the knowledge from one generation to the other. They play a crucial role in our lives. Thus I was both excited and nervous while editing this book. I was pleased by the thought of being able to make a mark but I was also nervous to do it right because the future of students depends upon it. Hence, I took a few months to research further into the discipline, revise my knowledge and also explore some more aspects. Post this process, I begun with the editing of this book.

The urinary tract includes the kidneys, urethra, ureters and bladder. They work together to eliminate waste from the body and regulate blood volume, blood pH and blood pressure. A urinary tract infection affects a part of the urinary tract. It is known as a bladder infection when it infects the lower urinary tract. When it affects the upper urinary tract, it is referred to as a kidney infection. The symptoms of the infection in the lower urinary tract involve pain with urination and frequent urination. A kidney infection shows symptoms like fever and flank pain. The major cause of infection is a bacterium known as Escherichia coli. It can also be caused by fungi and other bacteria. The risk factors for this infection are diabetes, obesity and genetics. This book presents researches and studies performed by experts across the globe. It brings forth some of the most innovative concepts and elucidates the unexplored aspects of urinary tract infections. Those in search of information to further their knowledge will be greatly assisted by this book.

I thank my publisher with all my heart for considering me worthy of this unparalleled opportunity and for showing unwavering faith in my skills. I would also like to thank the editorial team who worked closely with me at every step and contributed immensely towards the successful completion of this book. Last but not the least, I wish to thank my friends and colleagues for their support.

Editor

The impact of trimethoprim-sulfamethoxazole as *Pneumocystis jiroveci* pneumonia prophylaxis on the occurrence of asymptomatic bacteriuria and urinary tract infections among renal allograft recipients

Ramandeep Singh[1*], Frederike J. Bemelman[1], Caspar J. Hodiamont[2], Mirza M. Idu[3], Ineke J. M. ten Berge[1] and Suzanne E. Geerlings[4]

Abstract

Background: The international guidelines recommend the administration of trimethoprim-sulfamethoxazole (TMP-SMX) as *Pneumocystis jiroveci* pneumonia (PJP) prophylaxis for six months after transplantation. The aim of this study is to evaluate the influence of TMP-SMX prophylaxis on the occurrence of asymptomatic bacteriuria (ASB) and urinary tract infections (UTIs) as cystitis and allograft pyelonephritis (AGPN) and its impact on the antimicrobial resistance pattern of causative microorganisms.

Methods: We have conducted a retrospective before-after study in adult renal allograft recipients with one year follow-up after transplantation. We compared the ("after") group that received TMP-SMX as PJP prophylaxis to the ("before") group that did not receive it.

Results: In total, 343 renal allograft recipients were analysed, of whom 212 (61.8 %) received TMP-SMX as PJP prophylaxis. In this study, 63 (18.4 %) did only develop ASB without UTI, 26 (7.6 %) developed cystitis and 43 (12.5 %) developed AGPN. The remaining 211 (61.5 %) renal allograft recipients did not develop any bacteriuria at all. Multivariable Cox proportional regression analysis indicated that TMP-SMX as PJP prophylaxis was not associated with reduced prevalence of ASB (Hazard ratio (HR) = 1.52, 95 % CI = 0.79–2.94, *p* = 0.213), nor with reduced incidence of cystitis (HR = 2.21, 95 % CI = 0.76–6.39, *p* = 0.144), nor AGPN (HR = 1.12, 95 % CI = 0.57–2.21, *p* = 0.751). Among the group receiving TMP-SMX as PJP prophylaxis there was a trend was observed in increase of both amoxicillin (86 % versus 70 %) and TMP-SMX (89 % versus 48 %) resistance which already appeared within the first 30 days after TMP-SMX exposure.

(Continued on next page)

* Correspondence: r.singh@amc.uva.nl
[1]Department of Internal Medicine, Renal transplant Unit, Division of Nephrology, Academic Medical Center – University of Amsterdam, PO box 22660 ,1100 DD Amsterdam, The Netherlands
Full list of author information is available at the end of the article

(Continued from previous page)

Conclusions: Among renal allograft recipients, administration of TMP-SMX as PJP prophylaxis does not prevent ASB nor UTI, however it is associated with tendency towards increased amoxicillin and TMP-SMX resistance.

Keywords: Asymptomatic bacteriuria, Urinary tract infections, Renal transplantation, Trimethoprim-sulfamethoxazole, *Pneumocystis jiroveci* pneumonia prophylaxis

Background

Bacteriuria which is the most common infectious complication after renal transplantation [1] is categorised in asymptomatic bacteriuria (ASB) and urinary tract infections (UTIs) as cystitis and allograft pyelonephritis (AGPN). The incidence of bacteriuria is the highest within the first three months after renal transplantation [2] and many risk factors for bacteriuria in general and for both ASB and UTI separately have been described in the medical literature [3]. Administration of low dose antibiotics as UTI prophylaxis is commonly implemented within different patient groups. For example, among non-pregnant women experiencing recurrent UTIs, low dose antimicrobial prophylaxis has been shown to be effective in preventing UTIs [4]. Renal allograft recipients also receive low dose antibiotics, which is trimethoprim-sulfamethoxazole (TMP-SMX) intended as *Pneumocystis jiroveci* pneumonia (PJP) prophylaxis for six months after transplantation as recommended by international guidelines [2, 5].

The aim of this study is to evaluate the influence of TMP-SMX intended as PJP prophylaxis on both the prevalence of ASB and incidence of UTIs among renal allograft recipients. In addition to this, we also evaluate the impact of TMP-SMX as PJP prophylaxis on the antimicrobial resistance pattern of the microorganisms causing these bacteriuria events.

Methods

Study design

Retrospective before-after study with adult renal allograft recipients. The administration of TMP-SMX as PJP prophylaxis was implemented in June 2007. The "before" group consisted of those renal allograft recipients that did not receive TMP-SMX and the "after" group consisted of those who did receive it. We compared the group that received TMP-SMX as PJP prophylaxis to the group that did not receive it. Renal allograft recipients transplanted between July 2005 (start of implementing external stented ureterocystostomy) and 2009 were analysed, with one year follow-up after transplantation for developing bacteriuria.

Definitions

ASB was defined as a bacteriuria event (at least 10^5 colony-forming units (CFU)/ml) without any clinical symptoms suggestive for UTI [2, 6]. UTI was categorised into cystitis and AGPN. Cystitis was defined as the presence of leukocyturia (≥ 10 leukocytes per high power field microscopy analysis), bacteriuria ($\geq 10^4$ CFU/ml) with symptoms of the lower urinary tract (urgency, frequency and dysuria) without fever. AGPN was defined as the presence of leukocyturia, bacteriuria ($\geq 10^4$ colony-forming units (CFU)/ml) and fever (>38.0 °C) [2] with exclusion of other infectious cause for fever.

Delayed graft function was defined as the requirement of dialysis within the first week after transplantation [7]. Acute rejection episode was diagnosed through a renal allograft biopsy.

Cytomegalovirus (CMV) disease was defined as a positive quantitative polymerase chain reaction (PCR) with end organ involvement resulting in fever, gastrointestinal disease, pneumonia, hepatitis nephritis and/or retinitis as described by the guidelines [8, 9].

Renal allograft surgery procedures and medications

The renal allograft was positioned into the iliac fossa through an extraperitoneal approach. Cephamandole was routinely administered as peroperative antimicrobial prophylaxis. All renal allograft recipients received external stented ureterocystostomy with an 8 French catheter. This stent was inserted in the bladder through a suprapubic puncture and positioned in the pelvis of the renal allograft and was routinely removed after five days. The Foley catheter, which was inserted pre-operatively, was removed after seven days if urine leakage was excluded by cystography on that same day.

All renal allograft recipients receive triple immunosuppressive therapy which includes steroids combined with mycophenolate mofetil or mycophenolic acid and a calcineurin inhibitor, mostly tacrolimus but alternatively cyclosporine. If necessary, induction therapy with basiliximab was given pre-operatively according to the international guidelines [10].

Valganciclovir was provided for a period of six months after renal transplantation. Trimethoprim-sulfamethoxazole as PJP prophylaxis at a daily dose of 480 mg was implemented in June 2007. After transplantation, all renal allograft recipients received this prophylaxis for a period of six months. Recipients being allergic for, or having other contraindications for TMP-SMX did not receive TMP-SMX prophylaxis.

Patient follow-up after transplantation

After discharge from the renal transplantation ward, all renal transplant recipients were frequently followed within our outpatient clinics. During the first three months after transplantation, all renal allograft recipients were seen twice per week on average. Hereafter, renal allograft recipients were seen once a month within the first year after transplantation.

Surveillance for bacteriuria occurred through screening for leukocyturia within the urine sediment. In case of leukocyturia, a urine culture was taken. A urine culture was also taken in case of fever or urinary tract symptoms. On average, every renal allograft recipient received 22 urine sediment analyses/urine cultures within the first year after transplantation. Only ASB episodes occurring within the first three months after transplantation were treated. Hereafter, ASB was not systematically treated since the international guideline does not give a consensus of management [2, 11].

Susceptibility testing

Susceptibility testing was performed either using disk diffusion according to EUCAST criteria or using the VITEK2® system (BioMérieux, France). Interpretation of susceptibility results was performed using EUCAST breakpoints. Microorganisms were classified as "resistant" against a certain antimicrobial agent if the MIC reported by the VITEK2® system or the zone diameter using disk diffusion exceeded the breakpoint for susceptibility.

Antimicrobial resistance pattern and TMP-SMX exposure

To evaluate the impact of TMP-SMX as PJP prophylaxis on the antimicrobial resistance pattern of the causative microorganisms, we determined the frequency of resistance to amoxicillin, TMP-SMX, amoxicillin-clavulanic acid, ciprofloxacin and nitrofurantoin among *E. coli* isolates according to TMP-SMX exposure. These *E. coli* isolates were subcategorised in three arbitrary time-frames according to the time between transplantation and urine culture. The "early" time-frame consisted of *E. coli* isolates cultured within the first 30 days after transplantation, those cultured between 31 and 180 days were categorised within the "intermediate" time-frame. The third time-frame consisted of *E. coli* isolates cultured between 181 and 365 days were categorised into "late" time-frame.

Each UTI was considered as a unique episode. Multiple ASB episodes in one renal allograft recipient were considered as unique in case of different genus of the cultured causative microorganism. In case of multiple ASB episodes with the same causative microorganism; these cultures were considered as unique if there was at least one negative urine culture between them.

Statistical analysis

Statistical analysis was performed by using SPSS version 21 software (IBM SPSS Statistics for Windows, Version 21.0. Armonk, NY: IBM Corp.). Figures were made with GraphPad Prism version 5.00 for windows, GraphPad Software, San Diego California USA.

Continuous variables were expressed as the mean with its standard deviation in case of normal distribution. In case of non-normal distribution, the median and (25–75 %) interquartile range (IQR) were noted. In case of normal distribution, Student's t-test was used to compare continuous variables between two groups. In case of non-normal distribution Mann Whitney-U test was used. Categorical variables were expressed as proportion (n) and percentage (%), and were compared using Chi-square test.

To determine the risk factors for ASB and UTI (cystitis or AGPN), we compared the group that did not develop any bacteriuria at all (reference group) to the group that developed respectively only ASB, cystitis or AGPN. These events were analysed separately with Cox proportional hazard model analysis.

To determine the hazard of developing respectively ASB or UTI according to TMP-SMX as PJP prophylaxis use, we first performed univariable Cox proportional hazard model in which ASB or UTI were the dependent variable and TMP-SMX the independent variable. In the first multivariable model we adjusted for the group differences stratified according to TMP-SMX use. In the second multivariable model we adjusted for both the group differences according to TMP-SMX use and also for variables significantly associated with developing respectively ASB or UTI obtained by the univariable COX proportional hazard model. The results of these analysis were reported as hazard ratio (HR) with its 95 % confidence interval (95 % CI). The hazards were proportional over time, we tested this by defining the two groups as a function over time variable, which we divided into two equal periods. A p value smaller than 0.05 was considered as statistically significant.

Results

Comparison of the group without and with TMP-SMX as PJP prophylaxis

Table 1 gives an overview of the entire group according to TMP-SMX as PJP prophylaxis use. In total, 343 renal allograft recipients with one-year follow-up were analysed, 212 (61.8 %) received TMP-SMX as PJP prophylaxis in the "after" group. In total 17 renal allograft recipients transplanted after June 2007 did not receive TMP-SMX as result of allergy/intolerance and were classified in the "no TMP-SMX" group.

There were three significant differences between the group without and with TMP-SMX as PJP prophylaxis; diabetes mellitus ($p = 0.007$), indwelling urological catheters

Table 1 Comparison between the group without and with TMP-SMX as PJP prophylaxis

	Total $N = 343$ (100 %)	No TMP-SMX $N = 131$ (38.2 %)	TMP-SMX $N = 212$ (61.8 %)	P value
Variables				
Age recipient	52 (40–61)	52 (40–59)	52 (39–61)	0.420
BMI recipient	25.2 +/−4.5	24.7 +/− 4.2	25.5 +/−4.6	0.128
Female gender	152 (44.3)	65 (49.6)	87 (41.0)	0.120
Diabetes Mellitus (a)	94 (27.4)	25 (19.1)	69 (32.5)	0.007
Age donor	50 (40–57)	49 (39–57)	51 (41–57)	0.232
Allograft from deceased donor	215 (62.7)	83 (63.4)	132 (62.3)	0.839
Delayed graft function	109 (31.8)	42 (32.1)	67 (31.6)	0.930
Acute rejection	80 (23.3)	31 (23.7)	49 (23.1)	0.925
Indwelling urological catheter (b)	53 (15.5)	10 (7.6)	43 (20.3)	0.002
First transplantation	294 (85.7)	113 (86.3)	181 (85.4)	0.821
CMV disease	26 (7.6)	13 (9.9)	13 (6.1)	0.197
Maintenance therapy				<0.001
Tacrolimus-MMF-steroids	205 (59.8)	49 (37.4)	156 (73.2)	
MMF-cyclosporine-steroids	38 (11.1)	28 (21.4)	10 (4.7)	
MA-cyclosporine-steroids	100 (29.2)	54 (41.2)	46 (21.7)	
Induction therapy				
Basiliximab	216 (63.0)	82 (62.6)	134 (63.2)	0.909
Primary renal disease				
Hypertension	88 (25.7)	23 (17.6)	65 (30.7)	
Cystic renal disease	49 (14.3)	18 (13.7)	31 (14.6)	
IgA nephropathy	28 (8.2)	15 (11.5)	13 (6.1)	
Diabetes	20 (5.8)	7 (5.3)	13 (6.1)	
Focal segmental glomerulosclerosis	27 (7.9)	11 (8.4)	16 (7.5)	
Reflux and anatomical abnormalities	25 (7.3)	11 (8.4)	14 (6.6)	
Glomerulonephritis	26 (7.6)	10 (7.6)	16 (7.5)	
Unknown origin	27 (7.9)	12 (9.2)	15 (7.1)	
Others	53 (15.5)	24 (18.3)	29 (13.7)	
Bacteriuria outcomes:				
No bacteriuria	211 (61.5)	94 (71.7)	117 (55.2)	0.002
Bacteriuria	132 (38.5)	37 (28.2)	95 (44.8)	
Subtype of bacteriuria				
- only ASB	63 (18.4)	17 (13.0)	46 (21.7)	
- cystitis	26 (7.6)	5 (3.8)	21 (9.9)	
- AGPN	43 (12.5)	15 (11.5)	28 (13.2)	

Continuous variables are depicted as mean with +/− standard deviation or as median with (25–75 %) interquartile range. Nominal variables are depicted as the total number analysed with its percentage (%). *AGPN* allograft pyelonephritis, *ASB* asymptomatic bacteriuria, *CI* confidence interval, *CMV* cytomegalovirus, *MA* mycophenolic acid, *MMF* mycophenolate mofetil, *TMP-SMX* trimethoprim-sulfamethoxazole
a: The variable "diabetes mellitus" includes type 1, type 2 diabetes and new onset of diabetes after transplantation (NODAT), irrespective of whether it was the primary disease which led to renal failure. b: The variable "Indwelling urological catheter" represents Foley catheter, nephrostomy catheter and intermittent self-catheterisation

$(p = 0.002)$ and tacrolimus based immunosuppressive therapy $(p < 0.001)$ were more prevalent in the group receiving TMP-SMX as PJP prophylaxis in comparison to the group without it.

ASB and UTI rate according to TMP-SMX administration
Table 1 also displays the amount of bacteriuria according to TMP-SMX exposure. Within one year after transplantation, 211 (61.5 %) out of 343 renal allograft recipients did

The impact of trimethoprim-sulfamethoxazole as Pneumocystis jiroveci pneumonia prophylaxis...

5

not develop any episode of bacteriuria at all, 63 (18.4 %) recipients developed only ASB, 26 (7.6) developed cystitis and 43 (12.5) developed AGPN. In comparison to the group without TMP-SMX as PJP prophylaxis, bacteriuria more prevalent among the group that did receive it (44.8 % versus 28.2 %, $p = 0.002$).

Within one year after transplantation, the cumulative amount of unique bacteriuria episodes was 316 within the entire study group; 79 episodes (25.2 %) occurred in the group without TMP-SMX prophylaxis and 236 episodes (74.9 %) occurred in the group with this prophylaxis.

Risk factors for ASB and UTIs

Table 2 displays the univariable analysis of the variables associated with developing ASB, cystitis or AGPN respectively compared to the reference group that did not developed any bacteriuria at all. Risk factors for ASB were advanced age of the recipient (HR = 1.02, 95 % CI = 1.00–1.04, $p = 0.029$), female gender (HR = 2.01, 95 % CI = 1.22–3.33, $p = 0.007$) advanced age of the donor (HR = 1.03, 95 % CI = 1.01–1.05, $p = 0.010$) and indwelling urological catheters (HR = 12.94, 95 % CI = 7.76–21.57, $p < 0.001$).

Risk factors for cystitis were diabetes mellitus (HR = 1.13, 95 % CI = 1.45–6.75, $p = 0.004$), BMI of recipient (HR = 1.09, 95 % CI = 1.01–1.17, $p = 0.027$), receiving a renal allograft obtained from deceased donor (HR = 5.28, 95 % CI = 1.59–17.60, $p = 0.007$), delayed graft function (HR = 2.41, 95 % CI = 1.12–5.21, $p = 0.025$) and indwelling urological catheters (HR = 8.22, 95 % CI = 3.09–21.90, $p < 0.001$). The only identified risk factor for AGPN was the presence of an indwelling urological catheter (HR = 11.24, 95 % CI = 5.92–21.33, $P < 0.001$).

Influence of TMP-SMX as PJP prophylaxis on the occurrence of ASB and UTIs

Since the group without and with TMP-SMX as PJP prophylaxis were not comparable to each other on the variables diabetes mellitus, the presence of urological catheters and the subtype of the immunosuppressive therapy (Table 1), we performed multivariable Cox proportional hazard regression analysis in which we also adjusted for these three variables (Tables 3, 4 and 5).

In the univariable Cox proportional hazard regression analysis TMP-SMX was associated with developing ASB (HR = 2.03, 95 % CI = 1.17–3.55, $p = 0.012$) as shown in Table 3. After correcting for both the group differences according to TMP-SMX prophylaxis administration and for univariable risk factors for ASB (Table 3), TMP-SMX was not associated with reduced occurrence of ASB (HR = 1.52, 95 % CI = 0.79–2.94, $p = 0.213$).

In the univariable Cox proportional regression analysis, TMP-SMX was associated with developing cystitis (HR = 3.12, 95 % CI = 1.18–8.28, $p = 0.022$), however after adjustment for both the group differences according to TMP-SMX prophylaxis administration and univariable risk factors for developing cystitis (Table 4), TMP-SMX did not prevent cystitis (HR = 2.21, 95 % CI = 0.76–6.39, $p = 0.144$).

Administration of TMP-SMX as PJP prophylaxis was not associated with reduced incidence of AGPN in both univariable model (HR = 1.46, 95 % CI = 1.78–2.73, $p = 0.239$) nor in the adjusted model (HR = 1.12, 95 % CI = 0.57–2.21, $p = 0.751$) (Table 5).

To illustrate this, we additionally analysed the subgroup that did not develop diabetes, and never had indwelling urological catheter in situ ($n = 217$). For this subgroup, time between transplantation and respectively ASB, cystitis and AGPN is displayed in Fig. 1.

Causative microorganisms and antimicrobial resistance pattern

In total 315 unique bacteriuria episodes were identified within one year after transplantation. The majority of the causative microorganisms of the bacteriuria events were by *Escherichia coli* (*E. coli*) and *Enterococcus* spp. (Table 6).

Figure 2a displays the percentage of resistance for the five antibiotics among *E. coli* isolates. Among the *E. coli* isolates cultured from the group that received TMP-SMX as PJP prophylaxis, there was a tendency towards higher resistance rate for both amoxicillin (86 % versus 70 %) and TMP-SMX (89 % versus 48 %) compared to the group that did not receive it. No differences in resistance rates of amoxicillin-clavulanic acid, ciprofloxacin or nitrofurantoin were observed.

To evaluate the change in amoxicillin and TMP-SMX resistance in course of time after transplantation, we compared the percentage of resistance against these two antibiotics among *E. coli* isolates cultured within the first 30 days after transplantation ("early" time-frame), between 31 and 180 days ("intermediate" time-frame) and finally within 181–365 days ("late" time-frame) after transplantation (Fig. 2b and c). Among the group with TMP-SMX as PJP prophylaxis, the *E. coli* isolates cultured within the first 30 days after transplantation, had a higher resistance rate to amoxicillin (80 % versus 50 %) and TMP-SMX (83 % versus 13 %), in comparison to *E. coli* isolates within the same time frame but without TMP-SMX exposure.

Discussion

We were particularly interested whether TMP-SMX as PJP prophylaxis had any influence on the occurrence of ASB and UTI after renal transplantation. The administration of TMP-SMX as PJP prophylaxis was not associated with lower ASB prevalence nor lower UTI incidence. Furthermore, after TMP-SMX exposure, a tendency

Table 2 Univariable comparison between the group that did not develop any bacteriuria at all and the group that developed respectively only ASB, cystitis or AGPN

Variables	No bacteriuria versus only ASB				No bacteriuria versus cystitis			No bacteriuria versus AGPN		
	No bacteriuria (REF) N = 211 (61.5 %)	Only ASB N = 63 (18.4 %)	Univariable analysis HR (95 % CI)	P value	Cystitis N = 26 (7.6 %)	Univariable analysis HR (95 % CI)	P value	AGPN N = 43 (12.5 %)	Univariable analysis HR (95 % CI)	P value
TMP-SMX prophylaxis	117 (55.5)	46 (73.0)	2.03 (1.17–3.55)	0.012	21 (80.8)	3.12 (1.18–8.28)	0.022	28 (65.1)	1.46 (0.78–2.73)	0.239
Age of recipient	51 (38–59)	54 (46–64)	1.02 (1.00–1.04)	0.029	56 (44–60)	1.03 (1.00–1.06)	0.108	54 (38–62)	1.01 (0.99–1.04)	0.282
Female gender	85 (40.3)	38 (60.3)	2.01 (1.22–3.33)	0.007	13 (50.0)	1.43 (0.67–3.10)	0.357	16 (37.2)	1.18 (0.63–2.18)	0.610
Diabetes Mellitus (a)	49 (23.2)	19 (30.2)	1.37 (0.80–2.35)	0.250	13 (50.0)	3.13 (1.45–6.75)	0.004	13 (30.2)	1.39 (0.73–2.67)	0.320
BMI of recipient	25.0 +/–4.30	25.3 +/–4.35	1.02 (0.96–1.08)	0.576	27.0 +/–6.7	1.09 (1.01–1.17)	0.027	25.0 +/–3.9	1.00 (0.94–1.08)	0.932
Age of donor	49 (40–56)	53 (43–65)	1.03 (1.01–1.05)	0.010	51 (40–58)	1.00 (0.97–1.03)	0.738	48 (37–57)	1.00 (0.98–1.02)	0.992
Allograft from deceased donor	122 (57.8)	50 (79.4)	1.22 (0.73–2.03)	0.453	23 (88.5)	5.28 (1.59–17.60)	0.007	30 (69.8)	1.61 (0.84–3.09)	0.152
Delayed graft function	60 (28.4)	19 (30.2)	1.08 (0.63–1.84)	0.790	13 (50.0)	2.41 (1.12–5.21)	0.025	17 (39.5)	1.56 (0.85–2.87)	0.156
Acute rejection	43 (20.4)	19 (30.2)	1.56 (0.91–2.67)	0.109	8 (30.8)	1.64 (0.71–3.78)	0.244	10 (23.3)	1.12 (0.55–2.28)	0.751
Indwelling urological catheter (b)	5 (2.4)	28 (44.4)	12.94 (7.76–21.57)	<0.001	5 (19.2)	8.22 (3.09–21.90)	<0.001	15 (34.9)	11.24 (5.92–21.33)	<0.001
First transplantation	180 (85.3)	54 (85.7)	1.04 (0.52–2.11)	0.907	22 (84.6)	0.97 (0.34–2.83)	0.961	38 (88.4)	1.27 (0.50–3.22)	0.619
CMV disease	16 (7.6)	6 (9.5)	1.26 (0.54–2.92)	0.592	1 (3.8)	0.50 (0.07–3.66)	0.491	3 (7.0)	0.88 (0.28–2.87)	0.842
Maintenance therapy										
Tacrolimus + MMF + steroids	122 (57.8)	41 (65.1)	1.00		18 (69.2)	1.00		24 (55.8)	1.00	
MMF + cyclosporine + steroids	22 (10.4)	8 (12.7)	1.02 (0.48–2.19)	0.851	2 (7.7)	0.65 (0.15–2.81)	0.567	6 (14.0)	1.30 (0.53–3.19)	0.563
MA + cyclosporine + steroids	67 (31.8)	14 (22.2)	0.65 (0.35–1.19)	0.164	6 (23.1)	0.63 (0.25–1.57)	0.319	13 (30.2)	0.97 (0.49–1.90)	0.919
Induction therapy										
Basiliximab	134 (63.5)	39 (61.9)	0.94 (0.56–1.56)	0.805	43 (52.3)	0.58 (0.27–1.24)	0.159	30 (69.8)	1.28 (0.67–2.46)	0.455

Continuous variables are depicted as mean with +/− standard deviation or as median with (25–75 %) interquartile range. Nominal variables are depicted as the total number analysed with its percentage (%). *AGPN* allograft pyelonephritis, *ASB* asymptomatic bacteriuria, *CI* confidence interval, *CMV* cytomegalovirus, *MA* mycophenolic acid, *MMF* mycophenolate mofetil, *NA* not applicable, *HR* hazard ratio, *REF* reference, *TMP-SMX* trimethoprim-sulfamethoxazole

a: The variable "diabetes mellitus" includes type 1, type 2 diabetes and new onset of diabetes after transplantation (NODAT), irrespective of whether it was the primary disease which led to renal failure

b: The variable "Indwelling urological catheter" represents Foley catheter, nephrostomy catheter and intermittent self-catheterisation

Table 3 Univariable and multivariable Cox regression analysis for developing ASB within one year after transplantation according to TMP-SMX prophylaxis administration

	Outcome ASB HR (95 % CI)	P value
TMP-SMX: univariable model (a)	2.03 (1.17–3.55)	0.012
TMP-SMX: first multivariable model (b)	1.18 (0.63–2.20)	0.600
TMP-SMX: second multivariable model (c)	1.52 (0.79–2.94)	0.213

a: Univariable model: adjusted for only TMP-SMX use
b: First multivariable analysis: adjusted for diabetes mellitus, subtype of immunosuppressive therapy and indwelling urological catheters
c: Second multivariable analysis: adjusted for diabetes mellitus, subtype of immunosuppressive therapy, indwelling urological catheters, age of recipient and donor and female gender

Table 5 Univariable and multivariable Cox regression analysis for developing AGPN within one year after transplantation according to TMP-SMX prophylaxis administration

	Outcome AGPN HR (95 % CI)	P value
TMP-SMX: univariable model (a)	1.46 (0.78–2.73)	0.239
TMP-SMX: first multivariable model (b)	1.12 (0.57–2.21)	0.751

a: Univariable model: adjusted for only TMP-SMX use
b: First multivariable analysis: adjusted for diabetes mellitus, subtype of immunosuppressive therapy and indwelling urological catheters. Since indwelling urological catheters were the only risk factors for AGPN no second multivariable analysis has been performed

towards increased amoxicillin and TMP-SMX resistance was observed.

In this study, we observed that 18.4 % developed only ASB and 20.1 % developed UTI; of which 7.6 % developed cystitis and 12.5 % AGPN. In the medical literature, the incidence of bacteriuria shows a great variety as result of large differences in the used diagnostic criteria and frequency of routine urine culture testing [1, 12] The prevalence of ASB ranges between 17 % [13] and 40 % [14] within the first year after transplantation. Cystitis incidence has been reported at 12.2 % during three year follow-up [15] while the AGPN incidence ranges between 13 % [16] and 16.5 % [17] during four to ten year follow-up time.

Compared to the group without TMP-SMX as PJP prophylaxis, the group receiving TMP-SMX prophylaxis had significantly more bacteriuria as result of higher prevalence of diabetes and indwelling urological catheters. Increased diabetes prevalence in the group receiving TMP-SMX prophylaxis can most likely be explained by the more frequently administration of tacrolimus, which has decreased insulin sensitivity as a common side effect [18]. In addition to this, indwelling urological

Table 4 Univariable and multivariable Cox regression analysis for developing cystitis within one year after transplantation according to TMP-SMX prophylaxis administration

	Outcome cystitis HR (95 % CI)	P value
TMP-SMX: univariable model (a)	3.12 (1.18–8.28)	0.022
TMP-SMX: first multivariable model (b)	2.29 (0.79–6.67)	0.127
TMP-MSX: second multivariable model (c)	2.21 (0.76–6.39)	0.144

a: Univariable model: adjusted for only TMP-SMX use
b: First multivariable analysis: adjusted for diabetes mellitus, subtype of immunosuppressive therapy and indwelling urological catheters
c: Second multivariable analysis: adjusted for diabetes mellitus subtype of immunosuppressive therapy, indwelling urological catheters, BMI of recipient, type of renal allograft (obtained from a deceased versus living donor) and delayed graft function

catheters are a great risk factor for bacteriuria; it has been estimated that there is a daily risk of 5 % for developing bacteriuria after catheterisation and approximately 70 % of catheterised patients develop bacteriuria after 14 days [19, 20]. As result of these three differences, we performed multivariable Cox regression analysis in which we adjusted for these three variables and for the variables associated with developing respectively ASB, cystitis or AGPN. Within these multivariable models, administration of TMP-SMX as PJP prophylaxis was not associated with reduced occurrence of ASB, cystitis or AGPN. Comparable outcome has been observed by another research group which reported that the use of one double-strength tablet of TMP-SMX three times a week did not prevent UTI defined as cystitis and pyelonephritis [21]. However, another study [22] demonstrated that the addition of 30-day of ciprofloxacin to TMP-SMX prophylaxis lowered the incidence of UTI in comparison to TMP-SMX prophylaxis alone. Interestingly, no difference was observed in the incidence of pyelonephritis.

The observation that TMP-SMX does not prevent ASB nor UTIs could likely be explained by the great potency of gram negative bacteria for developing TMP-SMX resistance after exposure to it. Indeed, it has been shown that TMP-SMX exposure results in TMP-SMX resistance in *E. coli*, which is even observed after one month of TMP-SMX administration [23].

The first clinical trials evaluating the effect of antimicrobial prophylaxis on the incidence of bacteriuria among renal allograft recipients were performed in late eighties and early nineties of the last millennium [24–26]. In these studies, TMP-SMX was used as prophylaxis. The intervariability of TMP-SMX dose between these studies was large and ranged between 480 mg once a day to 960 mg twice a day. Also the duration of antimicrobial prophylaxis administration differed. A systematic review [27] which also included these studies concluded that antimicrobial prophylaxis indeed reduces bacteriuria and bacteraemia. However the analysed original intervention studies did not mention the clinical symptoms associated with

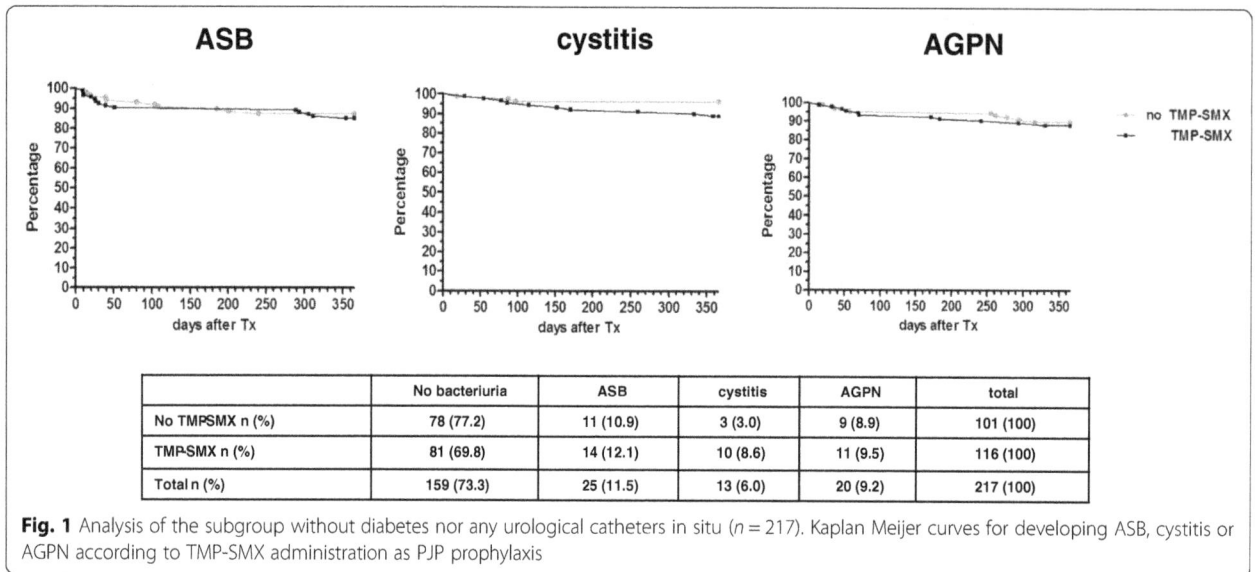

	No bacteriuria	ASB	cystitis	AGPN	total
No TMPSMX n (%)	78 (77.2)	11 (10.9)	3 (3.0)	9 (8.9)	101 (100)
TMP-SMX n (%)	81 (69.8)	14 (12.1)	10 (8.6)	11 (9.5)	116 (100)
Total n (%)	159 (73.3)	25 (11.5)	13 (6.0)	20 (9.2)	217 (100)

Fig. 1 Analysis of the subgroup without diabetes nor any urological catheters in situ ($n = 217$). Kaplan Meijer curves for developing ASB, cystitis or AGPN according to TMP-SMX administration as PJP prophylaxis

bacteriuria. Therefore in these studies, it is difficult to determine whether TMP-SMX at prophylactic dose prevents ASB or UTI, or possibly both.

The second aim of our study was to evaluate the impact of TMP-SMX as PJP prophylaxis on the antimicrobial resistance pattern of the causative microorganisms. Among *E. coli* isolates cultured within the first 30 days after transplantation, there was an increase in both amoxicillin and TMP-SMX resistance after TMP-SMX exposure. This co-resistance of TMP-SMX with amoxicillin has also been described in other studies [23, 28] and is a common finding, since the resistance genes of these antimicrobials are located on the same plasmid [28–30]. However as a limitation, our study was not powered to observe statistical significant differences in antimicrobial resistance according to TMP-SMX exposure, therefore no statistical tests were performed in this analysis.

We also observed that the difference in amoxicillin resistance with and without TMP-SMX did not differ anymore

among *E. coli* isolates cultured between 181 and 365 days after renal transplantation reflecting the antimicrobial resistance drift, since the likelihood of exposure to antibiotics increases in course of time. Indeed, excessive exposure to antibiotics is the greatest contributing factor for developing antimicrobial resistance [31]. However, among the *E. coli* isolates cultured between 181 and 365 days after transplantation, there was still a difference noticeable in TMP-SMX resistance with and without TMP-SMX exposure, indicating that TMP-SMX resistance developed after subsequent six months of TMP-SMX exposure might be able to persist for a longer period of time after discontinuation.

In this study we analysed renal allograft recipients transplanted between 2005 and 2009; a possibility exist that the increase of amoxicillin and TMP-SMX resistance according to TMP-SMX exposure could be influenced by an increase in antimicrobial resistance rate in course of time (background resistance). To evaluate this, we compared our data about the increase in amoxicillin and TMP-SMX resistance among *E. coli* isolates within this study, to those *E. coli* isolates cultured within unselected hospital departments across the Netherlands between 2005 and 2009. Within this time span, amoxicillin resistance rate among *E. coli* steadily increased from 44 to 48 % [32]. The background TMP-SMX resistance did not increase above 30 % in 2009 [32]. This increase in background antimicrobial resistance is smaller than the increase in antimicrobial resistance observed in our study population, which could be attributed to the six months exposure to TMP-SMX as PJP prophylaxis.

The unique aspect of this study is the comparison of a relative large group of renal allograft recipients who received TMP-SMX intended as PJP prophylaxis to a group who did not receive it. The limitations of our study are

Table 6 Causative microorganisms of the unique bacteriuria episode according to TMP-SMX prophylaxis administration

	Entire cohort	No TMP-SMX	TMP-SMX
	$N = 315$ (100 %)	$N = 79$ (25.2 %)	$N = 236$ (74.9 %)
Escherichia coli	128 (40.6)	31 (39.2)	97 (41.1)
Enterococcus spp.	70 (22.2)	18 (22.8)	52 (22.0)
Enterobacter spp.	15 (4.8)	7 (8.9)	8 (3.4)
Klebsiella spp.	20 (6.3)	2 (2.5)	18 (7.6)
Proteus spp.	12 (3.8)	6 (7.6)	6 (2.6)
Pseudomonas spp.	38 (12.1)	7 (8.9)	31 (13.1)
Others	32 (10.2)	8 (10.1)	24 (10.2)

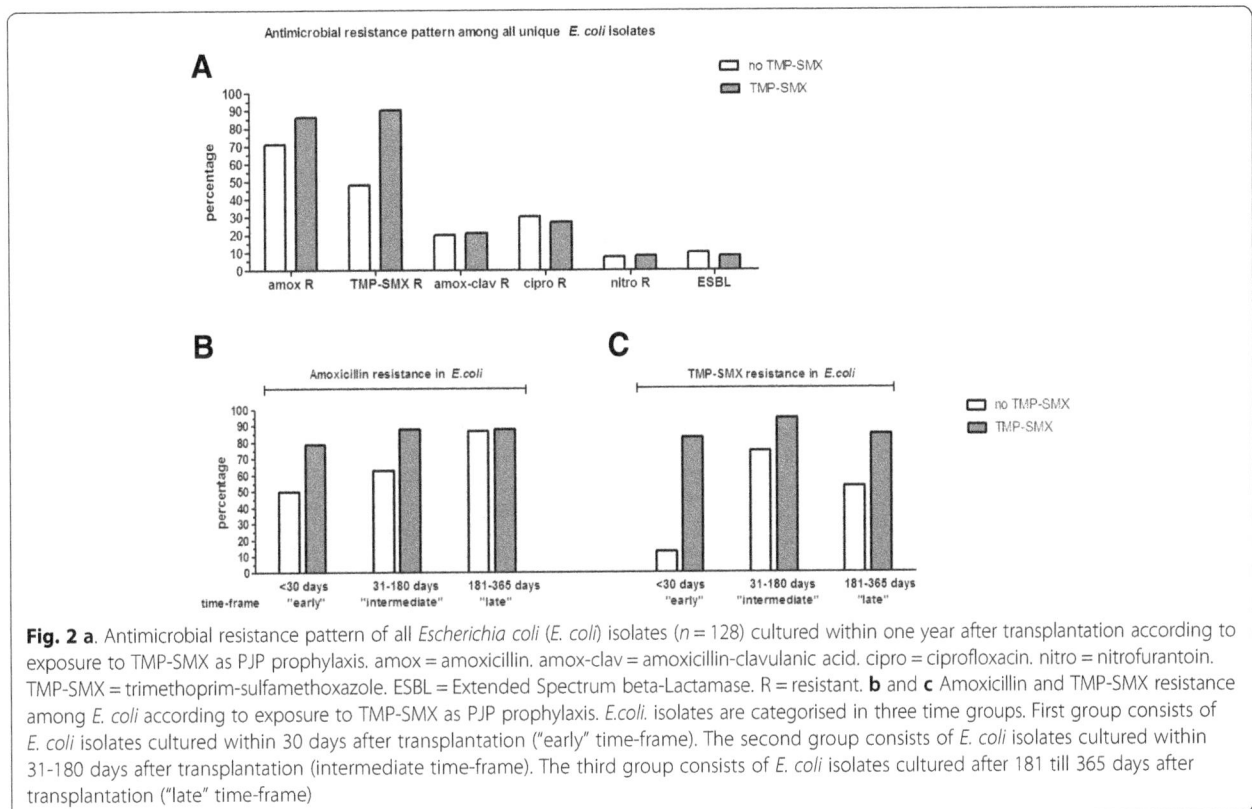

Fig. 2 a. Antimicrobial resistance pattern of all *Escherichia coli* (*E. coli*) isolates (*n* = 128) cultured within one year after transplantation according to exposure to TMP-SMX as PJP prophylaxis. amox = amoxicillin. amox-clav = amoxicillin-clavulanic acid. cipro = ciprofloxacin. nitro = nitrofurantoin. TMP-SMX = trimethoprim-sulfamethoxazole. ESBL = Extended Spectrum beta-Lactamase. R = resistant. **b** and **c** Amoxicillin and TMP-SMX resistance among *E. coli* according to exposure to TMP-SMX as PJP prophylaxis. *E.coli*. isolates are categorised in three time groups. First group consists of *E. coli* isolates cultured within 30 days after transplantation ("early" time-frame). The second group consists of *E. coli* isolates cultured within 31-180 days after transplantation (intermediate time-frame). The third group consists of *E. coli* isolates cultured after 181 till 365 days after transplantation ("late" time-frame)

related to the retrospective and non-interventional setup. In retrospective studies, the determination of ASB prevalence is less accurate than determining UTI incidence because UTI is diagnosed by the presence of predefined clinical UTI symptoms accompanied by bacteriuria, while the rate of ASB is heavily influenced by the frequency of routine urine culturing [33]. Therefore, the likelihood for ASB detection increases by frequent urine culturing. To exclude potential bias caused by the frequency of testing, we analysed each ASB patient only once to determine risk factors for ASB. Another limitation of this study may be the policy of not systematically treating ASB episodes occurring three months after transplantation. Due to the retrospective setup, it is difficult to determine which circumstances resulted in the decision to treat a certain ASB episode occurring after three months transplantation.

Conclusions

Our retrospective before-after study indicates that TMP-SMX prophylaxis does not have an additional bacteriuria preventive property besides PJP prevention. However it may have a certain contribution to an increase in amoxicillin and TMP-SMX resistance. Despite great advances made in renal transplantation medicine, there is still a need for effective UTI preventive measures among renal allograft recipients.

Ethical consent

Due to the retrospective study setup, ethics approval was waived by the Medical Ethics Review Committee of the Academic Medical Center (Amsterdam, the Netherlands), where this study was performed.

Abbreviations

AGPN: allograft pyelonephritis; ASB: asymptomatic bacteriuria; CFU: colony forming unit; CI: confidence interval; CMV: cytomegalovirus; E. coli: *Escherichia coli*; HR: hazard ratio; PJP: *Pneumocystis jiroveci* pneumonia; TMP-SMX: trimethoprim-sulfamethoxazole; Tx: transplantation; UTI: urinary tract infection.

Competing interests

The authors declare that they have no competing interests.

Authors' contributions

RS study setup, data collection, data analysis and interpretation. Contribution in writing the manuscript. FJB study setup, data analysis and interpretation. Contribution in writing the manuscript. Supervisor of the project. CJH data collection, data analysis. Contribution in writing the manuscript. MMI data analysis and interpretation. Contribution in writing the manuscript. Transplant surgeon of the analysed patients. IJMtB data analysis and interpretation. Contribution in writing the manuscript. SEG study setup, data analysis and interpretation. Contribution in writing the manuscript. Supervisor of the project. All authors have read the final manuscript and approved the contents.

Author details
[1]Department of Internal Medicine, Renal transplant Unit, Division of Nephrology, Academic Medical Center – University of Amsterdam, PO box 22660 ,1100 DD Amsterdam, The Netherlands. [2]Department of Medical Microbiology, Academic Medical Center – University of Amsterdam, PO box 226601100 DD Amsterdam, The Netherlands. [3]Department of Surgery, Division of Vascular Surgery, Academic Medical Center – University of Amsterdam, PO box 226601100 DD Amsterdam, The Netherlands. [4]Department of Internal Medicine, Division of Infectious Diseases, Academic Medical Center-University of Amsterdam, PO box 226601100 DD Amsterdam, The Netherlands.

References

1. Alangaden G. Urinary tract infections in renal transplant recipients. Curr Infect Dis Rep. 2007;9(6):475–9.
2. Parasuraman R, Julian K. Urinary tract infections in solid organ transplantation. Am J Transplant. 2013;13 Suppl 4:327–36.
3. Singh R, Geerlings SE, Bemelman FJ. Asymptomatic bacteriuria and urinary tract infections among renal allograft recipients. Curr Opin Infect Dis. 2015; 28(1):112–6.
4. Albert X, Huertas I, Pereiro, II, Sanfelix J, Gosalbes V, Perrota C. Antibiotics for preventing recurrent urinary tract infection in non-pregnant women. Cochrane Database Syst Rev. 2004(3):Cd001209.
5. Kasiske BL, Zeier MG, Chapman JR, Craig JC, Ekberg H, Garvey CA, Green MD, Jha V, Josephson MA, Kiberd BA et al. KDIGO clinical practice guideline for the care of kidney transplant recipients: a summary. Kidney Int. 2010; 77(4):299–311.
6. Nicolle LE, Bradley S, Colgan R, Rice JC, Schaeffer A, Hooton TM. Infectious Diseases Society of America guidelines for the diagnosis and treatment of asymptomatic bacteriuria in adults. Clin Infect Dis. 2005;40(5):643–54.
7. Halloran PF, Hunsicker LG. Delayed graft function: state of the art, November 10–11, 2000. Summit meeting, Scottsdale, Arizona, USA. Am J Transplant. 2001; 1(2):115–20.
8. Ljungman P, Griffiths P, Paya C. Definitions of cytomegalovirus infection and disease in transplant recipients. Clin Infect Dis. 2002;34(8):1094–7.
9. Preiksaitis JK, Brennan DC, Fishman J, Allen U. Canadian society of transplantation consensus workshop on cytomegalovirus management in solid organ transplantation final report. Am J Transplant. 2005;5(2):218–27.
10. Kasiske BL, Zeier MG, Craig JC, Ekberg H, Garvey CA, Green MD, et al. KDIGO clinical practice guideline for the care of kidney transplant recipients. Am J Transplant. 2009;9(Suppl 3):S1–155.
11. Rice JC, Safdar N. Urinary tract infections in solid organ transplant recipients. Am J Transplant. 2009;9 Suppl 4:S267–72.
12. Saemann M, Horl WH. Urinary tract infection in renal transplant recipients. Eur J Clin Investig. 2008;38 Suppl 2:58–65.
13. Green H, Rahamimov R, Goldberg E, Leibovici L, Gafter U, Bishara J, Mor E, Paul M. Consequences of treated versus untreated asymptomatic bacteriuria in the first year following kidney transplantation: retrospective observational study. Eur J Clin Microbiol Infect Dis. 2013;32(1):127–31.
14. Golebiewska JE, Debska-Slizien A, Rutkowski B. Treated asymptomatic bacteriuria during first year after renal transplantation. Transpl Infect Dis. 2014;16(4):605–15.
15. Fiorante S, Fernandez-Ruiz M, Lopez-Medrano F, Lizasoain M, Lalueza A, Morales JM, San-Juan R, Andres A, Otero JR, Aguado JM . Acute graft pyelonephritis in renal transplant recipients: incidence, risk factors and long-term outcome. Nephrol Dial Transplant. 2011;26(3):1065–73.
16. Giral M, Pascuariello G, Karam G, Hourmant M, Cantarovich D, Dantal J, Blancho G, Coupel S, Josien R, Daguin P et al. Acute graft pyelonephritis and long-term kidney allograft outcome. Kidney Int. 2002;61(5):1880–6.
17. Kamath NS, John GT, Neelakantan N, Kirubakaran MG, Jacob CK. Acute graft pyelonephritis following renal transplantation. Transpl Infect Dis. 2006;8(3):140–7.
18. Chen QJ, Li J, Zuo SR, Zhang YP, Jia SJ, Yuan H, Liu SK, Cheng K, Ming YZ, Zuo XC, et al. Tacrolimus decreases insulin sensitivity without reducing fasting insulin concentration: a 2-year follow-up study in kidney transplant recipients. Ren Fail. 2015;1–6.
19. Pickard R, Lam T, Maclennan G, Starr K, Kilonzo M, McPherson G, Gillies K, McDonald A, Walton K, Buckley B, et al. Types of urethral catheter for reducing symptomatic urinary tract infections in hospitalised adults requiring short-term catheterisation: multicentre randomised controlled trial and economic evaluation of antimicrobial- and antiseptic-impregnated urethral catheters (the CATHETER trial). Health Technol Assess (Winchester, England). 2012;16(47):1–197.
20. Haley RW, Hooton TM, Culver DH, Stanley RC, Emori TG, Hardison CD, Quade D, Shachtman RH, Schaberg DR, Shah BV, et al. Nosocomial infections in U.S. hospitals, 1975–1976: estimated frequency by selected characteristics of patients. Am J Med. 1981;70(4):947–59.
21. Vidal E, Torre-Cisneros J, Blanes M, Montejo M, Cervera C, Aguado JM, Len O, Carratala J, Cordero E, Bou G, et al. Bacterial urinary tract infection after solid organ transplantation in the RESITRA cohort. Transpl Infect Dis. 2012; 14(6):595–603.
22. Wojciechowski D, Chandran S. Effect of ciprofloxacin combined with sulfamethoxazole-trimethoprim prophylaxis on the incidence of urinary tract infections after kidney transplantation. Transplantation. 2013;96(4):400–5.
23. Beerepoot MA, ter Riet G, Nys S, van der Wal WM, de Borgie CA, de Reijke TM, et al. Lactobacilli vs antibiotics to prevent urinary tract infections: a randomized, double-blind, noninferiority trial in postmenopausal women. Arch Intern Med. 2012;172(9):704–12.
24. Fox BC, Sollinger HW, Belzer FO, Maki DG. A prospective, randomized, double-blind study of trimethoprim-sulfamethoxazole for prophylaxis of infection in renal transplantation: clinical efficacy, absorption of trimethoprim-sulfamethoxazole, effects on the microflora, and the cost-benefit of prophylaxis. Am J Med. 1990;89(3):255–74.
25. Maki DG, Fox BC, Kuntz J, Sollinger HW, Belzer FO. A prospective, randomized, double-blind study of trimethoprim-sulfamethoxazole for prophylaxis of infection in renal transplantation. Side effects of trimethoprim-sulfamethoxazole, interaction with cyclosporine. J Lab Clin Med. 1992;119(1):11–24.
26. Tolkoff-Rubin NE, Cosimi AB, Russell PS, Rubin RH. A controlled study of trimethoprim-sulfamethoxazole prophylaxis of urinary tract infection in renal transplant recipients. Rev Infect Dis. 1982;4(2):614–8.
27. Green H, Rahamimov R, Gafter U, Leibovitci L, Paul M. Antibiotic prophylaxis for urinary tract infections in renal transplant recipients: a systematic review and meta-analysis. Transpl Infect Dis. 2011;13(5):441–7.
28. den Heijer CD, Beerepoot MA, Prins JM, Geerlings SE, Stobberingh EE. Determinants of antimicrobial resistance in Escherichia coli strains isolated from faeces and urine of women with recurrent urinary tract infections. PLoS One. 2012;7(11), e49909.
29. Kahlmeter G, Menday P. Cross-resistance and associated resistance in 2478 Escherichia coli isolates from the Pan-European ECO.SENS Project surveying the antimicrobial susceptibility of pathogens from uncomplicated urinary tract infections. J Antimicrob Chemother. 2003;52(1):128–31.
30. Amyes SG. The success of plasmid-encoded resistance genes in clinical bacteria. An examination of plasmid-mediated ampicillin and trimethoprim resistance genes and their resistance mechanisms. J Med Microbiol. 1989;28(2):73–83.
31. Rao GG. Risk factors for the spread of antibiotic-resistant bacteria. Drugs. 1998;55(3):323–30.
32. Hoogkamp-Korstanje JAA, Mouton JW, Sande-Bruinsma N. NETHMAP 2011 Consumption of antimicrobial agents and antimicrobial resistance among medically important bacteria in the Netherlands. 2011.
33. Mitra S, Alangaden GJ. Recurrent urinary tract infections in kidney transplant recipients. Curr Infect Dis Rep. 2011;13(6):579–87.

Carbapenem resistance, inappropriate empiric treatment and outcomes among patients hospitalized with Enterobacteriaceae urinary tract infection, pneumonia and sepsis

Marya D. Zilberberg[1*], Brian H. Nathanson[2], Kate Sulham[3], Weihong Fan[3] and Andrew F. Shorr[4]

Abstract

Background: Drug resistance among gram-negative pathogens is a risk factor for inappropriate empiric treatment (IET), which in turn increases the risk for mortality. We explored the impact of carbapenem-resistant Enterobacteriaceae (CRE) on the risk of IET and of IET on outcomes in patients with Enterobacteriaceae infections.

Methods: We conducted a retrospective cohort study in Premier Perspective database (2009–2013) of 175 US hospitals. We included all adult patients with community-onset culture-positive urinary tract infection (UTI), pneumonia, or sepsis as a principal diagnosis, or as a secondary diagnosis in the setting of respiratory failure, treated with antibiotics within 2 days of admission. We employed regression modeling to compute adjusted association of presence of CRE with risk of receiving IET, and of IET on hospital mortality, length of stay (LOS) and costs.

Results: Among 40,137 patients presenting to the hospital with an Enterobacteriaceae UTI, pneumonia or sepsis, 1227 (3.1%) were CRE. In both groups, the majority of the cases were UTI (51.4% CRE and 54.3% non-CRE). Those with CRE were younger (66.6+/−15.3 vs. 69.1+/−15.9 years, $p < 0.001$), and more likely to be African-American (19.7% vs. 14.0%, $p < 0.001$) than those with non-CRE. Both chronic (Charlson score 2.0+/−2.0 vs. 1.9+/−2.1, $p = 0.009$) and acute (by day 2: ICU 56.3% vs. 30.4%, $p < 0.001$, and mechanical ventilation 35.8% vs. 11.7%, $p < 0.001$) illness burdens were higher among CRE than non-CRE subjects, respectively. CRE patients were 3× more likely to receive IET than non-CRE (46.5% vs. 11.8%, $p < 0.001$). In a regression model CRE was a strong predictor of receiving IET (adjusted relative risk ratio 3.95, 95% confidence interval 3.5 to 4.5, $p < 0.001$). In turn, IET was associated with an adjusted rise in mortality of 12% (95% confidence interval 3% to 23%), and an excess of 5.2 days (95% confidence interval 4.8, 5.6, $p < 0.001$) LOS and $10,312 (95% confidence interval $9497, $11,126, $p < 0.001$) in costs.

Conclusions: In this large US database, the prevalence of CRE among patients with Enterobacteriaceae UTI, pneumonia or sepsis was comparable to other national estimates. Infection with CRE was associated with a four-fold increased risk of receiving IET, which in turn increased mortality, LOS and costs.

Keywords: UTI, Pneumonia, Sepsis, Enterobacteriaceae, Antimicrobial resistance, Inappropriate empiric therapy, Hospital mortality, Hospital cost

* Correspondence: evimedgroup@gmail.com
[1]EviMed Research Group, LLC, PO Box 303, Goshen, MA 01032, USA
Full list of author information is available at the end of the article

Background

Initial antibiotic therapy affects outcomes in severe infection. For empiric therapy to have a benefit on patient outcomes, it must not only be given in a timely manner but must also be active in vitro against the infecting pathogen. Many studies indicate that either delaying antibiotic therapy or selecting a treatment to which the infecting pathogen is non-susceptible increases the risk for death 2–5-fold [1–13]. Therefore, clinicians must be aware of the common pathogens in specific infectious syndromes and of local antimicrobial susceptibility patterns in order to make appropriate choices for antimicrobial therapies. Unfortunately, rapidly rising rates of resistance and shifting resistance patterns render ensuring appropriate empiric coverage a challenge [14].

Recently, the Centers for Disease Control and Prevention have identified carbapenem-resistance among Enterobacteriaceae as an urgent threat in the US [15]. Though Enterobacteriaceae are common pathogens in pneumonia, urinary tract infections and sepsis and thus are often treated in most empiric coverage recommendations, the escalating frequency of carbapenem resistance in these pathogens makes ensuring initially appropriate antimicrobial treatment in areas where carbapenem-resistant Enterobacteriaceae (CRE) are prevalent nearly impossible [13, 14, 16–19]. Furthermore, administering broad-spectrum agents to all severely ill patients in order not to miss some individual with a rare highly resistant pathogen is not a sustainable practice, since the concerns for promoting further resistance may outweigh any potential benefit to patient-specific outcomes. In this way, the dilemma of CREs amplifies the tension between public (preservation of antimicrobial activity) and patient-level (optimizing clinical outcomes) health imperatives.

It remains unclear if the nexus between inappropriate therapy and outcomes seen with other pathogens exists in the case of infections due to CRE. Few analyses have specifically addressed this issue, while some that have attempted this lacked the ability to delineate the impact of inappropriate empiric therapy of CREs on attributable morbidity or on resources such as length of stay (LOS) [20, 21]. To understand better the relationship between carbapenem-resistance, choice of inappropriate empiric therapy (IET), and key hospital outcomes, we conducted a cohort study of patients admitted to the hospital with community-onset urinary tract infections (UTI), pneumonia and sepsis due to Enterobacteriaceae.

Methods

This was a multi-center retrospective cohort study of patients admitted to the hospital with pneumonia, sepsis and UTI (referred to from here on as "UTI"), or sepsis from another source in the Premier Research database in the years 2009–2013. We hypothesized that infection with a CRE phenotype increased the risk of receiving IET. In turn, we hypothesized that the receipt of IET is adversely associated with hospital mortality, LOS, and costs.

Because this study used already existing fully de-identified retrospective data, it was exempt from IRB review.

Since the data source was the same and methods utilized in this study were similar to those used in our previous study, please refer to that paper for details [22].

Patient population

Patients were included if they were adults (age ≥ 18 years) hospitalized with a UTI International Classification of Diseases, version 9, Clinical Modification (ICD-9-CM) codes (principal diagnosis 112.2, 590.1, 590.11, 590.2, 590.3, 590.8.590.81, 595, 597, 599 or 996.64, or principal sepsis diagnosis [see below] with UTI as a secondary diagnosis), pneumonia ICD-9-CM codes (principal diagnosis 481–486, or respiratory failure codes [518.81 or 518.84] with pneumonia as a secondary diagnosis) or sepsis codes from another source (principal diagnosis 038, 038.9, 020.0, 790.7, 995.92 or 785.52, or respiratory failure codes [518.81 or 518.84] with sepsis coded as a secondary diagnosis) [23–27]. In order to eliminate confounding of the outcomes by pre-infection onset hospital events, only patients with infection present on admission, as evidenced by antibiotic treatment beginning within the first 2 days of hospitalization and continuing for at least 3 consecutive days, or until discharge, were included [24–26]. Patients were excluded if they were transferred from another acute care facility, if they were diagnosed with cystic fibrosis, or if their hospital length of stay (LOS) was 1 day or less. Those who met criteria for both UTI and sepsis or pneumonia and sepsis were included in the UTI or pneumonia group, respectively. Those with both UTI and pneumonia were analyzed with the pneumonia group. Patients were followed until death in or discharge from the hospital.

Data source

The data for the study derived from Premier Research database, an electronic laboratory, pharmacy and billing data repository, for years 2009 through 2013, which contains approximately 15% of all hospitalizations nationwide. For detailed description of the dataset, please, refer to citation #22.

Baseline variables

We classified each community-onset infection (UTI, pneumonia or sepsis) as healthcare-associated (HCA) if one or more of the following risk factors was present: 1) prior hospitalization within 90 days of the index hospitalization, 2) hemodialysis, 3) admission from a long-term care facility, 4) immune suppression [3, 6, 16, 23–26]. All other infections were considered to be community-acquired (CA). For other patient factors and hospital-level variables, please see citation #22.

Microbiology and treatment variables and definitions

Urinary, blood and respiratory cultures had to be obtained within the first 2 days of hospitalization.

The following organisms were defined as Enterobacteriaceae of interest:

1. *Escherichia coli*
2. *Klebsiella pneumoniae*
3. *Klebsiella oxytoca*
4. *Enterobacter cloacae*
5. *Enterobacter aerogenes*
6. *Proteus mirabilis*
7. *Proteus spp.*
8. *Serratia marcescens*
9. *Citrobacter freundii*
10. *Morganella morganii*
11. *Providencia spp.*

Premier database receives organism susceptibility reports from individual institutions' laboratories as S (susceptible), I (intermediate) or R (resistant). Although no MIC data are available in the database, all microbiology testing was performed locally at the institutions contributing the data and conformed to the CLSI standards. Carbapenem-resistant Enterobacteriaceae were defined as one of the above organisms where susceptibility testing yielded an I or R result to at least one of the four carbapenems: imipenem, meropenem, ertapenem or doripenem.

IET was present if the antibiotic administered for the infection did not cover the organism or if appropriate coverage did not start within 2 days of the positive culture being obtained.

Statistical analyses

We compared characteristics of patients infected with CRE to those infected with carbapenem-susceptible Enterobacteriaceae (CSE) and those treated with IET to those treated with non-IET. All unadjusted comparisons were done using standard methods described in detail in citation #22.

We developed a generalized logistic regression model to explore the relationship between CRE and the risk of IET. Covariates in the model were identical to those in citation #22. We calculated the relative risk ratio with 95% confidence intervals of receiving IET for CRE vs. CSE based on Huber-White robust standard errors clustered at the hospital level [28]. Consistent with our prior study, we confirmed our results in a non-parse model and a propensity matched model with propensity for CRE derived from a logistic regression model using the non-parse model's predictors [22]. To explore the impact of IET on hospital mortality, LOS and costs, we developed hierarchical regression models with hospitals as random effects along with confirmatory propensity-matched models.

All tests were two-tailed, and a p value <0.05 was deemed a priori to represent statistical significance. All analyses were performed in Stata/MP 13.1 for Windows (StataCorp LP, College Station, TX).

Results

Among 230,086 patients presenting to the hospital with a UTI, pneumonia or sepsis, 40,137 (17.4%) met the inclusion criteria for Enterobacteriaceae of which the majority were UTI (54.2%), with the remainder either pneumonia (13.1%) or sepsis (32.7%). Among all patients with Enterobacteriaceae, 1227 (3.1%) had 1938 CRE organisms (Table 1). The prevalence of CRE among the Enterobacteriaceae ranged from 2.9% in UTI to 3.6% in pneumonia. Notably, over 85% of patients in both the

Table 1 Individual CRE organisms and their frequencies

CRE organism name	CRE organism Count	% of Total CRE	% of the Total patients[a]
	(N = 1938)	(N = 1938)	(N = 1227)
Klebsiella pneumoniae	724	37.4%	59.0%
Proteus mirabilis	370	19.1%	30.2%
Escherishia coli	294	15.2%	24.0%
Enterobacter cloacae	128	6.6%	10.4%
Providencia spp	94	4.9%	7.7%
Serratia marcescens	87	4.5%	7.1%
Morganella morganii	87	4.5%	7.1%
Enterobacter aerogenes	40	2.1%	3.3%
Proteus spp.	27	1.4%	2.2%
Citrobacter freundii	27	1.4%	2.2%
Klebsiella oxytoca	22	1.1%	1.8%
Enterobacter other	13	0.7%	1.1%
Citrobacter other	14	0.7%	1.1%
Serratia other	6	0.3%	0.5%
Klebsiella other	5	0.3%	0.4%

[a]Sum adds up to >100%, as some patients had >1 CRE organism

Table 2 Baseline characteristics

	CSE N = 38,910	%	CRE N = 1227	%	P-value
Mean age, years (SD)	69.1 (15.9)		66.6 (15.3)		<0.001
Gender: male	16,273	41.8%	642	52.3%	<0.001
Race					
White	28,295	72.7%	821	66.9%	<0.001
Black	5464	14.0%	242	19.7%	
Hispanic	1069	2.7%	32	2.6%	
Other	4082	10.5%	132	10.8%	
Admission Source					
Non-healthcare facility (including from home)	25,559	65.7%	776	63.2%	<0.001
Clinic	1285	3.3%	27	2.2%	
Transfer from ECF	3697	9.5%	266	21.7%	
Transfer from another non-acute care facility	473	1.2%	22	1.8%	
Emergency Department	7766	20.0%	132	10.8%	
Other	130	0.3%	4	0.3%	
Elixhauser Comorbidities					
Congestive heart failure	9623	24.7%	329	26.8%	0.096
Valvular disease	3112	8.0%	96	7.8%	0.825
Pulmonary circulation disease	2323	6.0%	93	7.6%	0.020
Peripheral vascular disease	4285	11.0%	169	13.8%	0.002
Paralysis	4085	10.5%	271	22.1%	<0.001
Other neurological disorders	8668	22.3%	348	28.4%	<0.001
Chronic pulmonary disease	11,035	28.4%	371	30.2%	0.151
Diabetes without chronic complications	11,616	29.9%	420	34.2%	0.001
Diabetes with chronic complications	3809	9.8%	141	11.5%	0.049
Hypothyroidism	6764	17.4%	224	18.3%	0.428
Renal failure	10,810	27.8%	446	36.3%	<0.001
Liver disease	2084	5.4%	65	5.3%	0.929
Peptic ulcer disease with bleeding	17	0.0%	1	0.1%	0.428
AIDS	12	0.0%	0	0.0%	1.000
Lymphoma	604	1.6%	21	1.7%	0.657
Metastatic cancer	1787	4.6%	40	3.3%	0.027
Solid tumor without metastasis	1569	4.0%	34	2.8%	0.026
Rheumatoid arthritis/collagen vascular	1721	4.4%	45	3.7%	0.204
Coagulopathy	5350	13.7%	139	11.3%	0.015
Obesity	6095	15.7%	191	15.6%	0.926
Weight loss	6855	17.6%	340	27.7%	<0.001
Fluid and electrolyte disorders	21,332	54.8%	378	30.8%	0.764
Chronic blood loss anemia	545	1.4%	24	2.0%	0.105
Deficiency anemia	15,154	38.9%	598	48.7%	<0.001
Alcohol abuse	1367	3.5%	33	2.7%	0.122
Drug abuse	923	2.4%	35	2.9%	0.278
Psychosis	2358	6.1%	81	6.6%	0.435
Depression	5854	15.0%	174	14.2%	0.404

Table 2 Baseline characteristics *(Continued)*

Hypertension	24,938	64.1%	781	63.7%	0.752
Charlson Comoribidity Score					
0	12,010	30.9%	334	27.2%	<0.001
1	7855	20.2%	230	18.7%	
2	7902	20.3%	244	19.9%	
3	5118	13.2%	180	14.7%	
4	2897	7.4%	146	11.9%	
5+	3128	8.0%	93	7.6%	
Mean (SD)	1.9 (2.1)		2.0 (2.0)		0.009
Median [IQR]	1 [0,3]		2 [0, 3]		<0.001
Hospital Characteristics					
Census region					
Midwest	10,531	27.1%	288	23.5%	<0.001
Northeast	5297	13.6%	336	27.4%	
South	16,203	41.6%	310	25.3%	
West	6879	17.7%	293	23.9%	
Number of Beds					
< 200	6589	16.9%	192	15.6%	<0.001
200 to 299	8779	22.6%	338	27.5%	
300 to 499	12,691	32.6%	421	34.3%	
500+	10,851	27.9%	276	22.5%	
Teaching	14,609	37.5%	566	46.1%	<0.001
Urban	35,079	90.2%	1167	95.1%	<0.001

CSE carbapenem sensitive Enterobacteriaceae, *CRE* carbapenem resistant Enterobacteriaceae, *SD* standard deviation, *ECF* extended care facility, *AIDS* acquired immune deficiency syndrome, *IQR* interquartile range

CRE and CSE groups had a sepsis diagnosis code at some point during the hospitalization.

Those with CRE were younger (66.6+/−15.3 vs. 69.1+/−15.9 years, $p < 0.001$), and more likely to be African-American (19.7% vs. 14.0%, $p < 0.001$) than those with CSE. Many of the individual chronic conditions were more prevalent in the CRE than CSE group, and the mean Charlson comorbidity index reflected this (2.0+/−2.0 vs. 1.9+/−2.1, $p = 0.009$) (Table 2). CRE was more common than CSE in the West and the Northeast, in urban hospitals, in those of medium size (200–499 beds) and in teaching hospitals ($p < 0.001$ for each comparison) (Table 2). Large hospitals (500+ beds) were less likely to have CRE than CSE (Table 2).

In both the CRE and CSE groups, over one-half the patients had the diagnosis of UTI, with the remaining divided between sepsis (33.3% CRE vs. 32.7% CSE) and pneumonia (15.2% CRE vs. 13.0% CSE) (Table 2). Patients infected with CRE were more likely to have a HCA infection (58.5% vs. 35.4%, $p < 0.001$) along with a greater illness severity by day 2 of admission (ICU 56.0% vs. 40.8%, $p < 0.001$; mechanical ventilation 35.6% vs. 15.7%, $p < 0.001$; though not vasopressors 16.7% vs. 14.9%, $p = 0.081$) than CSE patients (Table 3). Although among the CRE group there was a higher prevalence of empiric use of carbapenems, aminoglycosides and polymyxins than in those eventually found to be infected with a CSE, those with CRE infections were also significantly more likely to receive IET (52.8% vs. 11.1%, $p < 0.001$). Unadjusted hospital mortality median LOS and costs among CRE were also significantly greater than CSE, and these differences held across all infection types (Table 3).

Comparing the cohort of 37,694 patients (93.9% of all patients with Enterobacteriaceae) with valid antimicrobial treatment data, 32,710 (86.8%) received appropriate therapy (Table 4). While patients receiving appropriate empiric therapy were more likely to have UTI or sepsis than those in the IET group, the frequency of pneumonia was higher among patients on IET (20.0%) than those on appropriate treatment (12.0%) ($p < 0.001$) (Table 4). As for the unadjusted hospital outcomes, mortality was higher in patients receiving IET than appropriate therapy (12.2% vs. 9.9%, $p < 0.001$). Both LOS and costs were

Table 3 Infection characteristics, treatment and outcomes

	CSE N = 38,910	%	CRE N = 1227	%	P-value
Infection characteristics					
Sepsis	12,726	32.7%	409	33.3%	0.039
Pneumonia	5060	13.0%	187	15.2%	
UTI	21,124	54.3%	631	51.4%	
HCA	13,782	35.4%	718	58.5%	<0.001
Illness severity measures by day 2					
ICU admission	15,876	40.8%	687	56.0%	<0.001
Mechanical ventilation	6092	15.7%	437	35.6%	<0.001
Vasopressors	5798	14.9%	205	16.7%	0.081
Antibiotics administered by day 2					
Aminoglycosides	3843	9.9%	242	19.7%	<0.001
Antipseudomonal penicillins	6403	16.5%	313	25.5%	<0.001
Antipseudomonal floroquinolones	18,468	47.5%	406	33.1%	<0.001
Antipseudomonal penicillins with beta-lactamase inhibitors	19,727	50.7%	617	50.3%	0.775
Extended spectrum cephalosporins	13,327	34.3%	415	33.8%	0.755
Folate pathway inhibitors	251	0.6%	12	1.0%	0.155
Penicillins with beta-lactamase inhibitors	854	2.2%	26	2.1%	0.837
Polymyxins	126	0.3%	24	2.0%	<0.001
Tetracyclines	248	0.6%	6	0.5%	0.519
Tigecycline	586	1.5%	86	7.0%	<0.001
Aztreonam	1740	4.5%	56	4.6%	0.878
Empiric treatment appropriateness					
Non-IET	32,197	82.7%	513	41.8%	<0.001
IET	4336	11.1%	648	52.8%	
Indeterminate	2337	6.0%	66	5.4%	
Hospital outcomes					
Mortality	3958	10.2%	178	14.5%	<0.001
Mean (SD) LOS, days	9.6 (10.7)		15.6 (17.4)		<0.001
Median [IQR] LOS, days	7 [4, 11]		10 [6, 18]		<0.001
Mean (SD) costs, $	20,601 (29702)		38,494 (46,964)		<0.001
Median [IQR] costs, $	13,020 [7501, 24,237]		22,909 [12,988, 42,815]		<0.001
Hospital outcomes stratified by infection type					
UTI					
Mortality	1873	8.9%	78	12.4%	0.002
Mean (SD) LOS, days	9.0 (9.4)		14.6 (15.9)		<0.001
Median [IQR] LOS, days	7 [4, 11]		10 [6, 17]		<0.001
Mean (SD) costs, $	19,036 (24,494)		33,400 (37,662)		<0.001
Median [IQR] costs, $	12,082 [7104, 21,822]		21,154 [12,687, 39,374]		<0.001
Sepsis					
Mortality	1660	13.0%	81	19.8%	<0.001
Mean (SD) LOS, days	10.9 (12.6)		18.0 (20.8)		<0.001
Median [IQR] LOS, days	7 [4, 13]		11 [7, 21]		<0.001
Mean (SD) costs, $	26,793 (37,390)		50,038 (60,602)		<0.001

Carbapenem resistance, inappropriate empiric treatment and outcomes among patients hospitalized...

17

Table 3 Infection characteristics, treatment and outcomes (Continued)

Median [IQR] costs, $	15,614 [8584, 30,317]		27,264 [14,581, 57,825]		<0.001
Pneumonia					
Mortality	425	8.4%	19	10.2%	0.395
Mean (SD) LOS, days	9.2 (10.4)		13.4 (13.0)		<0.001
Median [IQR] LOS, days	7 [4, 10]		9 [6, 16]		<0.001
Mean (SD) costs, $	19,250 (25,743)		30,432 (35,089)		<0.001
Median [IQR] costs, $	11,826 [7076, 21,100]		19,820 [12,220, 35,713]		<0.001

CSE carbapenem sensitive Enterobacteriaceae, CRE carbapenem resistant Enterobacteriaceae, UTI urinary tract infection, HCA healthcare-associated, ICU intensive care unit, IET inappropriate empiric therapy

significantly higher in the IET group than in the group receiving non-IET (Table 4). These relationships generally held irrespective of the infection type (Table 4).

In a parse generalized regression model exploring the impact of CRE on the risk of IET, resistance was the single strongest predictor of receiving IET (adjusted relative risk ratio 3.95, 95% confidence interval 3.51, 4.46, $p < 0.001$) (Table 5). The confirmatory analyses produced similar risk ratios (Table 5).

In a hierarchical regression model adjusting for all confounders (demographics, comorbidities, severity of illness measures, hospital characteristics) IET was associated with an increased risk of in-hospital mortality (adjusted relative risk ratio 1.12; 95% confidence interval 1.03, 1.23, $p = 0.013$) (Table 5). In other hierarchical models, the excess LOS and costs associated with IET exposure were 5.2 days (95% confidence interval 4.8, 5.6, $p < 0.001$) and $10,312 (95% confidence interval $9497, $11,126, $p < 0.001$). Propensity-matched analyses produced similar estimates (Table 5).

An interaction term suggested a greater impact on mortality of IET in the setting of sepsis, which prompted a sensitivity analysis in the group whose organisms were cultured from blood. In this set of analyses, including 12,807 patients (186 CRE, 1.5%), the impact of IET on mortality was indeed greater (relative risk ratio 1.55, 95% confidence interval 1.18 to 2.03) than in the overall cohort.

Discussion

We demonstrate in this large multicenter observational cohort that among patients admitted from the community with a UTI, sepsis or pneumonia, over 17% have an infection with Enterobacteriaceae, of which approximately 3% are CRE. Although infrequent, the presence of CRE increases the risk of receiving IET substantially. In turn, receiving IET is associated with a rise in hospital mortality, LOS and costs, a rise particularly pronounced in patients with sepsis.

Multiple studies have noted an increase in the prevalence of CRE among patients with serious infections in the hospital. A recent US surveillance study reported the annual population incidence of CRE infections to be nearly 3 cases per 100,000 population [28]. A US Centers for Disease Control and Prevention study noted a rise in CRE prevalence from 1.2% in 2001 to 4.2% in 2011 [29]. The same study analyzing a different database, however, noted an increase in CRE from 0 in 2001 to 1.4% in 2010, echoing findings of other investigators [19, 30, 31]. Our findings are generally in agreement with these numbers. Although CRE incidence and prevalence are far lower than such common pathogens as methicillin-resistant *Staphylococcus aureus* or *Clostridium difficile*, there are few treatment alternatives for CRE, which underscores the need for more precise information about the epidemiology and outcomes related to CRE infections [32, 33]. Consequently, this study helps to address this need for more granular information regarding this pathogen. In addition we confirm that at this point, CRE is encountered most often as a urinary pathogen, which may mediate the otherwise high mortality rate associated with CRE infections. Despite this, the increasing frequency of this organism as a cause of sepsis indicates that CRE is poised to become a major contributor to infectious disease related mortality in the US.

Though thought of mostly as healthcare-associated pathogens, our data suggest that this may be too narrow a view. Namely, in our cohort, over 40% of patients with CRE did not have an identifiable exposure to the healthcare system. There are several potential sources for misclassifying this burden, one of which may be the 90-day period for prior hospitalization as a risk factor for HCA infection. Though it remains unclear how long the impact of prior hospitalization persists on the risk of resistance, and 90 days is a standard interval used in many other studies, in some investigations this period is longer [34]. Although a probable overestimate due to misclassification and because of limitations in the patient records, our data

Table 4 Characteristics of the cohort based on the receipt of inappropriate empiric treatment

	Non-IET N = 32,710	%	IET N = 4984	%	P-value
Baseline characteristics					
Mean age, years (SD)	69.0 (16.0)		69.4 (15.3)		0.094
Gender: male	13,680	41.8%	2169	43.5%	0.024
Race					
White	23,921	73.1%	3443	69.1%	<0.001
Black	4384	13.4%	862	17.3%	
Hispanic	919	2.8%	163	3.3%	
Other	3486	10.7%	516	10.4%	
Admission Source					
Non-healthcare facility (including from home)	21,450	65.6%	3034	60.9%	<0.001
Clinic	1093	3.3%	138	2.8%	
Transfer from ECF	2996	9.2%	759	15.2%	
Transfer from another non-acute care facility	379	1.2%	77	1.5%	
Emergency Department	6688	20.4%	959	19.2%	
Other	104	0.3%	17	0.3%	
Elixhauser Comorbidities					
Congestive heart failure	7836	24.0%	1509	30.3%	<0.001
Valvular disease	2594	7.9%	425	8.5%	0.148
Pulmonary circulation disease	1912	5.8%	358	7.2%	<0.001
Peripheral vascular disease	3564	10.9%	577	11.6%	0.152
Paralysis	3289	10.1%	770	15.4%	<0.001
Other neurological disorders	7227	22.1%	1269	25.5%	<0.001
Chronic pulmonary disease	9079	27.8%	1663	33.4%	<0.001
Diabetes without chronic complications	9695	29.6%	1623	32.6%	<0.001
Diabetes with chronic complications	3152	9.6%	524	10.5%	0.052
Hypothyroidism	5645	17.3%	942	18.9%	0.004
Renal failure	9024	27.6%	1540	30.9%	<0.001
Liver disease	1774	5.4%	245	4.9%	0.138
Peptic ulcer disease with bleeding	15	0.0%	2	0.0%	1.000
AIDS	8	0.0%	4	0.1%	0.063
Lymphoma	508	1.6%	74	1.5%	0.716
Metastatic cancer	1543	4.7%	182	3.7%	0.001
Solid tumor without metastasis	1335	4.1%	163	3.3%	0.006
Rheumatoid arthritis/collagen vascular	1422	4.3%	215	4.3%	0.914
Coagulopathy	4626	14.1%	540	10.8%	<0.001
Obesity	5079	15.5%	822	16.5%	0.081
Weight loss	5583	17.1%	1117	22.4%	<0.001
Fluid and electrolyte disorders	17,961	54.9%	2702	54.2%	0.357
Chronic blood loss anemia	459	1.4%	79	1.6%	0.313
Deficiency Anemia	12,735	38.9%	2096	42.1%	<0.001
Alcohol abuse	1139	3.5%	163	3.3%	0.446
Drug abuse	789	2.4%	103	2.1%	0.135
Psychosis	1979	6.1%	294	5.9%	0.676

Table 4 Characteristics of the cohort based on the receipt of inappropriate empiric treatment *(Continued)*

Depression	4859	14.9%	806	16.2%	0.018
Hypertension	20,987	64.2%	3154	63.3%	0.229
Charlson Comoribidity Score					
0	10,353	31.7%	1239	24.9%	<0.001
1	6517	19.9%	1072	21.5%	
2	6595	20.2%	1047	21.0%	
3	4223	12.9%	757	15.2%	
4	2400	7.3%	465	9.3%	
5+	2622	8.0%	404	8.1%	
Mean (SD)	1.9 (2.1)		2.0 (2.0)		<0.001
Median [IQR]	1 [0, 3]		2 [1 3]		<0.001
Infection characteristics and treatment					
Infection characteristics					
Sepsis	10,736	32.8%	1468	29.5%	<0.001
Pneumonia	3936	12.0%	995	20.0%	
UTI	18,038	55.1%	2521	50.6%	
HCA	11,413	34.9%	2221	44.6%	<0.001
CRE	513	1.6%	648	13.0%	<0.001
Illness severity					
ICU admission	13,524	41.3%	2074	41.6%	0.720
Mechanical ventilation	5064	15.5%	1062	21.3%	<0.001
Vasopressors	4929	15.1%	709	14.2%	0.111
Antibiotics administered					
Aminoglycosides	3694	11.3%	351	7.0%	<0.001
Antipseudomonal penicillins	6199	19.0%	347	7.0%	<0.001
Antipseudomonal floroquinolones	15,995	48.9%	2480	49.8%	0.258
Antipseudomonal penicillins with beta-lactamase inhibitors	16,874	51.6%	2008	40.3%	<0.001
Extended spectrum cephalosporins	12,174	37.2%	1134	22.8%	<0.001
Folate pathway inhibitors	225	0.7%	36	0.7%	0.809
Penicillins with beta-lacatamase inhibitors	681	2.1%	147	2.9%	0.005
Polymyxins	102	0.3%	32	0.6%	<0.001
Tetracyclines	210	0.6%	15	0.3%	0.004
Tigecycline	485	1.5%	110	2.2%	<0.001
Aztreonam	1319	4.0%	258	5.2%	<0.001
Hospital Characteristics					
Area					
Midwest	8848	27.0%	1133	22.7%	<0.001
Northeast	4397	13.4%	950	19.1%	
South	13,579	41.5%	1951	39.1%	
West	5886	18.0%	950	19.1%	
Number of Beds					
< 200	5597	17.1%	744	14.9%	<0.001
200 to 299	7508	23.0%	1171	23.5%	
300 to 499	10,540	32.2%	1781	35.7%	
500+	9065	27.7%	1288	25.8%	

Table 4 Characteristics of the cohort based on the receipt of inappropriate empiric treatment *(Continued)*

Teaching	12,096	37.0%	1988	39.9%	0.217
Urban	29,418	89.9%	4574	91.8%	<0.001
Hospital outcomes					
Mortality	3234	9.9%	607	12.2%	<0.001
Mean (SD) LOS, days	9.0 (8.5)		14.7 (19.4)		<0.001
Median [IQR] LOS, days	7 [4, 11]		9 [5, 16]		<0.001
Mean (SD) costs, $	20,227 (25,616)		33,216 (49,567)		<0.001
Median [IQR] costs, $	12,719 [7401, 23,275]		17,386 [9255, 35,625]		<0.001
Hospital outcomes stratified by infection type					
UTI					
Mortality	1548	8.6%	267	10.6%	<0.001
Mean (SD) LOS, days	8.5 (7.8)		13.3 (17.1)		<0.001
Median [IQR] LOS, days	6 [4, 10]		9 [5, 15]		<0.001
Mean (SD) costs, $	18,103 (21,440)		28,069 (40,490)		<0.001
Median [IQR] costs, $	11,862 [7015, 21,222]		16,209 [8828, 31,535]		<0.001
Sepsis					
Mortality	1356	12.6%	260	17.7%	<0.001
Mean (SD) LOS, days	9.9 (9.9)		18.9 (23.3)		<0.001
Median [IQR] LOS, days	7 [4, 12]		12 [6, 22]		<0.001
Mean (SD) costs, $	24,532 (32,043)		47,881 (64,812)		<0.001
Median [IQR] costs, $	15,048 [8312, 28,558]		25,121 [12,382, 55,529]		<0.001
Pneumonia					
Mortality	330	8.4%	80	8.0%	0.726
Mean (SD) LOS, days	8.5 (7.6)		12.0 (17.6)		<0.001
Median [IQR] LOS, days	7 [4, 10]		7 [4, 13]		<0.001
Mean (SD) costs, $	18,220 (21,710)		24,623 (38,753)		<0.001
Median [IQR] costs, $	11,742 [7125, 20,561]		13,040 [7393, 26,339]		<0.001

IET inappropriate empiric therapy, *SD* standard deviation, *ECF* extended care facility, *AIDS* acquired immune deficiency syndrome, *IQR* interquartile range, *HCA* healthcare-associated, *CSE* carbapenem sensitive Enterobacteriaceae, *CRE* carbapenem resistant Enterobacteriaceae, *UTI* urinary tract infection, *ICU* intensive care unit, *IQR* interquartile range 25–75%

are not the first to bring into question this assumption in a US population. In the surveillance study of CRE by Guh et al., 2/3 of the cultures derived from the outpatient setting [35]. More importantly, 8% lacked any markers of healthcare exposure [35]. In an additional small study by Tang et al., community-acquired CRE accounted for 30% of all CRE infections [36]. Though higher in our study, the fact remains that persons with no ongoing relevant exposure to the healthcare system may still contract an infection with this organism. This finding is troubling in that it parallels what has been observed with extended-spectrum beta-lactamase carrying pathogens and their increasing prevalence in community-acquired infections [37–40].

There is mounting evidence to demonstrate that rising antimicrobial resistance impedes clinical efforts at instituting appropriate empiric treatment [14]. We confirm the important role resistance plays in thwarting the ability to choose appropriately, whereby the risk of receiving IET in the setting of CRE rose 4-fold compared to CSE. In turn, though modest, IET's adverse impact on hospital mortality is consistent with what has been reported in other infections [1–13]. The more pronounced impact of IET on hospital LOS (~5 excess days) and costs (~additional $10,000) is a novel finding for infections with CRE, and provides a sound rationale for investing in technologies that identify patients at risk for CRE more rapidly, particularly given that this is approximately double the attributable burden reported in infections caused by other resistant organisms [41]. Moreover, having a precise estimate of the attributable costs of these infections helps put into perspective the potential value of various prevention and treatment paradigms. It is methodologically challenging to estimate the attributable impact of carbapenem resistance on cost

Carbapenem resistance, inappropriate empiric treatment and outcomes among patients hospitalized...

21

Table 5 Adjusted risk of inappropriate empiric therapy, hospital mortality, excess LOS and costs

	Marginal effect, CSE	Marginal effect, CRE	Adjusted relative risk ratio/excess days or costs (95% confidence interval)	P-value
Risk of IET				
Parse Model	11.8%	47.7%	3.95 (3.51, 4.46)	<0.001
Propensity score (based on 100% CRE cases matched to CSE 1:1)	13.1%	55.8%	4.27 (3.64, 5.00)	<0.001
Non-parse model	11.9%	47.7%	4.00 (3.48, 4.59)	<0.001
	Marginal effect, non-IET	Marginal effect, IET	Adjusted relative risk ratio/excess days or costs (95% confidence interval)	P-value
Risk of death				
Hierarchical model	9.8%	11.0%	1.12 (1.03, 1.23)	0.013
Propensity score (based on 96.4% IET cases matched to non-IET 1:1)	10.5%	11.9%	1.13 (1.01, 1.27)	0.030
Length of stay (days)				
Hierarchical model	8.2	13.4	5.2 (4.8, 5.6)	<0.001
Propensity score (based on 96.4% IET cases matched to non-IET 1:1)	9.6	14.6	5.0 (4.4, 5.6)	<0.001
Hospital costs				
Hierarchical model	$20,508	$30,819	$10,312 ($9497, $11,126)	<0.001
Propensity score (based on 96.4% IET cases matched to non-IET 1:1)	$22,005	$32,837	$10,831 ($9254, $12,409)	<0.001

IET inappropriate empiric therapy, *CSE* carbapenem sensitive Enterobacteriaceae, *CRE* carbapenem resistant Enterobacteriaceae

and LOS in nosocomial CRE infections since those outcomes are confounded by the cause of the initial hospitalization. Therefore, our findings help clarify this issue.

Our study has a number of strengths and limitations. The limitations that are common to both the current and previous studies are discussed in citation #22. Specific to the current analysis, a potential source of misclassification is a relatively high prevalence of *Proteus mirabilis* as a pathogen, as this microbe may have naturally occurring higher MICs for imipenem (Table 1) [42, 43]. Since susceptibility data in Premier are reported not by the MIC, but by susceptibility designation (S, I, R, see above in Methods), for the purpose of this analysis we had to presume that clinical adjudication occurred at each individual institution. However, this type of misclassification, if present, is likely to lead to an underestimate of the impact of CRE on outcomes, thus suggesting that in fact, CRE, when determined without this potential misclassification, may have an even greater effect on the risk of IET exposure.

Conclusions

In summary, CRE is an uncommon but important pathogen in community-onset UTI, pneumonia and sepsis. We confirm that, similar to other resistant organisms, it evades appropriate empiric treatment and exposure to IET worsens both clinical and economic outcomes. Although the true extent of the problem requires further study, our data confirm that a substantial proportion of CRE may be acquired in the community irrespective of exposure to the healthcare system. In sum, our study provides compelling evidence to hasten development of rapid identification methods and new antibiotic treatments in order to optimize empiric therapy among hospitalized patients with serious infections.

Abbreviations
CA: Community-acquired; CRE: Carbapenem-resistant Enterobaceriaceae; CSE: Carbapenem-sensitive Enterobaceriaceae; HCA: Healthcare-associated; ICU: Intensive care unit; IET: Inappropriate empiric therapy; LOS: Length of stay; UTI: Urinary tract infection

Acknowledgements
No one other than the listed authors participated in the study design, analysis, interpretation or manuscript drafting or revision.

Funding
Funding: This study was funded by a grant from The Medicines Company. Ms. Sulham and Ms. Fan are employees of The Medicines Company. Sponsor role: Although Ms. Sulham and Ms. Fan are employees of the sponsor and participated in the study as co-investigators, the larger sponsor had no role in study design, data analysis or interpretation or publication decisions.

Authors' contributions
MDZ contributed substantially to the study design, data interpretation, and the writing of the manuscript. BHN contributed substantially to the study

design, data interpretation, and the writing of the manuscript. He had full access to all of the data in the study and takes responsibility for the integrity of the data and the accuracy of the data analysis. KS contributed substantially to the study design, data interpretation, and the writing of the manuscript. WF contributed substantially to the study design, data interpretation, and the writing of the manuscript. AFS contributed substantially to the study design, data interpretation, and the writing of the manuscript. All authors read and approved the final manuscript.

Competing interests
This study was supported by The Medicines Company.
Dr. Zilberberg is a consultant to The Medicines Company. Her employer, EviMed Research Group, LLC, has received research grant support from The Medicines Company.
Dr. Nathanson is an employee of OptiStatim, LLC, who received grant support from EviMed Research Group, LLC, for conducting this study.
Ms. Fan and Ms. Sulham are employees of and stockholders in The Medicines Company.
Dr. Shorr is a consultant and has received research grant support from The Medicines Company.
Drs. Zilberberg and Shorr have received grant support and have served as consultants to Pfizer, Merck, Inc., Tetraphase, Melinta, Asahi Kasei, Shionogi, Archaogen and Theravance.

Consent for publication
Not applicable.

Disclosure
This study was funded by The Medicines Company, Parsippany, NJ, USA. The data from this study were in part presented at ID Week 2016 meeting. I certify that all coauthors have seen and agree with the contents of the manuscript. I certify that the submission is not under review by any other publication.

Author details
[1]EviMed Research Group, LLC, PO Box 303, Goshen, MA 01032, USA. [2]OptiStatim, LLC, PO Box 60844, Longmeadow, MA 01116, USA. [3]The Medicines Company, 8 Sylvan Way, Parsippany, NJ 07054, USA. [4]Washington Hospital Center, 110 Irving St. NW, Washington, DC 20010, USA.

References
1. National Nosocomial Infections Surveillance (NNIS) System Report. Am J Infect Control. 2004;32:470. https://www.cdc.gov/nhsn/pdfs/datastat/nnis_2004.pdf.
2. Obritsch MD, Fish DN, MacLaren R, Jung R. National surveillance of antimicrobial resistance in Pseudomonas aeruginosa isolates obtained from intensive care unit patients from 1993 to 2002. Antimicrob Agents Chemother. 2004;48:4606–10.
3. Micek ST, Kollef KE, Reichley RM, et al. Health care-associated pneumonia and community-acquired pneumonia: a single-center experience. Antimicrob Agents Chemother. 2007;51:3568–73.
4. Iregui M, Ward S, Sherman G, et al. Clinical importance of delays in the initiation of appropriate antibiotic treatment for ventilator-associated pneumonia. Chest. 2002;122:262–8.
5. Alvarez-Lerma F, ICU-acquired Pneumonia Study Group. Modification of empiric antibiotic treatment in patients with pneumonia acquired in the intensive care unit. Intensive Care Med. 1996;22:387–94.
6. Zilberberg MD, Shorr AF, Micek MT, Mody SH, Kollef MH. Antimicrobial therapy escalation and hospital mortality among patients with HCAP: a single center experience. Chest. 2008;134:963–8.
7. Dellinger RP, Levy MM, Carlet JM, Bion J, Parker MM, Jaeschke R, Reinhart K, Angus DC, Brun-Buisson C, Beale R, Calandra T, Dhainaut JF, Gerlach H, Harvey M, Marini JJ, Marshall J, Ranieri M, Ramsay G, Sevransky J, Thompson BT, Townsend S, Vender JS, Zimmerman JL, Vincent JL. Surviving sepsis campaign: international guidelines for management of severe sepsis and septic shock: 2008. Crit Care Med. 2008;36:296–327.
8. Shorr AF, Micek ST, Welch EC, Doherty JA, Reichley RM, Kollef MH. Inappropriate antibiotic therapy in gram-negative sepsis increases hospital length of stay. Crit Care Med. 2011;39:46–51.
9. Kollef MH, Sherman G, Ward S, Fraser VJ. Inadequate antimicrobial treatment of infections: a risk factor for hospital mortality among critically ill patients. Chest. 1999;115:462–74.
10. Garnacho-Montero J, Garcia-Garmendia JL, Barrero-Almodovar A, Jimenez-Jimenez FJ, Perez-Paredes C, Ortiz-Leyba C. Impact of adequate empirical antibiotic therapy on the outcome of patients admitted to the intensive care unit with sepsis. Crit Care Med. 2003;31:2742–51.
11. Harbarth S, Garbino J, Pugin J, Romand JA, Lew D, Pittet D. Inappropriate initial antimicrobial therapy and its effect on survival in a clinical trial of immunomodulating therapy for severe sepsis. Am J Med. 2003;115:529–35.
12. Ferrer R, Artigas A, Suarez D, Palencia E, Levy MM, Arenzana A, Pérez XL, Sirvent JM. Effectiveness of treatments for severe sepsis: a prospective, multicenter, observational study. Am J Respir Crit Care Med. 2009;180:861–6.
13. Sievert DM, Ricks P, Edwards JR, Schneider A, Patel J, Srinivasan A, Kallen A, Limbago B, Fridkin S, National Healthcare Safety Network (NHSN) Team and Participating NHSN Facilities. Antimicrobial-resistant pathogens associated with healthcare-associated infections: summary of data reported to the National Healthcare Safety Network at the Centers for Disease Control and Prevention, 2009–2010. Infect Control Hosp Epidemiol. 2013;34:1–14.
14. Zilberberg MD, Shorr AF, Micek ST, Vazquez-Guillamet C, Kollef MH. Multi-drug resistance, inappropriate initial antibiotic therapy and mortality in gram-negative severe sepsis and septic shock: a retrospective cohort study. Crit Care. 2014;18(6):596.
15. Centers for Disease Control and Prevention. Antibiotic Resistance Threats in the United States, 2013. Available at https://www.cdc.gov/drugresistance/threat-report-2013/pdf/ar-threats-2013-508.pdf. Accessed 29 May 2014.
16. Kollef MH, Shorr A, Tabak YP, et al. Epidemiology and outcomes of health-care-associated pneumonia: results from a large US database of culture-positive pneumonia. Chest. 2005;128:3854–62.
17. Hospital-Acquired Pneumonia Guideline Committee of the American Thoracic Society and Infectious Diseases Society of America. Guidelines for the management of adults with hospital-acquired pneumonia, ventilator-associated pneumonia, and healthcare-associated pneumonia. Am J Respir Crit Care Med. 2005;171:388–416.
18. Dellinger RP, Levy MM, Rhodes A, et al. Surviving sepsis campaign: international guidelines for management of severe sepsis and septic shock: 2012. Crit Care Med. 2013;41:580–637.
19. Zilberberg MD, Shorr AF. Secular trends in gram-negative resistance among urinary tract infection hospitalizations in the United States, 2000-2009. Infect Control Hosp Epidemiol. 2013;34:940–6.
20. Daikos GL, Petrikos P, Psichogiou M, Kosmidis C, Vryonis E, Skoutelis A, Georgousi K, Tzouvelekis LS, Tassios PT, Bamia C, Petrikkos G. Prospective observational study of the impact of VIM-1 metallo-beta-lactamase on the outcome of patients with Klebsiella Pneumoniae bloodstream infections. Antimicrob Pagents Chemother. 2009;53:1868–73.
21. Ben-David D, Kordevani R, Keller N, Tal I, Marzel A, Gal-Mor O, Maor Y, Rahav G. Outcome of carbapenem resistant Klebsiella pneumoniae blood stream infections. Clin Microbiol Infect. 2012;18:54–60.
22. Zilberberg MD, Nathanson BH, Sulham K, Fan W, Shorr AF. Multidrug resistance, inappropriate empiric therapy, and hospital mortality in Acinetobacter baumannii pneumonia and sepsis. Crit Care. 2016 Jul 11;20:221.
23. Meddings J, Saint S, McMahon LF. Hospital-acquired catheter-associated urinary tract infection: documentation and coding issues may reduce financial impact of Medicare's new payment policy. Infect Control Hosp Epidemiol. 2010;31:627–33.
24. Rothberg MB, Pekow PS, Priya A, Zilberberg MD, Belforti R, Skiest D, Lagu T, Higgins TL, Lindenauer PK. Using highly detailed administrative data to predict pneumonia mortality. PLoS One. 2014 Jan 31;9(1):e87382.
25. Rothberg MB, Haessler S, Lagu T, Lindenauer PK, Pekow PS, Priya A, Skiest D, Zilberberg MD. Outcomes of patients with healthcare-associated pneumonia: worse disease or sicker patients? Infect Control Hosp Epidemiol. 2014;35(Suppl 3):S107–15.
26. Rothberg MB, Zilberberg MD, Pekow PS, Priya A, Haessler S, Belforti R, Skiest D, Lagu T, Higgins TL, Lindenauer PK. Association of guideline-based antimicrobial therapy and outcomes in healthcare-associated pneumonia. J Antimicrob Chemother 2015 Jan 3. pii: dku 533. [Epub ahead of print]

27. Martin GS, Mannino DM, Eaton S, Moss M. The epidemiology of sepsis in the United States from 1979 through 2000. N Engl J Med. 2003;348:1546–54.
28. Williams RL. A note on robust variance estimation for cluster-correlated data. Biometrics. 2000;56:645–6.
29. Centers for Disease Control and Prevention (CDC). Vital signs: carbapenem-resistant enterobacteriaceae. MMWR Morb Mortal Wkly Rep. 2013;62:165–70.
30. Braykov NP, Eber MR, Klein EY, Morgan DJ, Laxminarayan R. Trends in resistance to carbapenems and third-generation cephalosporins among clinical isolates of *Klebsiella pneumoniae* in the United States, 1999–2010. Infect Control Hosp Epidemiol. 2013;34:259–68.
31. Zilberberg MD, Shorr AF. Prevalence of multidrug-resistant *Pseudomonas aeruginosa* and carbapenem-resistant Enterobacteriaceae among specimens from hospitalized patients with pneumonia and bloodstream infections in the United States from 2000 to 2009. J Hosp Med. 2013;8:559–63.
32. Dantes R, Mu Y, Belflower R, et al. Emerging infections program–active bacterial Core surveillance MRSA surveillance investigators. National burden of invasive methicillin-resistant *Staphylococcus aureus* infections, United States, 2011. JAMA Intern Med. 2013;173:1970–8.
33. Lessa FC, Mu Y, Bamberg WM, et al. Burden of *Clostridium difficile* infection in the United States. N Engl J Med. 2015;372:825–34.
34. Herold BC, Immelgluck LC, MAranan MC, Lauderdale DS, Gaskin RE, Boyle-Vavra S, Leitch CD, Daum RS. Community-acquired methicillin-resistant Staphylococcus Aureus in children with no identified predisposing risk. JAMA. 1998;279:593–8.
35. Guh AY, Bulens SN, Mu Y, et al. Epidemiology of Carbapenem-resistant Enterobacteriaceae in 7 US communities, 2012-2013. JAMA. 2015;314:1479–87.
36. Tang HJ, Hsieh CF, Chang PC, Chen JJ, Lin YH, Lai CC, Chao CM, Chuang YC. Clinical significance of community- and healthcare-acquired Carbapenem-resistant Enterobacteriaceae isolates. PLoS One. 2016;11(3):e0151897.
37. Doi Y, Park YS, Rivera JI, et al. Community-associated extended-spectrum β-lactamase-producing *Escherichia coli* infection in the United States. Clin Infect Dis. 2013;56:641–8.
38. Pitout JD, Nordmann P, Laupland KB, Poirel L. Emergence of Enterobacteriaceae producing extended-spectrum beta-lactamases (ESBLs) in the community. J Antimicrob Chemother. 2005;56:52–9.
39. Rodríguez-Baño J, Alcalá J, Cisneros JM, et al. *Escherichia coli* producing SHV-type extended-spectrum beta-lactamase is a significant cause of community-acquired infection. J Antimicrob Chemother. 2009;63:781–4.
40. Banerjee R, Strahilevitz J, Johnson JR, et al. Predictors and molecular epidemiology of community-onset extended-spectrum β-lactamase-producing *Escherichia coli* infection in a Midwestern community. Infect Control Hosp Epidemiol. 2013;34:947–53.
41. Shorr AF, Micek ST, Kollef MH. Inappropriate therapy for methicillin-resistant Staphylococcus Aureus: resource utilization and cost implications. Crit Care Med. 2008;36:2335–40.
42. Bouchillon SK, Badal RE, Hoban DJ, Hawser SP. Antimicrobial susceptibility of inpatient urinary tract isolates of gram-negative bacilli in the United States: results from the study for monitoring antimicrobial resistance trends (SMART) program: 2009–2011. Clin Ther. 2013;35:872–7.
43. Hawser SP, Badal RE, Bouchillon SK, Hoban DJ, Hackel MA, Biedenbach DJ, Goff DA. Susceptibility of gram-negative aerobic bacilli from intra-abdominal pathogens to antimicrobial agents collected in the United States during 2011. J Inf Secur. 2014;68:71–6.

A single center observational study on emergency department clinician non-adherence to clinical practice guidelines for treatment of uncomplicated urinary tract infections

Catherine Zatorski[1], Mark Zocchi[2], Sara E. Cosgrove[3], Cynthia Rand[4], Gillian Brooks[1] and Larissa May[5*]

Abstract

Background: The Emergency Department (ED) is a frequent site of antibiotic use; poor adherence with evidence-based guidelines and broad-spectrum antibiotic overuse is common. Our objective was to determine rates and predictors of inappropriate antimicrobial use in patients with uncomplicated urinary tract infections (UTI) compared to the 2010 International Clinical Practice Guidelines (ICPG).

Methods: A single center, prospective, observational study of patients with uncomplicated UTI presenting to an urban ED between September 2012 and February 2014 that examined ED physician adherence to ICPG when treating uncomplicated UTIs. Clinician-directed antibiotic treatment was compared to the ICPG using a standardized case definition for non-adherence. Binomial confidence intervals and student's t-tests were performed to evaluate differences in demographic characteristics and management between patients with pyelonephritis versus cystitis. Regression models were used to analyze the significance of various predictors to non-adherent treatment.

Results: 103 cases met the inclusion and exclusion criteria, with 63.1 % receiving non-adherent treatment, most commonly use of a fluoroquinolone (FQ) in cases with cystitis (97.6 %). In cases with pyelonephritis, inappropriate antibiotic choice (39.1 %) and no initial IV antibiotic for pyelonephritis (39.1 %) where recommended were the most common characterizations of non-adherence. Overall, cases of cystitis were no more/less likely to receive non-adherent treatment than cases of pyelonephritis (OR 0.9, 95 % confidence interval 0.4–2.2, $P = 0.90$). In multivariable analysis, patients more likely to receive non-adherent treatment included those without a recent history of a UTI (OR 3.8, 95 % CI 1.3–11.4, $P = 0.02$) and cystitis cases with back or abdominal pain only (OR 11.4, 95 % CI 2.1–63.0, $P = 0.01$).

Conclusions: Patients with cystitis with back or abdominal pain only were most likely to receive non-adherent treatment, potentially suggesting diagnostic inaccuracy. Physician education on evidence-based guidelines regarding the treatment of uncomplicated UTI will decrease broad-spectrum use and drug resistance in uropathogens.

Keywords: Antimicrobial stewardship, Urinary tract infection (UTI), Broad-spectrum antibiotics, Cystitis, Pyelonephritis

* Correspondence: Larissa.may@gmail.com
[5]Department of Emergency Medicine, UC Davis Medical Center, 4150 V Street, Suite 2100, Sacramento, CA 95817, USA
Full list of author information is available at the end of the article

Background

The burden of increasingly resistant bacterial infections strains our healthcare system and is a major global public health challenge [1]. Antimicrobial stewardship programs aim to improve antimicrobial use and reduce emergence of resistance through a variety of mechanisms, but few systematic efforts to date have been made to perform antimicrobial stewardship in the emergency department (ED) setting [2]. The ED is a frequent site of antibiotic use and thus, provides a unique opportunity for antimicrobial stewardship. Up to half of all antimicrobial prescriptions are inappropriate [3], with poor adherence with evidence based guidelines (EBG) for infectious diseases [4, 5] and overuse of broad spectrum antibiotics [6, 7]; however, this has not been quantified in an ED setting.

Urinary tract infections (UTI) are one of the most common complaints diagnosed in the ED and accounted for approximately 2.4 million visits in 2010 [8]. Uncomplicated UTIs encompass acute, uncomplicated cystitis and pyelonephritis in outpatient, nonpregnant women [9]. Given that nearly half of all ED visits are by patients with non-life-threatening problems [10], emergency physicians must be adept at treating these illnesses. However, the natural limitations of the ED setting, such as inadequate microbiological testing and follow up, necessitates the use of treatment recommendations based on clinical findings in EBGs to minimize antimicrobial resistance and adverse events associated with broad spectrum antibiotic use.

The 2010 International Clinical Practice Guidelines (ICPG) established by the Infectious Diseases Society of America (IDSA) and the European Society for Microbiology and Infectious Diseases (ESCMID) updated the previous 1999 recommendations to account for changes in resistance, the increased adverse effects of antimicrobial therapy, and new antimicrobial agents available. It remains the most current guideline regarding treatment of uncomplicated UTI endorsed by the IDSA. In the absence of fever, flank pain, or other symptoms of pyelonephritis, fluoroquinolones are no longer first-line due to the increase in resistance and the propensity for side effects, a major departure from the 1999 guidelines [11]. Nitrofurantoin, fosfomycin, and trimethoprim-sulfamethoxazole (TMP-SMX) where community resistance rates are <20 % are recommended as first-line therapy for cystitis. Ciprofloxacin is preferred for pyelonephritis [9].

Our study objective was to determine proportions and predictors of inappropriate antimicrobial use as defined by 2010 ICPG established by the IDSA and the ESMID in emergency department patients presenting with a urinary tract infection.

Methods

This was a prospective, observational study that was reviewed and approved by the Institutional Review Board at The George Washington University. We enrolled non-pregnant women, between the ages of 18 and 49 years, in an urban, academic ED in a tertiary care hospital in Washington, DC, USA with approximately 75,000 patient visits per year between September 2012 and February 2014. All participants provided informed consent in accordance with standards set forth by HHS regulations 45 CFR 46.11a and FDA regulations 21 CFR 50.25. IDSA guidelines are endorsed by hospital infection control for antibiotic choice and a hospital-wide antibiogram is not readily available to ED clinicians and is not specific to uropathogens. Inclusion criteria included complaints of symptoms consistent with a UTI, including dysuria, increased frequency of urination, and hesitancy to urinate, those who had a urine dipstick, urinalysis with microscopy, and/or urine culture ordered. Results of the urine culture were not available to the clinical staff during the course of patient care and were used exclusively for research purposes or clinical follow up. Women were excluded if they were previously treated for a UTI within the past month due to the possibly of treatment failure from the previous infection [12–14], were currently on antibiotics, had severe comorbidities (diabetes mellitus, end stage renal disease, or immunocompromised) or had a recent urologic procedure or indwelling catheter. Enrollment occurred Monday to Friday, 8 am–7 pm, and Saturday to Sunday, 9 am–5 pm, due to the presence of department research assistants. Consecutive enrollment was attempted during this time. Clinical decision-making was at the discretion of the individual healthcare provider. At our site care for uncomplicated UTIs is primarily performed in the ED ambulatory care track by emergency medicine (EM) trained physicians and physician assistants (PA); however, EM residents (Post Graduate Years 1 through 4) and non-EM residents who rotate in the ED and also provide care. All clinical decisions made by physician assistants and EM residents are reviewed and approved by a board-certified EM physician prior to patient discharge. Pharmacists do not approve antibiotic prescriptions prior to administration or discharge.

Potential participants were screened for eligibility using the ED's electronic medical record (EMR) and, if eligible, were approached for participation. Those who gave informed consent had demographic, behavioral, clinical, and treatment information collected through structured interview with the patient and clinician. Treatment information was collected by interview right after the clinical encounter. Urine cultures were prospectively collected to ascertain pathogen type and susceptibility information. Urine dipstick, urinalysis with microscopy, and culture results were collected via chart abstraction of the EMR.

Clinician-directed antibiotic treatment was compared to the guideline recommendations, and took into account allergy. No attempt was made to familiarize treating providers with guideline recommendations. We developed a standard case definition for non-adherence. Antibiotic use was not considered consistent with guidelines if the patient received a FQ in the absence of fever and/or flank pain and did not have a documented allergy to nitrofurantoin or to sulfonamides, received less than the recommended dose or duration according to the IDSA guidelines, or had a regimen longer than 2 days over the recommended duration. Clinical and demographic characteristics were collected via structured data form and chart abstraction was performed for verification. Given our institution does not have an outpatient or ED specific antibiogram and the hospital wide antibiogram is not widely distributed in this setting, we assumed the use of TMP-SMX as guideline adherent since providers may assume lower resistance for patients with uncomplicated infection. Final International Classification of Disease 9 (ICD9) diagnosis was reviewed by an independent emergency physician to ensure that diagnosis correlated with signs and symptoms recorded in the patient's electronic medical record. We categorized cases as pyelonephritis or cystitis through direct interview of the clinician as well as review of the electronic medical record of the patient's symptoms and the treating provider's clinical impression as documented on the chart. Our case definition of pyelonephritis included the presence of fever or flank pain as per patient report. In instances where our case definitions did not match the clinical diagnosis we evaluated adherence per the clinician diagnosis ($n = 11$). We conduct a sensitivity analysis with these cases excluded and compare our results.

Results were summarized using proportions (%) for categorical data with binomial confidence intervals. Categorical variables were compared using either Pearson's Chi-squared or Fisher's exact test, where appropriate. To determine the predictors of non-adherence, univariate followed by multivariable logistic regression analysis were performed. Predictors included: patients' age, race (black, white, or other), provider type (resident vs. attending or PA), current sexual activity (yes/no), prior history of UTI outside the 1-month exclusion, diagnosis of pyelonephritis, decreased urine output, frequent urination, dysuria, abdominal pain, back pain, nausea/vomiting, vaginal discharge, days since onset of symptoms and urine analysis result. All variable was considered potentially significant and further analyzed in a stepwise multivariate logistic regression model using the backward selection method for determining significant independent factors at $P < 0.2$. While these are a large

number of variables to include, prior research demonstrates a variety of factors leading to overprescribing of broad spectrum antibiotics in cases of diagnostic uncertainty or clinical presentation, thus we felt it important to include demographic, clinical and test factors in our model [15, 16]. To reduce the number of variables included in the regression analyses, we collapsed urinary symptoms together (dysuria, frequent urination, and decreased urination) and non-urinary clinical symptoms together (back pain, abdominal pain, nausea/vomiting, and vaginal discharge). Odds ratios with 95 % confidence intervals were calculated. Predictors with a p-value of less than 0.05 were considered statistically significant. The final model was tested for fit using a Hosmer-Lemeshow X^2 (1.84, $P = 0.97$). Stata, v.13 (College Station, TX, USA) was used for all analyses.

Results

A total of 103 of 445 patients met the inclusion and exclusion criteria. Of these, a total of 65 (63.1 %) received treatment that did not adhere to the ICPG guidelines. Sixty-seven patients were identified as cystitis, of which 42 received treatment non-adherent to the guidelines (62.7 %). The most common characterization of non-adherence in cystitis was inappropriate use of a FQ, which occurred in 97.6 % (41/42) of the non-adherent cases. Thirty-six patients were identified as Pyelonephritis, of which 23 received treatment non-adherent to the guidelines (63.9 %). The most common description of non-adherence in pyelonephritis was inappropriate antibiotic choice and no initial IV antibiotic, which both occurred in 39.1 % (9/23) of the non-adherent cases. We found that 22.2 % of E. coli isolates from patients with uncomplicated UTI in our study were resistant to TMP-SMX, and 8.0 % to FQ (data not shown).

Baseline characteristics of patients with pyelonephritis compared to cystitis are presented in Table 1. Patients with pyelonephritis had higher prevalence of abdominal pain (75.0 % vs. 43.3 %, $P < 0.01$), back pain (69.4 % vs. 28.4 %, $P < 0.01$), nausea/vomiting (36.1 % vs 11.9 %, $P < 0.01$) than patients with cystitis. They were also more likely to have had symptoms for more than 4 days (58.3 vs 28.8 %, $P < 0.01$).

Characteristics of patient management and diagnostic results of patients with pyelonephritis versus cystitis are shown in Table 2. Residents were more likely to treat patients with pyelonephritis compared to cystitis (52.8 vs 25.4 %; $P < 0.01$). Non-adherence to guidelines was similar for patients with pyelonephritis and cystitis (63.9 % vs. 62.7 %; $P = 0.90$).

In the univariate analysis, patients with cystitis with back or abdominal pain had increased odds of receiving non-adherent treatment compared to patients with cystitis but no other non-urinary symptoms (OR 8.8,

Table 1 Patient demographic and clinical characteristics of 103 adults treated for uncomplicated UTI

Characteristics	Overall ($n = 103$)		Pyelonephritis ($n = 36$)		Cystitis ($n = 67$)		P-value
	%	(95 % CI)	%	(95 % CI)	%	95 % CI	
Race/ethnicity							
Black, non-Hispanic	51.5	(41.4–61.4)	55.6	(38.1–72.1)	49.3	(36.8–61.8)	0.74
White, non-Hispanic	31.1	(22.3–40.9)	30.6	(16.3–48.1)	31.3	(20.6–43.8)	
Hispanic or other race	17.5	(10.7–26.2)	13.9	(4.7–29.5)	19.4	(10.8–30.9)	
Age, y							
18–29	64.1	(54.0–73.3)	47.2	(30.4–64.5)	73.1	(60.9–83.2)	**<0.01**
30–39	25.2	(17.2–34.8)	44.4	(27.9–61.9)	14.9	(7.4–25.7)	
40+	10.7	(5.5–18.3)	8.3	(1.8–22.5)	11.9	(5.3–22.2)	
Clinical history							
Sexually active	83.5	(74.9–90.1)	77.8	(60.8–89.9)	86.6	(76.0–93.7)	0.25
No recent history of UTI	38.8	(29.4–48.9)	36.1	(20.8–53.8)	40.3	(28.5–53.0)	0.68
Clinical symptoms							
Dysuria	78.6	(69.5–86.1)	75.0	(57.8–87.9)	80.6	(87.5–99.1)	0.51
Frequent urination	83.5	(74.9–90.1)	83.3	(67.2–93.6)	83.6	(72.5–91.5)	0.97
Decreased urine output	37.9	(28.5–48.0)	47.2	(30.4–64.5)	32.8	(21.8–45.4)	0.15
Nausea/vomiting	20.4	(13.1–29.5)	36.1	(20.8–53.8)	11.9	(5.3–22.2)	**<0.01**
Vaginal discharge	13.6	(7.6–21.8)	11.1	(3.1–26.1)	14.9	(7.4–25.7)	0.59
Abdominal pain	54.4	(44.3–64.2)	75.0	(57.8–87.9)	43.3	(31.2–56.0)	**<0.01**
Back pain	42.7	(33.0–52.8)	69.4	(51.9–83.7)	28.4	(18.0–40.7)	**<0.01**
Onset of symptoms							
< 4 days	60.8	(50.6–70.3)	41.7	(25.5–59.2)	71.2	(58.7–81.7)	**0.01**
4–7 days	29.4	(20.8–39.3)	41.7	(25.5–59.2)	22.7	(13.3–34.7)	
> 7 days	9.8	(4.8–17.3)	16.7	(6.4–32.8)	6.1	(1.7–14.8)	

P-Values that appear in **bold** are significant at $p < 0.05$

95 % CI 1.7–45.9) as were patients with no recent history of an UTI (OR 2.4, 95 % CI 1.0–5.7) (Table 3). Patients with nausea or vomiting symptoms (any diagnosis) had reduced odds of receive guideline non-adherent treatment compared to patients without those symptoms (OR 0.3; 95 % CI 0.1–0.9). The multivariable model included, no recent history of UTI, type of UTI with symptoms, and nausea/vomiting. (Table 4). Physicians were more likely to be guideline non-adherent for patients with no recent history of UTI (OR 3.8; 95 % CI 1.3–11.4) –0.9), had cystitis with back or abdominal symptoms only (OR 11.4; 95 % CI 2.1–63.0), or had cystitis with vaginal discharge (OR 12.1; 95%CI 1.1–137.5). The wide confidence intervals of the clinical subgroups with small numbers of patients should be interpreted with caution. In a sensitivity analysis excluding patients where the clinician diagnosis did not match our case definition ($n = 11$) nausea/vomiting was dropped from the model and cystitis with vaginal discharge was no longer a significant predictor of non-adherence ($p = 0.07$).

Cystitis with back or abdominal pain only and no recent history of UTI remained significant.

Discussion

We found a high degree of non-adherence to current guidelines for the treatment of UTI; namely, the overuse of FQ in patients with uncomplicated cystitis and inappropriate antibiotic choice and no initial IV antibiotic for pyelonephritis. Interestingly, providers were more likely to be non-adherent with guidelines for cystitis cases where patients only had back or abdominal pain and for cases without a recent history of UTI. Providers were also more likely to be guideline non-adherent for patients with vaginal discharge, however this result was not statistically significant in our sensitivity analysis. The results potentially suggest diagnostic inaccuracy as well as overuse of broad spectrum antibiotics for patients with vaginal discharge and prior UTI. Only 19.4 % of our patients with uncomplicated cystitis received the first line agent of nitrofurantoin, despite the low rate of resistance compared to other antimicrobial agents.

Table 2 Clinical treatment, test results, and adherence to IDSA guidelines for 103 adults with uncomplicated UTI

Characteristics	Overall (n = 103)		Pyelonephritis (n = 36)		Cystitis (n = 67)		P-value
	%	(95 % CI)	%	(95 % CI)	%	(95 % CI)	
Provider							
Attending or PA	65.0	(55–74.2)	47.2	(30.4–64.5)	74.6	(62.5–84.5)	0.01
Resident	35.0	(25.8–45)	52.8	(35.5–69.6)	25.4	(15.5–37.5)	
Antibiotics prescribed							
Ciprofloxacin	59.2	(49.1–68.8)	47.2	(30.4–64.5)	65.7	(53.1–76.8)	0.09
Nitrofurantoin	20.4	(13.1–29.5)	22.2	(10.1–39.2)	19.4	(10.8–30.9)	
TMP-SMX	18.4	(11.5–27.3)	25.0	(12.1–42.2)	14.9	(7.4–25.7)	
Other	1.9	(0.2–6.8)	5.6	0.7–18.7)	0.0	(0.0–5.4)	
Urinalysis results							
Positive	76.7	(67.3–84.5)	72.2	(54.8–85.8)	79.1	(67.4–88.1)	0.43
Negative	23.3	(15.5–32.7)	27.8	(14.2–45.2)	20.9	(11.9–32.6)	
Culture results [a]							
Escherichia coli	60.6	(42.1–77.1)	50.0	(24.7–75.3)	70.6	(44–89.7)	0.23
Other pathogen	39.4	(22.9–57.9)	50.0	(24.7–75.3)	29.4	(10.3–56)	
Non-adherence to guidelines	63.1	(53.0–72.4)	63.9	(46.2–79.2)	62.7	(50–74.2)	0.90

[a] Only includes cultures that had pathogen growth (n = 42)

Reasons for this might include the perception that FQ are more effective, or the shorter treatment duration of FQ, which providers may perceive as more convenient for patients. Furthermore, 22.2 % of patients with symptoms of pyelonephritis received this medication, despite recommendations not to use nitrofurantoin for patients with pyelonephritis. Other studies have documented inappropriate antibiotic use for common infections in the ED and other settings [2, 3]. It is also possible that our structured interview detected symptoms consistent with pyelonephritis whereas the clinician was basing their assessment on different criteria, including physical examination. It is nonetheless concerning that there is a potential for misdiagnosis of these cases.

While UTIs are a common diagnosis and account for more than 2 million patient visits per year in hospital based settings alone, overall adherence to treatment guidelines has been historically low. In a 2011 cross-sectional study of lower UTIs in a general practice clinic (n = 658) performed over a 3-month period, researchers found that antibiotic treatment was given in 634 (96.4 %) cases and only 92 (17.7 %) of these received first line antibiotics [17].

Although definitive diagnosis of cystitis is made with clinical symptoms and bacteriuria, dysuria, frequency, and urgency have all been associated with the diagnosis of UTI [17, 18]. While the urine dipstick may be helpful in diagnosing UTI, it is unable to effectively rule it out with moderate clinical suspicion. Positive leukocyte esterase or nitrate has been found to have a positive

likelihood ratio of 2.5 for the diagnosis of UTI [19]. We found that a negative urinalysis increased the odds of non-adherence by more than 2-fold, although this was not statistically significant. This may be because patients with atypical features or negative results were treated with antibiotics for other conditions, or because clinicians were more likely to use broad spectrum antibiotics, such as FQ, for an uncertain diagnosis.

There were several limitations to our study. First, we enrolled participants at a single urban academic center using a convenience sample, which may not be representative of other sites. Given the small number of physicians sampled, individual errors or differing practice styles can influence the study greatly. Nonetheless, we found similar proportions of FQ use compared to other studies in and outside the ED setting [15, 20]. Furthermore, while proportions of antibiotic prescribing could potentially vary between academic and community based centers, we found no significant prescribing differences between attending physicians and residents. In addition, we did not directly ascertain providers' reasoning regarding antibiotic selection, which may have yielded additional insight into empiric antibiotic selection, such as coverage for other suspected etiologies. While we used a clinical diagnosis rather than microbiologic culture to confirm the diagnosis of UTI, we think our strategy of reviewing charts for inclusion of patients with uncomplicated cystitis and pyelonephritis based on clinical signs and symptoms as well as change prescribing practices documented diagnosis is appropriate given

Table 3 Univariate logistic regression of non-adherence to antibiotic guidelines for uncomplicated UTI

Variable	Non-Adherent %	OR	95 % CI	P-value
Race				
Black, non-Hispanic	66.0	1		
White, non-Hispanic	59.4	0.8	0.3–1.9	0.54
Hispanic or other race	61.1	0.8	0.3–2.4	0.71
Age				
18–29	63.6	1		
30–39	61.5	0.9	0.4–2.3	0.85
40+	63.6	1.0	0.3–3.8	1.00
Clinical history				
Sexually active	62.8	0.9	0.3–2.7	0.88
No recent history of UTI	75.0	2.4	1.0–5.7	**0.05**
Onset of symptoms				
< 4 days	67.7	1		
4–7 days	56.7	0.6	0.3–1.5	0.30
> 7 days	60.0	0.7	0.2–2.8	0.63
Provider				
Attending or PA	64.2	1		
Resident	61.1	0.9	0.4–2.0	0.76
Clinical symptoms				
Dysuria	64.2	1.2	0.5–3.3	0.66
Frequent urination	61.6	0.7	0.2–2.1	0.49
Decreased urination	61.5	0.9	0.4–2.0	0.80
Nausea/vomiting	42.9	0.3	0.1–0.9	**0.04**
Vaginal discharge	85.7	4.1	0.9–19.3	0.08
Back pain	61.4	0.9	0.4–2.0	0.75
Abdominal pain	62.5	0.9	0.4–2.1	0.90
Type of UTI				
Pyelonephritis	62.8	1		
Cystitis	55.6	0.9	0.4–2.2	0.90
Type of UTI with clinical symptom combinations				
Cystitis, no other non-urinary symptoms	52.0	1		
Cystitis, with back or adnominal pain symptoms only	90.5	8.8	1.7–45.9	**0.01**
Cystitis, with vaginal discharge	90.0	8.3	0.9–75.7	0.06
Cystitis, with other combinations of non-urinary symptoms	9.1	0.1	0.0–0.8	**0.03**
Pyelonephritis (any fever or flank pain present)	63.9	1.6	0.6–4.6	0.36
Urinalysis results				
Positive	58.2	1		
Negative	79.2	2.7	0.9–8.0	0.07

P-Values that appear in **bold** are significant at p < 0.05
Non-urinary symptoms include: back pain, abdominal pain, fever, flank pain, vaginal discharge, or nausea/vomiting

recommendations for empiric treatment without culture in most cases with uncomplicated infection [9]. The inclusion of pyelonephritis secondary to untreated cystitis or resistant pathogen was minimized by not enrolling women who were treated for urinary complaints within 1 month of presentation. However, we cannot eliminate it as a possibility and thus it represents an important limitation to our study. We also recognize the small

Table 4 Multivariable logistic regression analysis of non-adherence to antibiotic guidelines for uncomplicated UTI

Variable	OR	95 % CI	P-value
Clinical history			
No recent history of UTI	3.8	1.3–11.4	**0.02**
Clinical symptoms			
Nausea/vomiting	0.4	0.1–1.4	0.14
Type of UTI, symptoms			
Cystitis, no other non-urinary symptoms	1		
Cystitis, with back or adnominal pain symptoms only	11.4	2.1–63.0	**0.01**
Cystitis, with vaginal discharge	12.1	1.1–137.5	**0.05**
Cystitis, with other combinations of non-urinary symptoms	0.1	0.0–1.1	0.06
Pyelonephritis (fever or flank pain present)	2.7	0.8–9.3	0.12

P-Values that appear in **bold** are significant at $p < 0.05$
Non-urinary symptoms include: back pain, abdominal pain, fever, flank pain, vaginal discharge, or nausea/vomiting

sample size may have limited our ability to identify significant predictors of non-adherence. Odds ratios for clinical symptoms have wide confidence intervals and should be interpreted with caution. While we assumed adherence with TMP-SMX, microbiologic results show that > 20 % of isolates from patients with uncomplicated UTI are resistant to TMP-SMX, however this was not known to the treating providers during the study enrollment period. Finally, we cannot know whether providers made antibiotic treatment decisions based on prior microbiologic culture.

There were several cases where the clinician diagnosis differed from our case definition. For example, in seven cases the clinician diagnosis was cystitis in patients with documented fever or flank pain and in four cases the clinician diagnosis was pyelonephritis without documented fever or flank pain. While it is possible that clinicians based their diagnosis of cystitis versus pyelonephritis based on physical examination findings, this calls to question whether patients with symptoms consistent with pyelonephritis such as flank pain and fever, may be undertreated, and warrants further investigation.

Finally, we did not distribute guidelines surrounding UTI to our clinicians, but we cannot be certain that awareness of the study did not change prescribing practices to be more adherent to the recommended guidelines.

The ED is a unique care setting where physicians must make quick treatment decisions about prescribing antibiotics for UTIs with often incomplete information and limited opportunity for follow up. A previous study conducted by our group showed that clinical decision making regarding antibiotics for patients is complex and is

affected by limited environmental resources, lack of access to decision making tools including locally relevant guidelines, clinical inertia, and perceptions that broad spectrum antibiotics are superior in cases where follow up is not feasible [17]. In the case of uncomplicated UTI, however, this overuse of broad-spectrum antibiotics is in fact counterproductive, given the increasing resistance rates to FQ.

A primary cause of provider non-adherence is a lack of knowledge of antimicrobial guidelines. A 2000 cross-disciplinary survey of 92 delegates with an interest in UTIs showed that <3 % answered correctly [21]. While guidelines can be useful to guiding prescribing [22], many ED providers are skeptical as they feel the ED is a special population and that guidelines should be locally tailored. Lack of knowledge surrounding guidelines is also common [21]. Strategies to implement ED interventions in the form of validated clinical decision rules have yielded mixed results [23, 24]. However, there are unique facilitators to successful practice change in the ED, including interest in novel tools and acceptance of new responsibilities [26]. Interventions to address barriers to change in the ED include educational outreach, formal feedback to the clinical care team, and process change [25]. Best practices solutions utilize a multifaceted approach [27, 28]. Novel strategies include embedding guidelines in the electronic health record [29]. A recent study found that a stewardship intervention that included an electronic order set with audit and feedback found that adherence to UTI guidelines increased from 44 % at baseline to 82 % while use of FQ for uncomplicated cystitis decreased from 44 to 13 % overall [30]. Given the frequency of visits for uncomplicated UTI in the ED, and the importance of FQ in contributing to increasing trends in resistance, efforts should focus specifically on the use of FQ in the ED for patients with uncomplicated infections. However, it remains uncertain if these effects can be sustained over time and further studies are urgently needed to help reduce inappropriate broad-spectrum antibiotic use and improve adherence to clinical practice guidelines in patients with uncomplicated UTI and other infections.

Conclusions

63.1 % of patients who were treated in the ED for uncomplicated UTI received antibiotics that did not adhere to ICPG. The most common characterization of non-adherence was use of FQ in cystitis, followed by an inappropriate duration, no initial IV antibiotic for pyelonephritis, and another inappropriate antibiotic choice. Interestingly, physicians were less likely to be guideline non-adherent when patient's reported back or abdominal pain.

Abbreviations

EBG: Evidence based guidelines; ED: Emergency department; EM: Emergency medicine; ESCMID: European Society of Microbiology and Infectious Diseases; FQ: Fluoroquinolone; ICPG: International Clinical Practice Guidelines; IDSA: Infectious Disease Society of America; PA: Physician assistant; STI: Sexually transmitted Infection; TMP-SMX: Trimethoprim-sulfamethoxazole; UTI: Urinary tract infections

Acknowledgements

This project was supported by Award Number UL1TR000075 from the NIH National Center for Advancing Translational Sciences. Its contents are solely the responsibility of the authors and do not necessarily represent the official views of the National Center for Advancing Translational Sciences.

Funding

This project was supported by Award Number UL1TR000075 from the NIH National Center for Advancing Translational Sciences.

Authors' contributions

CZ participated in the conception and design of the experiment, the acquisition of data, and manuscript preparation. MZ carried out the statistical analysis and participated in the interpretation of the data and manuscript preparation. SEC participated in study conception and design, as well as helped to draft the manuscript. CR participated in study conception and design, as well as helped to draft the manuscript. GB participated in the conception and design of the experiment, the acquisition of data, and manuscript preparation. LM conceived of the study and participated in its design, coordination, and interpretation, as well as helped to draft the manuscript. All authors read and approved the final manuscript.

Authors' information

Deferred.

Competing interests

The listed authors do not have any financial or non-financial competing interested that would influence or alter the interpretation of data or presentation of the information provided.

Consent for publication

Not applicable.

Author details

[1]Department of Emergency Medicine, The George Washington University, 2120 L Street, NW Suite 4-450, Washington, DC 20037, USA. [2]Center for Healthcare Innovation & Policy Research, The George Washington University, 2100 Pennsylvania Avenue Suite 300, Washington, DC 20037, USA. [3]Department of Medicine, Division of Infectious Diseases, Johns Hopkins Medical Institutions, Osler 425, 600 N. Wolfe St., Baltimore, MD 21287, USA. [4]Division of Pulmonary and Critical Care Medicine, The Johns Hopkins Institutions, 5501 Hopkins Bayview Circle, Baltimore, MD 21224, USA. [5]Department of Emergency Medicine, UC Davis Medical Center, 4150 V Street, Suite 2100, Sacramento, CA 95817, USA.

References

1. Liberman JM. Appropriate antibiotic use and why it is important: the challenges of bacterial resistance. Ped Infect Dis. 2003;22(12):1143–51.
2. Drew RH. Antimicrobial stewardship programs: how to start and steer a successful progra. J Manag Care Pharm. 2009;15(2):S18–23.
3. Tamma PD, Cosgrove SE. Antimicrobial stewardship. Infect Dis Clin North Am. 2011;25(1):245–60.
4. Kane BG, Degutis LC, Sayward HK, D'Onofrio G. Compliance with the Centers for Disease Control and Prevention recommendations for the diagnosis and treatment of sexually transmitted diseases. Acad Emerg Med. 2004;11(4):371–7.
5. Schouten JA, Hulscher ME, Kullberg BJ, Cox A, Gyssens IC, van der Meer JW, et al. Understanding variation in quality of antibiotic use for community-acquired pneumonia: effect of patient, professional and hospital factors. J Antimicrob Chemother. 2005;56(3):575–82.
6. May L, Harter K, Yadav K, Strauss R, Abualenain J, Keim A, et al. Practice patterns and management strategies for purulent skin and soft-tissue infections in an urban academic ED. Am J Emerg Med. 2012;30(2):302–10.
7. Grover ML, Bracamonte JD, Kanodia AK, Bryan MJ, Donahue SP, Warner AM, et al. Assessing adherence to evidence-based guidelines for the diagnosis and management of uncomplicated urinary tract infection. Mayo Clin Proc. 2007;82(2):181–5.
8. Centers for Disease Control and Prevention, National Center for Health Statistics. National Hospital Ambulatory Medical Care Survey: 2010 Emergency Department Summary Tables. Atlanta: Centers for Disease Control and Prevention; 2010.
9. Gupta K, Hooton TM, Naber KG, Wullt B, Colgan R, Miller LG, et al. International clinical practice guidelines for the treatment of acute uncomplicated cystitis and pyelonephritis in women: A 2010 update by the Infectious Diseases Society of America and the European Society for Microbiology and Infectious Diseases. Clin Infect Dis. 2011;52(5):e103–20.
10. Tsai JC, Liang YW, Pearson WS. Utilization of emergency department in patients with non-urgent medical problems: patient preference and emergency department convenience. J Formos Med Assoc. 2010;109(7):533–42.
11. Warren JW, Abrutyn E, Hebel JR, Johnson JR, Schaeffer AJ, Stamm WE. Guidelines for antimicrobial treatment of uncomplicated acute bacterial cystitis and acute pyelonephritis in women. Infectious Diseases Society of America (IDSA). Clin Infect Dis. 1999;29(4):745–58.
12. Lawrenson RA, Logie JW. Antibiotic failure in the treatment of urinary tract infections in young women. J Antimicrob Chemother. 2001;48(6):895–901.
13. Bjerrum L, Dessau RB, Hallas J. Treatment failures after antibiotic therapy of uncomplicated urinary tract infections. A prescription database study. Scand J Prim Health Care. 2002;20(2):97–101.
14. Gagliotti C, Buttazzi R, Sforza S, Moro ML, Emilia-Romagna Antibiotic Resistance Study G. Resistance to fluoroquinolones and treatment failure/short-term relapse of community-acquired urinary tract infections caused by Escherichia coli. J Infect. 2008;57(3):179–84.
15. Stuck AK, Tauber MG, Schabel M, Lehmann T, Suter H, Muhlemann K. Determinants of quinolone versus trimethoprim-sulfamethoxazole use for outpatient urinary tract infection. Antimicrob Agents Chemother. 2012;56(3):1359–63.
16. Barlam TF, Soria-Saucedo R, Cabral HJ, Kazis LE. Unnecessary Antibiotics for Acute Respiratory Tract Infections: Association With Care Setting and Patient Demographics. Open Forum Infect Dis. 2016;3(1):ofw045.
17. Llor C, Rabanaque G, Lopez A, Cots JM. The adherence of GPs to guidelines for the diagnosis and treatment of lower urinary tract infection in women is poor. Fam Pract. 2011;28(3):294–99.
18. Shepherd AK, Pottinger PS. Management of urinary tract infections in the era of increasing antimicrobial resistance. Med Clin North Am. 2013;97(4):737–57. xii.
19. Giesen LG, Cousins G, Dimitrov BD, van de Laar FA, Fahey T. Predicting acute uncomplicated urinary tract infection in women: a systematic review of the diagnostic accuracy of symptoms and signs. BMC Fam Pract. 2010;11:78.
20. Deville WL, Yzermans JC, van Duijn NP, Bezemer PD, van der Windt DA, Bouter LM. The urine dipstick test useful to rule out infections. A meta-analysis of the accuracy. BMC Urol. 2004;4:4.
21. Naber KG. Survey on antibiotic usage in the treatment of urinary tract infections. J Antimicrob Chemother. 2000;46 Suppl 1:49–52. discussion 63-5.
22. Stiell IG, Clement CM, Grimshaw JM, Brison RJ, Rowe BH, Lee JS, et al. A prospective cluster-randomized trial to implement the Canadian CT Head Rule in emergency departments. CMAJ. 2010;182(14):1527–32.
23. Stiell IG, Clement CM, Grimshaw J, Brison RJ, Rowe BH, Schull MJ, et al. Implementation of the Canadian C-Spine Rule: prospective 12 centre cluster randomised trial. BMJ. 2009;339:b4146.

24. May L, Gudger G, Armstrong P, Brooks G, Hinds P, Bhat R, et al. Multisite exploration of clinical decision making for antibiotic use by emergency medicine providers using quantitative and qualitative methods. Infect Control Hosp Epidemiol. 2014;35(9):1114–25.

25. Clement CM, Stiell IG, Davies B, O'Connor A, Brehaut JC, Sheehan P, et al. Perceived facilitators and barriers to clinical clearance of the cervical spine by emergency department nurses: A major step towards changing practice in the emergency department. Int Emerg Nurs. 2011;19(1):44–52.

26. Grimshaw JM, Shirran L, Thomas R, Mowatt G, Fraser C, Bero L, et al. Changing provider behavior: an overview of systematic reviews of interventions. Med Care. 2001;39(8 Suppl 2):II2–II45.

27. Leblanc A, Legare F, Labrecque M, Godin G, Thivierge R, Laurier C, et al. Feasibility of a randomised trial of a continuing medical education program in shared decision-making on the use of antibiotics for acute respiratory infections in primary care: the DECISION+ pilot trial. Implement Sci. 2011;6:5.

28. Wanderer JP, Sandberg WS, Ehrenfeld JM. Real-time alerts and reminders using information systems. Anesthesiol Clin. 2011;29(3):389–96.

29. Westphal JF, Jehl F, Javelot H, Nonnenmacher C. Enhanced physician adherence to antibiotic use guidelines through increased availability of guidelines at the time of drug ordering in hospital setting. Pharmacoepidemiol Drug Saf. 2011;20(2):162–8.

30. Hecker MT, Fox CJ, Son AH, Cydulka RK, Siff JE, Emerman CL, et al. Effect of a stewardship intervention on adherence to uncomplicated cystitis and pyelonephritis guidelines in an emergency department setting. PLoS One. 2014;9(2):e87899.

Extended spectrum beta lactamase producing organisms causing urinary tract infections in Sri Lanka and their antibiotic susceptibility pattern

M. M. P. S. C. Fernando[1], W. A. N. V. Luke[2*], J. K. N. D. Miththinda[1], R. D. S. S. Wickramasinghe[1], B. S. Sebastiampillai[1], M. P. M. L. Gunathilake[1], F. H. D. S. Silva[1] and R. Premaratna[3]

Abstract

Background: Extended Spectrum Beta- Lactamase producing organisms causing urinary tract infections (ESBL-UTI) are increasing in incidence and pose a major burden to health care. While ESBL producing Klebsiella species seem to account for most nosocomial outbreaks, ESBL-producing *E. coli* have been isolated from both hospitalized and non-hospitalized patients. Although 95-100% ESBL organisms are still considered sensitive to meropenem, rapid emergence of carbapenem resistance has been documented in many countries. The objective of this study was to evaluate urinary tract infections caused by ESBL producers and the antibiotic susceptibility patterns in Sri Lanka.

Methods: Patients with confirmed ESBL-UTI admitted to Professorial Medical Unit, Colombo North Teaching Hospital from January – June 2015 were recruited to the study. Their urine culture and antibiotic susceptibility reports were evaluated after obtaining informed written consent.

Results: Of 61 culture positive ESBL-UTIs, *E. coli* caused 53 (86.8%), followed by Klebsiella in 8 (13.1%).30 (49.1%) had a history of hospitalization within the past three months and included 6/8(75%) of *Klebsiella* UTI and 24/53(45.2%) of *E.coli* UTI. Antibiotic susceptibility of ESBL organisms were; Meropenem 58 (95%), Imipenem 45 (73.7%), Amikacin 37 (60.6%) and Nitrofurantoin 28(45.9%). In 3(4.9%), *E.coli* were resistant to Meropenem. These three patients had received multiple antibiotics including meropenem in the recent past for recurrent UTI.

Conclusions: We observed a higher percentage of *E. coli* over Klebsiella as ESBL producing organisms suggesting most ESBL-UTIs to be community acquired, Carbapenems seem to remain as the first line therapy for majority of ESBL-UTIs in the local setting. However 4.9% prevalence of meropenem resistance is alarming compared to other countries.
Although prior antibiotic utilization and hospitalization may contribute to emergence of ESBL producing Klebsiella and *E.coli* in Sri Lanka, high prevalence of community acquired ESBL-*E. coli* needs further investigations to identify potential causes . Being a third world country with a free health care system, observed alarming rate of carbapenem resistance is likely to add a significant burden to health budget. We feel that treatment of infections in general needs a careful approach adhering to recommended antibiotic guidelines in order to prevent emergence of multi drug resistant organisms.

Keywords: ESBL producers, Urinary tract infections, Carbapenem resistance

* Correspondence: nathashaluke@gmail.com
[2]Department of Clinical Pharmacology, Faculty of Medicine, University of Kelaniya, Kelaniya, Sri Lanka
Full list of author information is available at the end of the article

Background

Infections caused by extended spectrum beta-lactamase (ESBL)-producing organisms are rising in epidemic proportions and poses a threat and a challenge to clinical practice around the World [1]. Although the exact global prevalence of ESBL producing organisms is not known, certain studies in the Indian subcontinent have found nearly 50% prevalence [2, 3].

ESBLs are a group of plasmid-mediated, diverse, complex and rapidly evolving enzymes which are capable of hydrolyzing penicillins, broad-spectrum cephalosporins and monobactams [1]. While ESBLs are generally derived from TEM and SHV-type enzymes, CTX –M type enzyme isolated from ESBL producers had been recognized as an important subtype leading to multi drug resistance [4]. ESBLs are commonly produced by *E. coli* and Klebsiella species [1]. The plasmids bearing genes-encoding ESBLs also frequently carry genes that encode resistance to other antimicrobial agents, such as aminoglycosides and quinolones [5]. Therefore, the selection of antibacterials against ESBL organisms in clinical practice is often complicated.

Infections caused by ESBL producing organisms range from uncomplicated urinary tract infections (UTIs) to life-threatening sepsis. Fluoroquinolones may be used for the treatment of uncomplicated UTIs when found susceptible, but emerging resistance has limited their role in todays' clinical practice [5]. Therefore, carbapenems are regarded as the drugs of choice in the treatment of severe infections caused by ESBL-producing organisms [5]. However carbapenem resistance has also been increasingly reported in many countries recently [5]. Therefore, antibiotic therapy of infections caused by ESBL producers including that of UTIs is challenging. The options of antibiotics are very limited, and require long term treatment with novel and costly antibiotics such as Fosfomycin and Colistin. Risk factors for urinary tract infections caused by ESBL producers include recent hospitalizations, recent antibiotic treatment, age over 60 years, diabetes, male gender, recent *Klebsiella pneumoniae* infection, previous use of second or third-generation cephalosporins, quinolones, and penicillins [6].

In Sri Lanka the ESBL producing organisms and their antibiotic susceptibility patterns have not been extensively studied. We conducted a hospital based study in order to identify the ESBL producing organisms and their antibiotic susceptibility patterns using patients diagnosed with ESBL-UTI.

Methods

A descriptive cross-sectional study was conducted over a period of six months among adult patients admitted to the Professorial Medical Unit of the Colombo North Teaching Hospital, Ragama, Sri Lanka. Consecutive adult patients who had a culture positive urinary tract infections caused by ESBL producers admitted during the study period fulfilled criteria for selection to the study. (Figure 1: Flow chart on recruitment of study participants) Of them urine cultures that had been performed in five selected private hospital laboratories that maintain quality control and function under the supervision of consultant microbiologists were selected. Patients who consented to provide demographic, clinical and laboratory data were enrolled for the study. In these selected laboratories, ESBL organisms were detected using CLSI or Stokes Disc Diffusion Techniques and carbapenem resistance among ESBL organisms were reported based on the diameter of the zone of inhibition. None of the laboratories routinely performed the modified Hodge test for this purpose. Severity assessment of patients were carried out using clinical parameters (fever >100^0 F, presence of chills, rigors, renal angle tenderness, reduced urine output) and laboratory parameters (white cell count > $11,000/mm^3$ with neutrophil predominance, high CRP, high serum creatinine and ultrasound evidence of acute parenchymal renal disease or pyelonephritis). Blood cultures were obtained from all severely ill patients based on management protocol for severe pyelonephritis or septicemia. Selections of antibiotics for the treatment of these patients were based on the antibiotic susceptibility patterns documented in the urine culture reports. Ethical clearance was obtained from the

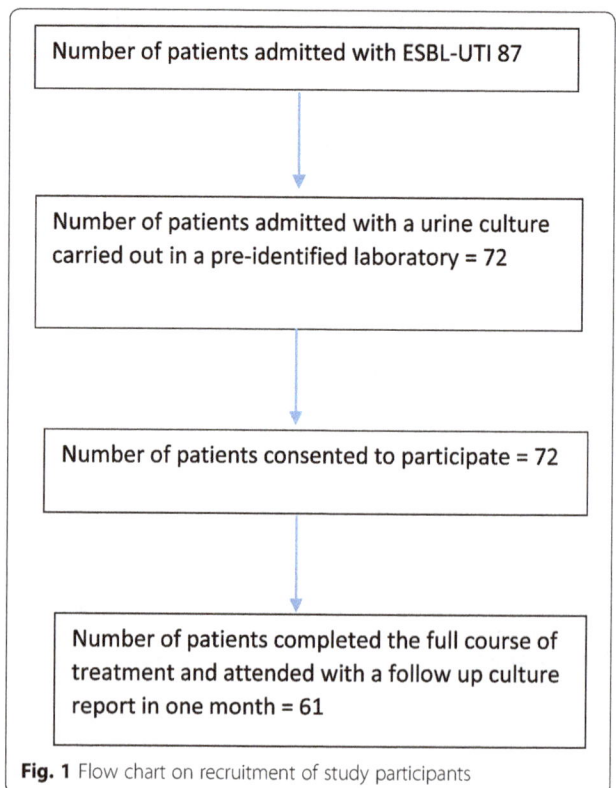

Fig. 1 Flow chart on recruitment of study participants

Ethics Review Committee, Faculty of Medicine, University of Kelaniya. Informed written consent was obtained from the patients prior to recruitment. The demographic and relevant clinical data was collected and recorded in a pre-tested interviewer administered questionnaire. Information related to past medical history, use of antibiotics and hospitalizations were collected from patients' follow up medical records. Relevant investigation results and data on treatment during current admission were obtained from ward bed head tickets (in ward patient management records). Data analysis was done using the SPSS software package (IBM Corporation, NY).

Results

Total of 61 patients consented for the study. Of the 61, 30 (49.1%) were male patients and the mean (SD) age was 64.1(12.6) years. *E.coli* accounted for 53(86.8%) of ESBL UTI's and Klebsiella was found in the rest 8 (13.1%). (Table 1) Thirty nine (63.9%) had received antibiotics in the past three months (11 were on prophylactic antibiotics);23(37.7%) penicillins (Amoxycillin and co-amoxyclav), 18 (29.5%) 3rd generation cephalosporins, 17 (27.8%) 2nd generation cephalosporins and 18 (29.5%) fluoroquinolones (Ciprofloxacin, Norfloxacin and levofloxacin). They included all 8 (100%) patients who had Klebsiella UTI and 31/53 (58.4%) who had UTI caused by *E. coli*. Of 61 patients, 30 (49.1%) had a history of hospitalization within the past three months and included 6/8(75%) of Klebsiella UTI and 24/53 (45.2%) of *E.coli* UTI (Table 2). Of the study population, 28 patients had blood cultures performed and of which 8 were bacteremic and had the same organism found in urine grown in the blood cultures.

Table 1 Characteristics of the study population

Gender	Male 30 (49.1%)
	Female 31 (50,8%)
Isolated organism	*E coli* 53 (86.8%)
	Klebsiella 8 (13.1%)
Co-morbidities	
Diabetes	54 (88.5%)
Hypertension	38 (62.2%)
Bronchial Asthma	8 (13.1%)
Chronic Liver Disease	10 (16.3%)
Renal Stones	3 (4.9%)
USS findings	
Acute pyelonephritis	21 (34.4%)
Chronic Kidney Disease	19 (31.1%)
Hydronephrosis	4 (6.5%)
Hydroureter	4 (6.5%)
Prostatomegaly	4 (6.5%)

Table 2 Associations with ESBL UITs

Associated factors	Yes (%)	No (%)
On Prophylactic Antibiotics	11 (18.0%)	50 (81.9%)
Hospitalization in last 3 months	30 (49.1%)	31 (50.8%)
Antibiotic treatment in last 3 months	39 (63.9%)	22 (36.0%)
Previous use of penicillin (Amoxycillin/co-amoxyclav)	23 (37.7%)	38 (62.2%)
Previous use of fluoroquinolones (Ciprofloxacin/Levofloxacin)	18 (29.5%)	43 (70.4%)
Previous use of 2G cephalosporins	17 (27.8%)	44 (72.1%)
Previous use of 3G cephalosporins	18 (29.5%)	43 (70.4%)

With regards to antibiotic susceptibility (Table 3), majority of ESBL organisms were susceptible to carbapenems; 58(95%) to Meropenem and 45(73.7%) to Imipenem, and 37(60.6%) were sensitive to Amikacin and 28(45.9%) to Nitrofurantoin. Therefore, resistance to Meropenem was found in 3 (4.9%) and to Imipenem in 16(26.2%). The three patients who had meropenem resistance had previously received multiple antibiotics including carbapenems for recurrent urinary tract infections and all three of them had diabetes. Two of these isolates were susceptible to amikacin and the other showed susceptibility to Piparacillin-tazobactum. All these patients were treated with respective antibiotics until they had a normal CRP level and required treatment for at least 10-14 days. All study participants had a repeat urine culture one month after the completion of treatment and remained negative for any growth.

Discussion

In this preliminary hospital based study, our objective was to identify the organisms causing ESBL-UTIs and their antibiotic susceptibility pattern. Therefore our study does not address issues such as incidence and prevalence of ESBL-UTI in the country. All of these patients had a special reference for admission to the unit, mainly based on non-availability or non- affordability of

Table 3 Antibiotic sensitivity pattern

Antibiotic	Yes	No
Meropenem	58 (96.1%)	3 (4.9%)
Imipenum	45 (73.7%)	16 (26.2%)
Nitrofurantoin	28 (45.9%)	33 (54%)
Amikacin	37 (60.6%)	24 (39.3%)
Gentamycin	30 (49.1%)	31 (50.8%)
Ceftrioxone	0	61 (100%)
Ceftazidime	0	61 (100%)
Ciprofloxacin	6 (9.8%)	55 (90.1%)
Piparacillin-tazobactum	12 (19.6%)	49 (80.3%)

expensive antibiotics or were considered too complicated for the management in peripheral hospitals.

In this study, majority (86.2%) of the ESBL producing isolates were *E.coli* and only 13.8% were Klebsiella. Similar pattern was found in South India in 2010 and a reversed pattern was found in North India in 2013 [3, 7]. Although we observed a higher percentage of *E. coli* over Klebsiella as ESBL producing organisms, it is difficult to conclude that most ESBLs in Sri Lanka are due to *E. coli*. This is because this study has a patient selection bias. Furthermore, ESBL-producing Klebsiella species are considered responsible for most nosocomial outbreaks and they are usually clonal and the strains are known to spread mainly through cross-transmission [2]. There is no evidence that hospital-acquired ESBL-producing *Klebsiellae* are decreasing in importance. Data from the Centers for Disease Control and Prevention show 47% increase of *Klebsiella pneumoniae* isolates from United States intensive care units in 2003 compared with the preceding 5 years [8]. On the other hand, an increase in the number of ESBL-producing *E. coli* is being described in several parts of the world [9–12]. In contrast to ESBL Klebsiella infections, many of the ESBL-producing *E. coli* have been isolated from non-hospitalized patients [9–12], and were less frequently clonally related and found to produce CTX-M enzymes [9–12]. These chromosomally encoded enzymes were found in some environmental bacteria, such as *Kluyvera* species [13], that colonize in farm animals [14, 15], and subsequently in a significant proportion of people in the community [16, 17]. In a study carried out in Netherlands ESBL producing *E. coli* were found in meat and poultry and were similar to strains isolated in rectal swabs and blood cultures of patients with ESBL sepsis, suggesting transmission of ESBL through the food chain [18]. Furthermore, some patients with infections caused by ESBL-producing Enterobacteriaceae did not have any previous significant health care contact suggesting they acquired ESBL producing *E coli* in the community. Similarly, in our study, we found 75% patients with Klebsiella ESBL had hospitalization and 100% of them were treated with an antibiotic during past three months compared to only 49% with *E coli* UTI had hospital admissions and 58% received antibiotics. This may suggest that patients with Klebsiella ESBL would have been nosocomial in origin and majority of *E. coli* would have been community acquired. However, this speculation needs confirmation by genetic studies.

In this cohort of patients with ESBL UTIs, 39 (63.9%) had received antibiotics during the three months prior to admission and out of the antibiotics received, penicillin group (amoxicillin and co-amoxyclav) was the commonest followed by 2nd generation cephalosporins, 3rd generation cephalosporins and fluoroquinolones (ciprofloxacin,

levofloxacin and norfloxacin) similar to that had been documented in other studies [2, 19]. Furthermore, 11(18%) were on prophylactic antibiotics for recurrent urinary tract infections and they developed ESBL-UTI while on antibiotics. Today, use of prophylactic antibiotics in recurrent urinary tract infections is no longer recommended as it enhances emergence of resistant strains [20]. Although whether use of prophylactic antibiotic per se, is a risk factor for emergence of ESBL producers is not clear [21], past use of antibiotics has been previously described in association with emergence of ESBL producers [6, 22]. Furthermore, inappropriate use of antimicrobials has been shown to play a pivotal role in the emergence of multi drug resistant organisms. Selection of resistant forms can occur during or after such antimicrobial treatment. In addition, surface antibacterials that are used for disinfection of many household products may play a role in development of antibacterial resistance [23]. Therefore clinicians should ensure the use of appropriate antibiotics for recommended periods in adequate doses in order to prevent emergence of multidrug resistant organisms such as ESBLs.

Furthermore, hospitals should implicate strategies to minimize the spread of ESBL producing organisms by observing universal precautions and minimizing contact among hospitalized patients [24]. This might reduce the spread of ESBL producing organisms in the community. Siegel *et al* recommended that patients infected with multi drug resistant organisms should have restricted contact with other patients [24]. Therefore, although it can be controversial, early discharge of not so seriously ill patients, such as those with ESBL UTIs, with view to home based treatment with potent and effective antibiotics which can be introduced once a day such as Ertapenem [25] or aminoglycosides such as amikacin may be considered in order to prevent spread of ESBL organisms within institutions. Furthermore, adherence to recommended hand washing techniques or use of hand rubs may help to prevent transmission of these infections from one patient to the other [26].

The carbapenems (imipenem, meropenem, ertapenem, doripenem) are still the first choice of treatment for serious infections with ESBL-producing *E. coli* and *K. pneumoniae*. It has been reported that >98% of the ESBL-producing *E. coli*, *K. pneumonia* and *P. mirabilis* are still susceptible to these drugs [27]. But with the emergence of the carbapenem-resistant Enterobacteriaceae, some older drugs were found effective against ESBL-producing *E. coli* or *K. pneumonia* infections. Fosfomycin was reported of having in vitro activity against the ESBL-producing *E. coli* or *K. pneumoniae*. In Hong Kong, most of the ESBL-producing *E. coli* isolates were reported to be sensitive to fosfomycin [28]. Colistin, Tigecycline, Polymyxins and some aminoglycosides are considered effective in the treatment of carbapenem re-sistant organisms [27]. The role of aminoglycosides should not be forgotten as some species will be sensitive and re-spond to aminoglycoside therapy. In a Spanish study pub-lished in 2014, 50 cases of Carbapenem resistant Klebsiella infections were treated with aminoglycosides showing a statistically significant reduction in mortality [29]. The role of piperacillin-tazobactam (PTZ) for pa-tients infected with ESBL-producing pathogens remains unclear. Although ESBLs are generally inhibited by tazo-bactam, many organisms produce multiple ESBLs simul-taneously, which may reduce the effectiveness of PTZ [30]. In a study done by Tamma et al in 2015 found PTZ to be inferior to carbapenem therapy for the treatment of ESBL bacteremia and suggested early carbapenem therapy for patients at high risk of invasive ESBL infections [31].

In this study, 95% of ESBL organisms were sensitive to meropenem. However one crucial finding of this prelimin-ary study was the 3/61 (4.9%) prevalence of meropenem resistance among ESBL organisms. All these three patients were diabetics and had a history of recurrent urinary tract infections with multiple hospitalizations and received multiple antibiotics including meropenem. Although lit-erature on carbapenem resistant ESBL producers is lim-ited, available regional studies demonstrate substantially lower rates of carbapenem resistance. No carbapenem re-sistance has been documented in India among 167 pa-tients in 2014 [19] and in Bangladesh among 115 patients in 2008 [32]. However, 0.4% carbapenem resistance has been documented in Pakistan in 2007 [33].

Conclusions
E. coli and Klebsiella were found to be the main ESBL-UTI among the patients referred for further management in the study setting and occurrence of carbapenem resist-ance was observed within them. Although most ESBL-UTIs had an association with past hospitalization and antibiotic use similar to that is documented in other coun-tries, its significance needs to be confirmed with a proper control group. Occurrence of community acquired ESBL-UTI needs further study to identify the likely reasons and the sources of such infections. Sri Lanka, being a third world country with a free health care system, presence of infections caused by ESBL producers and occurrence of carbapenem resistance among them is likely to add a sig-nificant burden to health budget. We feel that treatment of infections in general needs a careful approach and stress upon the value of adherence to recommended anti-biotic guidelines in order to prevent emergence of multi drug resistant organisms. Furthermore, antibiotics for meropenem resistant ESBL producers such as Fosfomycin and Colistins should be made available while reserving them only for the treatment of life threatening infections caused by ESBL producers.

Abbreviations
ESBL: extended spectrum Beta-lactamase; UTI: urinary tract infection

Acknowledgements
Ward staff of Colombo North Teaching hospital Professorial unit of Medicine.

Funding
No funding body.

Authors' contributions
All authors contributed for the design of the study and data collection and management of patients. MMPSCF and JKNDM are responsible for data entry and analysis; WANL and RP are responsible for writing up the paper. All authors read and approved the final version.

Authors' information
M.M.P. Sanath.C. Fernando (MBBS, MD): Senior Registrar, Professorial Medical Unit, CNTH, Ragama, Sri Lanka and currently on overseas training at Basingstoke and North Hampshire Hospital, United Kingdom.
WANathasha Luke (MBBS): Registrar in Internal Medicine, and Lecturer Department of Clinical Pharmacology, Faculty of Medicine, Universitiy of Kelaniya, Sri Lanka.
J.K.N.D Miththinda (MBBS, MD) Senior Registrar, Professorial Medical Unit, CNTH, Ragama, Sri Lanka and currently on overseas training in Wide Bay Health Service, Queensland, Australia.
R.D.S.S Wikramasinghe (MBBS), B.S. Sebastiampillai (MBBS) and M.P.M.L Gunathilake (MBBS) are registrars in Internal Medicine at Professorial Medical Unit, CNTH, Ragama, Sri Lanka.
F.H.D. Shehan Silva (MBBS, MD): Senior Registrar, Professorial Medical Unit, CNTH, Ragama, Sri Lanka.
Ranjan Premaratna, (MD, FRCP) Professor in Medicine, Department of Medicine, Faculty of Medicine, University of Kelaniya and Honorary consultant physician, CNTH, Ragama, Sri Lanka.

Competing interests
None declared.

Consent for publication
Not applicable.

Declarations
No financial support to this study.

Author details
[1]Professorial Medical Unit, North Colombo Teaching Hospital, Ragama, Sri Lanka. [2]Department of Clinical Pharmacology, Faculty of Medicine, University of Kelaniya, Kelaniya, Sri Lanka. [3]Department of Medicine, Faculty of Medicine, University of Kelaniya, Kelaniya, Sri Lanka.

References
1. Bradford PA. Extended-spectrum beta-lactamases in the 21st century: characterization, epidemiology, and detection of this important resistance threat. Clin Microbiol Rev [Internet]. 2001;14(4):933–51.
2. Ali AM, Rafi S, Qureshi AH. Frequency of extended spectrum beta lactamase producing gram negative bacilli among clinical isolates at clinical laboratories of Army Medical College, Rawalpindi. J Ayub Med Coll Abbottabad. 2004;16:35–7.
3. Sharma M, Pathak S, Srivastava P. Prevalence and antibiogram of Extended Spectrum Beta -lactamase (ESBL) producing Gram negative bacilli and

further molecular characterization of ESBL producing Escherichia coli and klebsiella spp. J Clin Diagn Res. 2013;7:2173–7.

4. Jesus RB, Paterson DL. Change in the Epidemiology of Infections Due to Extended-Spectrum β-Lactamase—Producing Organisms. Clin Infect Dis. 2006;42(7):935–7.

5. Ruppé É, Woerther PL, Barbier F. Mechanisms of antimicrobial resistance in Gram-negative bacilli. Ann Intensive Care. 2015;5:61.

6. Coldner R, Rock W, Chazan B, Keller N, Guy N, Sakran W, Raz R. Risk Factors for the Development of Extended-Spectrum Beta-Lactamase-Producing Bacteria in Non-hospitalized Patients. Eur J Clin Microbiol Infect Dis. 2004; 23(3):163–7.

7. Bhilash KP, Veeraraghavan B, Abraham OC. Epidemiology and Outcome of Bacteremia Caused by Extended Spectrum Beta-Lactamase (ESBL)-producing Escherichia Coli and Klebsiella Spp. in a Tertiary Care Teaching Hospital in South India. J Assoc Physicians India. 2010;58 Suppl:13–7 [PubMed].

8. National Nosocomial Infections Surveillance (NNIS) System Report, data summary from January 1992 through June 2004-issued October 2004 A report from the NNIS System. Am J Infect Control. 2004;32:(8)470–85.

9. Pitout JD, Nordmann P, Laupland KB, Poirel L. Emergence of Enterobacteriaceaeproducingextended-spectrum beta-lactamases (ESBLs) in the community. J Antimicrob Chemother. 2005;56:52–9.

10. Pitout JD, Gregson DB, Church DL, Elsayed S, Laupland KB. Community-wide outbreaksof clonally related CTX-M-14 beta-lactamase—producing Escherichia coli strains inthe Calgary health region. J Clin Microbiol. 2005;43: 2844–9.

11. Woodford N, Ward ME, Kaufmann ME, et al. Community and hospital spread of Escherichiacoliproducing CTX-M extended-spectrumbeta-lactamases in the UK. J Antimicrob Chemother. 2004;54:735–43.

12. Rodriguez-Ban¯o J, Navarro MD, Romero L, et al. Epidemiology and clinical features ofinfections caused by extended-spectrum betalactamase—producing Escherichia coli in nonhospitalizedpatients. J Clin Microbiol. 2004;42:1089–9.

13. Bonnet R. Growing group of extended-spectrumbeta-lactamases: the CTX-M enzymes. Antimicrob Agents Chemother. 2004;48:1–14.

14. Brinas L, Moreno MA, Teshager T, et al. Monitoringand characterization of extended-spectrumbeta-lactamases in Escherichia coli strainsfrom healthy and sick animals in Spain in2003. Antimicrob Agents Chemother. 2005;49: 1262–4.

15. Shiraki Y, Shibata N, Doi Y, Arakawa Y. Escherichiacoliproducing CTX-M-2 beta-lactamasein cattle. Japan Emerg Infect Dis. 2004;10:69–75.

16. Prats G, Mirelis B, Miro E, et al. Cephalosporin-resistant Escherichia coli among summercamp attendees with salmonellosis. EmergInfectDis. 2003;9: 1273–80.

17. Valverde A, Coque TM, Sanchez-Moreno MP, Rollan A, Baquero F, Canton R. Dramatic increasein prevalence of fecal carriage of extended-spectrum beta-lactamase—producingEnterobacteriaceaeduring nonoutbreak situationsin Spain. J Clin Microbiol. 2004;42:4769–75.

18. Overdevestl WI, Rijnsburger M, et al. Extended-Spectrum B-Lactamase Genes of Escherichia coli in Chicken Meat and Humans, the Netherlands. Emerg Infect Dis. 2011;17:1216–22.

19. Shaikh S, Fatima J, Shakil S, Rizvi SMD, Kamal MA. Risk factors for acquisition of extended spectrum beta lactamase producing Escherichia coli and Klebsiellapneumoniae in North-Indian hospitals. Saudi J Biol Sci. 2015;22(1): 37–41.

20. Pallett A, Hand K. Complicated urinary tract infections: practical solutions for the treatment of multiresistant Gram-negative bacteria. J Antimicrob Chemother. 2010;65 Suppl(3):25–33.

21. Yüksel S, Oztürk B, Kavaz A, Ozçakar ZB, Acar B, Güriz H, Aysev D, Ekim M, Yalçinkaya F. Antibiotic resistance of urinary tract pathogens and evaluation of empirical treatment in Turkish children with urinary tract infections. Int J Antimicrob Agents. 2006;28:413–6.

22. Rodríguez-Baño J, Navarro MD, Romero L, Muniain MA, Perea EJ, Pérez-Cano R, Hernández JR, Pascual A. Clinical and molecular epidemiology of extended-spectrum beta-lactamase-producing Escherichia coli as a cause of nosocomial infection or colonization: implications for control. Clin Infect Dis. 2006;42:37–45.

23. Levy SB. Factors impacting on the problem of antibiotic resistance. J Antimicrob Chemother. 2002;49(1):25–30.

24. Siegel JD, Rhinehart E, Jackson M, Chiarello L. Healthcare Infection Control Practices Advisory Committee. Management of multidrug-resistant organisms in health care settings, 2006. Am J Infect Control. 2007;35(10 Suppl 2):S165–93 [PubMed].

25. Lye DC, Wijaya L, Chan J, Chew PT, Yee SL. Ertapenem for treatment of extended-spectrum beta-lactamase-producing and multidrug-resistant gram-negative bacteraemia. Ann Acad Med Singapore. 2008;37:831–4.

26. Trampuz A, Widmer AF. Hand hygiene: a frequently missed lifesaving opportunity during patient care. Mayo Clin Proc. 2004;79:109–16.

27. Perez F, Endimiani A, Hujer KM, Bonomo RA. The continuing challenge of ESBLs. Curr Opin Pharmacol. 2007;7(5):459–69. doi:10.1016/j.coph.2007.08.003.

28. Ho PL, Yip KS, Chow KH, Lo JYC, Que TL, Yuen KY. Antimicrobial resistance among uropathogens that cause acute uncomplicated cystitis in women in Hong Kong: a prospective multicenter study in 2006 to 2008. Diagn Microbiol Infect Dis. 2010;66:87–93.

29. Gonzalez-Padilla M, Torre-Cisneros J, Rivera-Espinar F, Pontes-Moreno A, Lopez-Cerero L, Pascual A, Natera C, Rodriguez M, Salcedo I, Rodriguez-Lopez F, Rivero A, Rodriguez-Bano J. Gentamicin therapy for sepsis due to carbapenem-resistant and colistin-resistant Klebsiella pneumoniae. J Antimicrob Chemother. 2015;70:905–13.

30. Paterson D, Bonomo R. Extended-spectrum β-lactamases: a clinical update. Clin Microbiol Rev. 2005;18:657–86.

31. Tamma PD, Han JH, Rock C, Harris AD, Lautenbach E, Hsu AJ, Avdic E, Cosgrove SE. Carbapenem therapy is associated with improved survival compared with piperacillin-tazobactam for patients with extended-spectrum β-lactamase bacteremia. Clin Infect Dis. 2015;60:1319–25.

32. Iraj A, Nilufar YN. Antibiogram of extended spectrum beta-lactamase (ESBL) producing Escherichia coli and Klebsiella pneumoniae isolated from hospital samples, Bangladesh. J Med Microbiol. 2010;4:32–3.

33. Khan E, Ejaz M, Zafar A, Jabeen K, Shakoor S, Inayat R, Hasan R. Increased isolation of ESBL producing Klebsiella pneumoniae with emergence of carbapenem resistant isolates in Pakistan: Report from a tertiary care hospital. J Pak Med Assoc. 2010;60:186–90.

Effect of prior receipt of antibiotics on the pathogen distribution and antibiotic resistance profile of key Gram-negative pathogens among patients with hospital-onset urinary tract infections

Monique R. Bidell[1], Melissa Palchak Opraseuth[2], Min Yoon[2], John Mohr[2] and Thomas P. Lodise[1*]

Abstract

Background: This retrospective cohort study characterized the impact of prior antibiotic exposure on distribution and nonsusceptibility profiles of Gram-negative pathogens causing hospital-onset urinary tract infections (UTI).

Methods: Hospital patients with positive urine culture for *Pseudomonas aeruginosa, Escherichia coli, Klebsiella pneumoniae,* and other Enterobacteriaceae ≥3 days after hospital admission were included. Assessment outcomes included the distribution of bacteria in urine cultures, antibiotic susceptibility patterns, and the effect of prior antibiotic exposure, defined as 0, 1, or ≥2 prior antibiotics, on the distribution and antibiotic susceptibility profiles of the Gram-negative organisms.

Results: The most commonly isolated pathogens from 5574 unique UTI episodes (2027 with and 3547 without prior antibiotic exposure) were *E. coli* (49.5%), *K. pneumoniae* (17.1%), and *P. aeruginosa* (8.2%). *P. aeruginosa* was significantly more commonly isolated in patients with ≥2 prior antibiotic exposures (12.6%) compared with no exposure (8.2%; $p = 0.036$) or 1 prior exposure (7.9%; $p = 0.025$). Two or more prior antibiotic exposures were associated with slightly higher incidences of fluoroquinolone nonsusceptibility, multidrug resistance, and extended-spectrum β-lactamase phenotype compared with 0 or 1 exposure, suggesting an increased risk for resistant Gram-negative pathogens among hospital patients with urinary tract infections occurring ≥3 days after admission.

Conclusions: Clinicians should critically assess prior antibiotic exposure when selecting empirical therapy for patients with hospital-onset urinary tract infections caused by Gram-negative pathogens.

Keywords: Antibiotic use, Antimicrobial resistance, Fluoroquinolones, Gram-negative pathogens, Multidrug resistant, Urinary tract infection

Background

Increasing antibiotic resistance among Gram-negative pathogens, particularly in the hospital setting, is well documented and constitutes a major public health concern [1, 2]. Gram-negative organisms are implicated in a number of hospital-acquired infections, with urinary tract infections (UTIs) particularly common [1, 3]. Antibiotic resistance among hospital-acquired infections owing to Gram-negative pathogens greatly complicates the administration of timely and appropriate therapy, placing patients at increased risk for deleterious outcomes [4–6]. Resources such as antibiograms can facilitate the empirical antimicrobial selection process [7] by characterizing local resistance patterns. However, reliance on a single collective isolate institutional antibiogram for empirical antibiotic selection is associated with several notable shortcomings. Collective isolate antibiograms developed by many institutions do not capture the distribution of pathogens associated with a particular infection, nor do they reflect the susceptibility profile of a particular pathogen at an infection site (eg, urinary tract).

* Correspondence: thomas.lodise@acphs.edu
[1]Albany College of Pharmacy and Health Sciences, 106 New Scotland Avenue, Albany 12208-3492, NY, USA
Full list of author information is available at the end of the article

Although culture site–specific antibiograms can ameliorate this issue, they do not indicate patient-specific factors that increase the likelihood of an antibiotic-resistant infection [7].

Two critical patient characteristics that modify the risk for antibiotic-resistant infection are recent antibiotic exposure and recent admission to, or current residence in, a health care institution [2, 8, 9]. Considering the limitations associated with an antibiogram-only approach to empirical antibiotic selection, this study was designed to characterize the impact of prior antibiotic exposure on the distribution and nonsusceptibility profiles of key Gram-negative pathogens among US inpatients with hospital-onset UTIs. We specifically focused on this single modifiable risk factor because it is readily identifiable and accessible in the medical record system for all patients. Other possible patient risk factors were not included in the analysis so that a simple and straightforward guide to empirical antibiotic selection could be created.

Methods
Study design and population
This retrospective, observational study used hospital discharge data from the Premier Healthcare Database, which at the time of this study contained data from more than 435 million patient encounters. Laboratory results were available from a subset of approximately 160 facilities in the Premier Healthcare Database. Patients were included in the study if all the following criteria were met: inpatient discharge between January 1, 2012, and March 31, 2013; positive urine culture for any of the prespecified Gram-negative bacteria ≥3 days after hospital admission; and receipt of an antibiotic with activity against Gram-negative pathogens on the index culture date or within the 3-day period thereafter. The first documented urine culture was included in the analysis. Duplicate isolates from subsequent urine cultures within 30 days were excluded. Duplicate isolates recovered from urine cultures >30 days after the index culture were included because we felt these to be representative of either recurrent or new infection. As such, we felt it was important to include these subsequent occurrences as unique episodes within the study.

The Gram-negative organisms of interest were *Escherichia coli*, *Klebsiella pneumoniae*, *Pseudomonas aeruginosa*, and other members of the Enterobacteriaceae family (excluding *E. coli* and *K. pneumoniae*). Prior antibiotic exposure was defined as administration of ≥1 prespecified agents with Gram-negative activity during the current hospitalization and before the index urine culture. Antibiotics included for assessment of prior exposure were those available in the working Premier data set: meropenem, doripenem, imipenem, ertapenem,

piperacillin/tazobactam, cefepime, ceftazidime, ceftriaxone, cefotaxime, ciprofloxacin, levofloxacin, gentamicin, tobramycin, amikacin, ampicillin/sulbactam, cefazolin, gatifloxacin, cefazolin, tigecycline, and ticarcillin/clavulanic acid (or clavulanate). Data for other groups of antibiotics, including second-generation cephalosporins and trimethoprim/sulfamethoxazole, were not available.

Outcomes
The first outcome measure was distribution and antibiotic susceptibility patterns among the prespecified Gram-negative organisms for patients meeting inclusion criteria. The second outcome measure was the association of prior antibiotic exposure, defined as 0, 1, or ≥2 prior exposures, with the distribution and antibiotic susceptibility profiles of the Gram-negative organisms of interest. Organisms were assessed for susceptibility to fluoroquinolones (ciprofloxacin, levofloxacin, gatifloxacin), carbapenems (meropenem, imipenem, doripenem, ertapenem), and piperacillin/tazobactam.

For the purposes of this analysis, antibiotic susceptibility was classified as susceptible versus nonsusceptible (ie, intermediate or resistant), based on the microbiology report. Multidrug resistance was defined as nonsusceptibility to ≥1 agents in ≥3 antibiotic classes [10]. For *P. aeruginosa*, only meropenem-, imipenem-, or doripenem-nonsusceptibility was used to define carbapenem resistance; *P. aeruginosa* isolates were considered nonsusceptible to third-generation cephalosporins if they were resistant to ceftazidime, or, if data were unavailable, to cefepime. For Enterobacteriaceae, isolates were considered nonsusceptible to a third-generation cephalosporin if they had documented resistance to at least two agents (ceftriaxone, ceftazidime, or cefotaxime). Nonsusceptibility to third-generation cephalosporins was considered indicative of an extended-spectrum beta-lacatmase (ESBL) phenotype. For patients with missing carbapenem, piperacillin/tazobactam, or MDR susceptibility data, isolates were considered carbapenem-susceptible, piperacillin/tazobactam-susceptible, or non-MDR if they were susceptible to a third-generation cephalosporin. Otherwise, carbapenem, piperacillin/tazobactam, and MDR susceptibility data were considered missing and were not included in the analyses that evaluated the relationship between prior antibiotic exposures and antibiotic susceptibility profiles.

Statistical analysis
Unadjusted descriptive analysis was used to characterize the distribution and antibiotic susceptibility patterns of the Gram-negative organisms of interest and the effect of prior antibiotic exposure on each of these patterns. Although the study was not powered for prespecified statistical analyses, possible significance between groups (≥2

prior exposures compared with 0 or 1 prior exposure) was calculated using the method of Miettinen and Nurminen.

Results

Overall pathogen distribution and resistance profile

Descriptive statistics of patient demographics and characteristics of hospital visits are provided (see Additional file 1). A total of 5574 unique UTI episodes were included in the analysis ($n = 2027$ prior antibiotic exposure; $n = 3547$ no prior exposure), from which 6093 pathogens were isolated ($n = 2227$ from patients with prior antibiotic exposure; $n = 3866$ from patients with no prior exposure). The most commonly isolated pathogens were *E. coli* ($n = 3013$; 49.5%), *K. pneumoniae* ($n = 1039$; 17.1%), and *P. aeruginosa* ($n = 502$; 8.2%) (Fig. 1). Among all pathogens, fluoroquinolone nonsusceptibility and multidrug resistance exceeded 19 and 21%, respectively (Fig. 2). The ESBL phenotype was noted in 4.1% of pathogens, and carbapenem nonsusceptibility was noted in <2%.

Effect of prior antibiotic exposure

The distribution of pathogens in relation to prior antibiotic exposure is shown in Fig. 1. *P. aeruginosa* was isolated significantly more often in patients with ≥2 prior antibiotic exposures (12.6%) than in patients with no prior antibiotic exposure (8.2%; 95% confidence intervals [CI] 0.2, 10.1; $p = 0.036$) or with 1 prior exposure (7.9%; 95% CI 0.5, 10.5; $p = 0.025$). For other pathogen groups, the presence or absence of prior antibiotic exposure did not substantially affect distribution trends, and differences were nonsignificant.

Nonsusceptibility characteristics with respect to 0, 1, or ≥2 prior antibiotic exposures are shown in Fig. 2 and Table 1. Among all pathogens, a trend toward slightly

higher incidences of fluoroquinolone nonsusceptibility and of multidrug-resistant and ESBL phenotypes wase seen with ≥2 prior antibiotic exposures than with 1 or 0 (Fig. 2); however, with the exception of ESBL phenotype in patients with ≥2 vs 1 prior antibiotic exposures (6.6% vs 3.6%; 95% CI 0.1, 7.7; $p = 0.041$), these differences in incidence were not statistically significant. This trend seemed to be driven largely by susceptibility pattern changes observed with *K. pneumoniae* (Table 1).

Discussion

The aim of this study was to characterize the distribution and antibiotic nonsusceptibility profiles of key Gram-negative organisms by the presence of antibiotic exposures among patients with hospital-onset UTIs. Although numerous patient factors can affect pathogen distribution and susceptibility trends, we focused on this one risk factor given that it is modifiable and easily evaluated by clinicians using the medical record. Antibiotic exposure is an important consideration given a recent multicenter prevalence study describing antibiotic use in 50% of inpatients on any given day during admission [11]. Therefore, our approach focusing on the number of exposures offers a simple and straightforward supplement to guide empirical antibiotic selection for hospital-onset UTI treatment.

Our study focusing on the single risk factor of antibiotic exposure produced several notable findings. Consistent with epidemiologic trends, *E. coli* (49.5%) was the most commonly isolated pathogen [8, 9, 12], and this was consistent across all categories of prior antibiotic exposure. Although the simple binary designation of prior antibiotic exposure did not seem to affect overall pathogen distribution or nonsusceptibility trends,

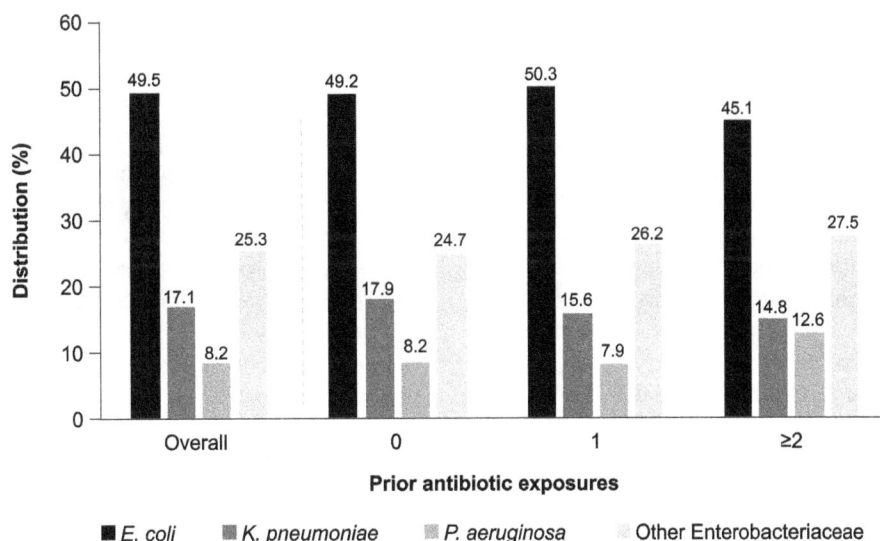

Fig. 1 Pathogen distribution by prior antibiotic exposure

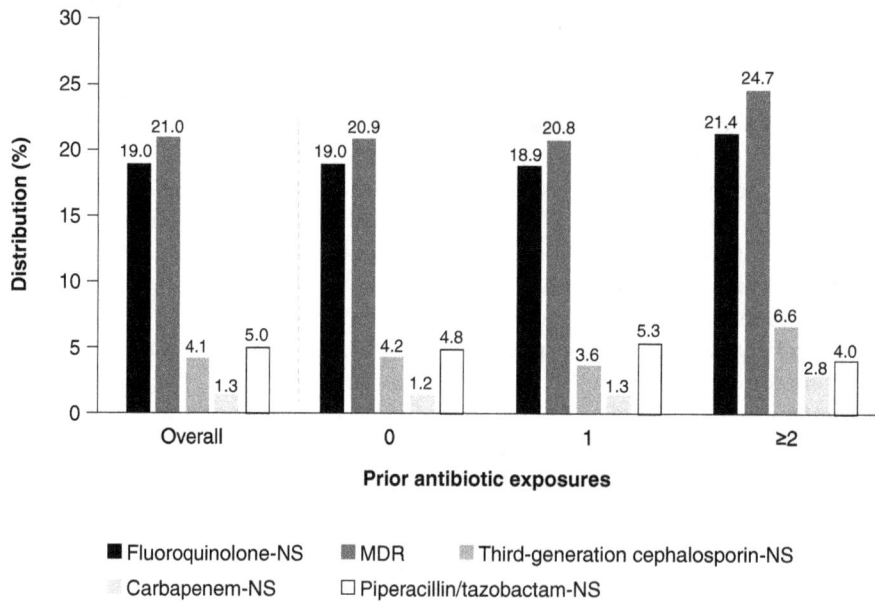

Fig. 2 Antibiotic nonsusceptibility phenotypes across all pathogens by prior antibiotic exposure. *MDR* multidrug resistant; *NS* nonsusceptible

differences became apparent on stratification by number of exposures. Prior receipt of ≥2 antibiotic regimens was associated with a significantly higher frequency of *P. aeruginosa* UTIs and with slightly higher incidences of fluoroquinolone-, carbapenem-, and third-generation cephalosporin-nonsusceptibility as well as multidrug resistance. Collectively, our findings suggest that previous exposure to ≥2 antibiotic regimens is associated with an alteration of the distribution and susceptibility profiles of Gram-negative pathogens among patients with hospital-onset UTIs.

Although antibiotic nonsusceptibility was highest among those with ≥2 prior exposures to antibiotics, fluoroquinolone nonsusceptibility rates were >18%, even in the absence of prior antibiotic exposure. This finding is not unexpected given the large-scale use of fluoroquinolones for UTIs in both community and health care settings. Emergence of resistance to these antibiotics is recognized by a number of world health agencies and is considered a major public health concern [1, 2, 12]. Because practice guidelines recommend empirical use of fluoroquinolones for UTIs only if local drug resistance rates do not exceed 10% [12], our findings suggest that caution should be exercised with empirical use of fluoroquinolones for hospital-onset UTIs, and strong consideration should be given to alternative therapies with broad-spectrum, Gram-negative coverage empirically.

Our findings also highlight the limitations associated with relying solely on antibiograms for patients with hospital-onset UTI, particularly those with ≥2 antibiotic exposures. Although antibiograms are a useful starting point in the empirical drug selection process, they reflect the cumulative susceptibility rates for the first recovered pathogen in a particular patient, regardless of current site, timing of collection (community vs hospital onset), or patient-specific risk factors for resistance (eg, prior exposure to antibiotics) [7]. Recent guidelines from the Infectious Diseases Society of America and the Society for Hospital Epidemiology of America acknowledge several of these limitations and encourage the development of enhanced antibiograms stratified by various parameters (eg, age, location within the institution, infection site, patient comorbidities, and site of acquisition) to improve empirical selection of antibiotics. Furthermore, these guidelines encourage the development of institution-specific clinical treatment guidelines for common infectious diseases [13]. Our findings that prior antibiotic exposure alters the distribution of pathogens and the susceptibility profiles of common Gram-negative organisms implicated in UTIs occurring ≥3 days after admission can easily be incorporated into clinical treatment guidelines to promote a more patient-specific approach to timely selection of appropriate empirical antibiotic therapy. In addition to guiding the selection of appropriately broad-spectrum empirical therapy for hospital-onset UTI, our findings may be helpful to institutional antimicrobial stewardship programs to target antibiotics likely to be inappropriate (eg, fluoroquinolones).

Some limitations should be considered when interpreting these findings. First, though we acknowledge that several factors may contribute to antibiotic-resistant infections, we purposefully did not assess multiple risk factors because data were not uniformly available for all patients. We also believed that inclusion of other patient factors would complicate our intent to create a simple, straightforward approach to guide empirical antibiotic

Table 1 Nonsusceptibility phenotypes by prior antibiotic exposure

Pathogen	Nonsusceptibility phenotype	Overall, % NS (n/N)	Prior antibiotic exposure		
			0	1	≥2
Escherichia coli (n = 3013)[a,b]	Fluoroquinolone-NS	25.4 (758/2990)	25.5 (482/1888)	24.8 (253/1020)	28.0 (23/82)
	Third-generation cephalosporin-NS	3.5 (105/3013)	3.8 (72/1903)	2.7 (28/1028)	6.1 (5/82)
	MDR	23.4 (705/3013)	24.1 (458/1903)	21.6 (222/1028)	30.5 (25/82)
	Carbapenem-NS	0.1 (4/3006)	0.2 (3/1900)	0.1 (1/1025)	0 (0/81)
	Piperacillin/tazobactam-NS	4.4 (131/2965)	4.6 (86/1871)	4.1 (42/1014)	3.8 (3/80)
Klebsiella pneumoniae (n = 1039)[a,c]	Fluoroquinolone-NS	6.8 (70/1036)	6.0 (41/689)	7.5 (24/320)	18.5 (5/27)
	Third-generation cephalosporin-NS	3.7 (38/1039)	2.7 (19/692)	5.0 (16/320)	11.1 (3/27)
	MDR	10.1 (105/1039)	9.2 (64/692)	11.3 (36/320)	18.5(5/27)
	Carbapenem-NS	1.5 (16/1035)	1.0 (7/690)	2.5 (8/319)	3.8 (1/26)
	Piperacillin/tazobactam-NS	7.1 (73/1021)	6.0 (41/685)	9.4 (29/310)	11.5 (3/26)
Pseudomonas aeruginosa (n = 502)[a,d]	Fluoroquinolone-NS	21.8 (109/499)	22.2 (70/316)	20.6 (33/160)	26.1 (6/23)
	Third-generation cephalosporin-NS	8.8 (44/502)	10.4 (33/318)	5.0 (8/161)	13.0 (3/23)
	MDR	8.8 (44/502)	10.4 (33/318)	5.0 (8/161)	13.0 (3/23)
	Carbapenem-NS	7.3 (36/496)	7.3 (23/314)	5.7 (9/159)	17.4 (4/23)
	Piperacillin/tazobactam-NS	4.0 (20/494)	4.1 (13/314)	4.4 (7/158)	0 (0/22)
Other Enterobacteriaceae (n = 1539)[a,e]	Fluoroquinolone-NS	14.1 (216/1531)	14.5 (137/947)	13.9 (74/534)	10.0 (5/50)
	Third-generation cephalosporin-NS	3.9 (60/1539)	4.0 (38/953)	3.9 (21/536)	2.0 (1/50)
	MDR	27.6 (424/1539)	26.4 (252/953)	29.9 (160/536)	24.0 (12/50)
	Carbapenem-NS	1.5 (23/1525)	1.5 (14/944)	1.7 (9/532)	0 (0/49)
	Piperacillin/tazobactam-NS	4.9 (75/1529)	4.8 (45/947)	5.4 (29/533)	2.0 (1/49)

MDR multidrug resistant, n number of nonsusceptible isolates, N total number of isolates, NS nonsusceptible

[a]For patients with missing susceptibility data, isolates were considered to be carbapenem-susceptible, piperacillin/tazobactam-susceptible, or non-MDR if they were susceptible to a third-generation cephalosporin. Otherwise, carbapenem, piperacillin/tazobactam, and MDR susceptibility data were considered missing, and isolates were not included in the analyses

[b]E. coli: 903 isolates were missing carbapenem susceptibility data, of which 896 were classified according to the rules described above and seven were excluded from the analysis due to missing data; 1412 isolates were missing piperacillin/tazobactam susceptibility data, of which 1364 were classified according to the rules and 48 were excluded

[c]K. pneumoniae: 317 isolates were missing carbapenem susceptibility data, of which 313 were classified according to the rules and four were excluded; 443 isolates were missing piperacillin/tazobactam susceptibility data, of which 425 were classified according to the rules and 18 were excluded

[d]P. aeruginosa: 97 isolates were missing carbapenem susceptibility data, of which 91 were classified according to the rules and six were excluded; 109 isolates were missing piperacillin/tazobactam susceptibility data, of which 101 were classified according to the rules and eight were excluded

[e]Other Enterobacteriaceae: 494 isolates were missing carbapenem susceptibility data, of which 480 were classified according to the rules and 14 were excluded; 721 isolates were missing piperacillin/tazobactam susceptibility data, of which 711 were classified according to the rules and ten were excluded

selection. Because we did not adjust for other factors, our findings cannot substantiate prior use of antibiotics as an independent risk factor for, or as a cause of, resistance, but our findings do show that prior use is an additional easily identifiable variable that can be used to guide empirical therapy. Second, the study was restricted to patients with UTIs occurring ≥3 days after hospital admission. Although we had access to detailed hospitalization data, information on antibiotic and health care exposure before admission was limited. As such, we focused on patients for whom complete, detailed data were available. The 3-day time frame after hospital admission fails to account for recent antibiotic use in outpatient or other institutional settings; therefore, the potential effects of these exposures on our findings are unknown. Third, this study did not specifically quantify the relationship between cumulative duration of

exposure to all or any given antibiotic and the presence of resistance. Given that the goal of the study was to provide clinicians with a straightforward, easily adaptable method for empirical antibiotic selection, we did not think it was necessary to specify with increased granularity the relationship between duration of prior antibiotic exposure and resistance. Although we were able to document prior receipt of many commonly used antibiotics with Gram-negative activity, data for other groups of antibiotics, including second-generation cephalosporins, and trimethoprim/sulfamethoxazole, were not available for this analysis. The relatively small number of patients with ≥2 prior antibiotic exposures might also limit the interpretation of findings regarding resistance, though increased rates observed among fewer pathogens is still of concern. In addition, though the statistical analysis suggests some significant differences between patients with ≥2 prior exposures and patients with 0 or 1 prior exposure, it should be noted that the numbers of patients in some of the groups were very small. As such, determination of the true statistical relevance of prior antibiotic exposure will require additional studies adequately powered to determine significance levels. Fourth, given that the presence of the ESBL phenotype among pathogens was not formally tested, the use of select third-generation cephalosporin resistance as a marker for ESBL may underestimate or overestimate the true incidence of ESBL. However, we believe third-generation cephalosporin resistance represented a practical surrogate because it is readily available to clinicians on urine culture susceptibility reports and that routine formal ESBL testing is not recommended by the Clinical and Laboratory Standards Institute (CLSI). Furthermore, given that culture susceptibility reports were from clinical and not reference laboratories, it can be assumed that third-generation cephalosporin resistance was reported using the US Food and Drug Administration–approved minimum inhibitory concentration breakpoint, which may better correlate with the presence of ESBL than CLSI breakpoints [14]. Finally, because findings are derived from positive urine cultures in the absence of a complete clinical picture, it is difficult to definitively distinguish between true infections and colonization. However, all patients received an antibiotic in response to a positive urine culture, which is suggestive of symptomatic infection for most patients.

Conclusions

Having received ≥2 prior antibiotic regimens was associated with increased risk for a resistant Gram-negative pathogen among patients with hospital-onset UTIs. In addition to considering the hospital antibiogram, which should be stratified for greater usefulness, hospital clinicians should critically assess prior exposure to antibiotics when selecting empirical therapy for patients with UTIs that occur ≥3 days after admission. Awareness of common pathogen distribution and nonsusceptibility trends among hospital patients with UTIs, combined with readily identifiable patient risk factors for infection with resistant pathogens, can provide a useful framework for clinicians during the empirical antibiotic selection process.

Abbreviations
CLSI: Clinical and Laboratory Standards Institute; ESBL: Extended-spectrum β-lactamase; MDR: Multidrug resistant; NS: Nonsusceptible; UTI: Urinary tract infection

Acknowledgments
Editorial support for this manuscript was provided by Sally Mitchell, PhD, and Meher Dustoor, PhD, of ApotheCom, Yardley, PA, USA, and was funded by Merck & Co., Inc., Kenilworth, NJ, USA.

Funding
This work was supported by Merck & Co., Inc., Kenilworth, NJ, USA.

Authors' contributions
MRB substantially contributed to the conception and design of the study, acquisition and analysis of data and interpretation of results, writing and critical review of the manuscript, gave approval of the final version of the manuscript to be published, and agreed to be accountable for the integrity of the data and the accuracy of the work. MPO substantially contributed to the conception and design of the study, acquisition and analysis of data and interpretation of results, writing and critical review of the manuscript, gave approval of the final version of the manuscript to be published, and agreed to be accountable for the integrity of the data and the accuracy of the work. MY substantially contributed to the conception and design of the study, acquisition and analysis of data and interpretation of results, writing and critical review of the manuscript, gave approval of the final version of the manuscript to be published, and agreed to be accountable for the integrity of the data and the accuracy of the work. JM substantially contributed to the conception and design of the study, acquisition and analysis of data and interpretation of results, writing and critical review of the manuscript, gave approval of the final version of the manuscript to be published, and agreed to be accountable for the integrity of the data and the accuracy of the work. TPL substantially contributed to the conception and design of the study, acquisition and analysis of data and interpretation of results, writing and critical review of the manuscript, gave approval of the final version of the manuscript to be published, and agreed to be accountable for the integrity of the data and the accuracy of the work. Employees of the study sponsor, in collaboration with the authors, were involved in the design, execution, analysis, and reporting of the research.

Authors' information
Not applicable.

Competing interests
MRB declares that she has no competing interests. MPO, MY, and JM were employees of Merck, Sharp & Dohme Corp., a subsidiary of Merck & Co., Inc., at the time of this study. TPL was a consultant for Merck, Sharp & Dohme Corp., a subsidiary of Merck & Co., Inc., at the time of the study.

Consent for publication
Not applicable.

Author details
[1]Albany College of Pharmacy and Health Sciences, 106 New Scotland Avenue, Albany 12208-3492, NY, USA. [2]Merck & Co., Inc., Kenilworth, NJ, USA.

References
1. World Health Organization. Antimicrobial resistance: global report on surveillance 2014. http://www.who.int/drugresistance/documents/surveillancereport/en/. Accessed 16 Sept 2016.
2. Jones RN. Resistance patterns among nosocomial pathogens: trends over the past few years. Chest. 2001;119:397S–404.
3. Zilberberg MD, Shorr AF. Secular trends in Gram-negative resistance among urinary tract infection hospitalizations in the United States, 2000-2009. Infect Control Hosp Epidemiol. 2013;34:940–6.
4. Mauldin PD, Salgado CD, Hansen IS, Durup DT, Bosso JA. Attributable hospital cost and length of stay associated with health care-associated infections caused by antibiotic-resistant Gram-negative bacteria. Antimicrob Agents Chemother. 2010;54:109–15.

5.   Thabit AK, Crandon JL, Nicolau DP. Antimicrobial resistance: impact on clinical and economic outcomes and the need for new antimicrobials. Exp Opin Pharmacother. 2015;16:159–77.

6.   Peralta G, Lamelo M, Alvarez-Garcia P, Velasco M, Delgado A, Horcajada JP, Montero M, Roiz MP, Fariñas MC, Alonso J, Martínez LM, Gutiérrez-Macías A, Alava JA, Rodríguez A, Fleites A, Navarro V, Sirvent E, Capdevila JA, Semi-Blee Study Group. Impact of empirical treatment in extended-spectrum beta-lactamase-producing Escherichia coli and Klebsiella spp. bacteremia: a multicentric cohort study. BMC Infect Dis. 2012;12:245.

7.   Pakyz AL. The utility of hospital antibiograms as tools for guiding empiric therapy and tracking resistance: insights from the Society of Infectious Diseases Pharmacists. Pharmacotherapy. 2007;27:1306–12.

8.   Hooton TM, Bradley SF, Cardenas DD, Colgan R, Geerlings SE, Rice JC, Saint S, Schaeffer AJ, Tambayh PA, Tenke P, Nicolle LE, Infectious Diseases Society of America. Diagnosis, prevention, and treatment of catheter-associated urinary tract infection in adults: 2009 International Clinical Practice Guidelines from the Infectious Diseases Society of America. Clin Infect Dis. 2010;50:625–63.

9.   Metlay JP, Strom BL, Asch DA. Prior antimicrobial drug exposure: a risk factor for trimethoprim-sulfamethoxazole-resistant urinary tract infections. J Antimicrob Chemother. 2003;51:963–70.

10. Magiorakos AP, Srinivasan A, Carey RB, Carmeli Y, Falagas ME, Giske CG, Harbarth S, Hindler JF, Kahlmeter G, Olsson-Liljequist B, Paterson DL, Rice LB, Stelling J, Struelens MJ, Vatopoulos A, Weber JT, Monnet DL. Multidrug-resistant, extensively drug-resistant and pandrug-resistant bacteria: an international expert proposal for interim standard definitions for acquired resistance. Clin Microbiol Infect. 2012;18:268–81.

11. Magill SS, Edwards JR, Beldavs ZG, Dumyati G, Janelle SJ, Kainer MA, Lynfield R, Nadle J, Neuhauser MM, Ray SM, Richards K, Rodriguez R, Thompson DL, Fridkin SK, Emerging Infections Program Healthcare-Associated Infections and Antimicrobial Use Prevalence Survey Team. Prevalence of antimicrobial use in US acute care hospitals, May-September 2011. JAMA. 2014;312:1438–46.

12. Gupta K, Hooton TM, Naber KG, Wullt B, Colgan R, Miller LG, Moran GJ, Nicolle LE, Raz R, Schaeffer AJ, Soper DE, Infectious Diseases Society of America; European Society for Microbiology and Infectious Diseases. International clinical practice guidelines for the treatment of acute uncomplicated cystitis and pyelonephritis in women: a 2010 update by the Infectious Diseases Society of America and the European Society for Microbiology and Infectious Diseases. Clin Infect Dis. 2011;52:e103–20.

13. Barlam TF, Cosgrove SE, Abbo LM, MacDougall C, Schuetz AN, Septimus EJ, Srinivasan A, Dellit TH, Falck-Ytter YT, Fishman NO, Hamilton CW, Jenkins TC, Lipsett PA, Malani PN, May LS, Moran GJ, Neuhauser MM, Newland JG, Ohl CA, Samore MH, Seo SK, Trivedi KK. Implementing an antibiotic stewardship program: guidelines by the Infectious Diseases Society of America and the Society for Healthcare Epidemiology of America. Clin Infect Dis. 2016;62:e51–77.

14. Mansury D, Motamedifar M, Sarvari J, Shirazi B, Khaledi A. Antibiotic susceptibility pattern and identification of extended spectrum beta-lactamases (ESBLs) in clinical isolates of *Klebsiella pneumoniae* from Shiraz, Iran. Iranian J Microbiol. 2016;8:55–61.

Use of antimicrobial resistance information and prescribing guidance for management of urinary tract infections: survey of general practitioners in the West Midlands

Dean Ironmonger[1*], Obaghe Edeghere[1], Savita Gossain[2] and Peter M. Hawkey[2,3*]

Abstract

Background: There is a marked variation in both antibiotic prescribing practice and urine sampling rates for diagnostic microbiology across general practices in England. To help understand factors driving this variation, we undertook a survey in 2012/13 to determine sampling protocols and antibiotic formularies used by general practitioners (GPs) for managing urinary tract infections (UTIs) in the West Midlands region of England.

Method: Cross-sectional survey of all eligible general practices in the West Midlands region of England undertaken in November 2012. GPs were invited to complete an online survey questionnaire to gather information on policies used within the practice for urine sampling for microbiological examination, and the source of antibiotic formularies used to guide treatment of UTIs. The questionnaire also gathered information on how they would manage five hypothetical clinical scenarios encountered in the community.

Results: The response rate was 11.3 % (409/3635 GPs), equivalent to a practice response rate of 26 % (248/950). Only 50 % of GPs reported having a practice policy for urine sampling. Although there was good agreement from GPs regarding collecting specimens in scenarios symbolising treatment failure (98 %), UTI in an adult male (98 %) and asymptomatic UTI in pregnancy (97 %), there was variation in GPs requesting a specimen for the scenarios involving a suspected uncomplicated urinary tract infection (UTI) and an asymptomatic catheterised elderly patient; with 40 and 38 % respectively indicating they would collect a specimen for microbiological examination.

Conclusion: Standardised evidence based clinical management policies and antibiotic formularies for GPs should be readily available. This will promote the rational use of diagnostic microbiology services, improve antimicrobial stewardship and aid the interpretation of ongoing antimicrobial resistance surveillance.

Keywords: Antimicrobial resistance, Antibiotic prescribing, Urinary tract infection, Community sampling

Background

Antimicrobial resistance (AMR) is a serious threat to health and the inappropriate use of antibiotics is central to the development of antibiotic resistance [1]. The UK five year AMR Strategy recommends the strengthening of AMR surveillance to inform local prescribing and

enable the monitoring of the impact of interventions aimed at reducing the burden of antibiotic resistance [2].

Antimicrobial susceptibility data from diagnostic microbiology laboratories can be used for surveillance to monitor trends in AMR [3]. This data is based on specimens submitted to laboratories and may be subject to selection bias due to over sampling of clinical specimens from patients with initial treatment failures, complicated clinical histories or severe infections [4, 5]. An English study in 2004 found a wide range for sampling urine specimens, from 29 to 266 urine samples/1000 patients/ year [5]. A Welsh study in 2006 found a similar range,

* Correspondence: dean.ironmonger@phe.gov.uk; Peter.Hawkey@
heartofengland.nhs.uk
[1]Field Epidemiology Service, Public Health England, 5 St Philips Place,
Birmingham, UK
[2]Public Health Laboratory, Public Health England, Heart of England NHS
Foundation Trust, Birmingham, UK
Full list of author information is available at the end of the article

with sampling rates varying from 0.6 to 237.3 urine samples/1000 patient/year [4], suggesting substantial variability in local sampling policies.

Studies in England and the United States have shown urine is the most frequent specimen sent for microbiological examination from non-hospitalised patients and urinary tract infection (UTI) is one of the most common diagnoses that results in antibiotic prescribing [6, 7]. In England in 2009, there was a fivefold difference in antibiotic prescribing volume between general practices [8], with 74 % of antibiotic prescribing occurring in community settings in 2014 [9].

There is a linear relationship between trends in antibiotic consumption and resistance [10, 11]. Variation in antibiotic prescribing rates in general practices have been shown to be negatively associated with variation in observed antibiotic resistance in the local population [12, 13]. National guidance for the management of infections and prescribing in the community has not reduced the variation in antibiotic prescribing across general practices in the UK, particularly in the management of upper respiratory and urinary tract infections [14].

In order to better understand some of the organisational and behavioural factors driving this variation in both antibiotic prescribing and specimen sampling for diagnostic microbiology, and thereby aid the interpretation of routine AMR surveillance data, we conducted a survey among general practitioners (GPs) in the West Midlands to examine the use of diagnostic microbiology services and empirical treatment for patients presenting with suspected UTI, and determine the source of prescribing advice.

Methods

Setting/population

The West Midlands is one of nine English administrative regions and in 2012 there were 950 general practices with a total of 3635 general practitioners responsible for 5.8 million registered patients [15]. Each practice had an average of 4 GPs with an average practice list size of just over 6,000 patients and 73 % of practices were located in Local Authority (English local administrative unit) areas designated as urban [15].

Survey of GPs in the West Midlands

We conducted a cross-sectional survey during November 2012 to February 2013 among GPs providing community healthcare in the West Midlands. Community healthcare was defined as ambulatory primary healthcare delivered by registered GPs working within practices in the West Midlands.

The survey questionnaire was developed using a template from an earlier Welsh study [4] and consisted of 17 questions divided into 3 sections (Additional file 1). Section 1 collected demographic data related to the

practice and GPs. Section 2 elicited information on policies employed for the management of UTI, with questions on the use and source of prescribing formularies, existence of practice policies for urine sampling; how microbiological results influenced antibiotic prescribing; and an estimate of the proportion of patients clinically suspected as having a UTI for which urine specimens were requested.

Section 3 described five hypothetical clinical scenarios (A to E) involving potential UTI presentations and GPs were asked whether they would request a specimen and/or prescribe antibiotics empirically (Table 1). Section 4 captured free text comments from the respondents.

We obtained a sampling frame of all eligible practices and GPs from NHS Primary Care Trusts (PCTs) (healthcare commissioners, now replaced by Clinical Commissioning Groups). This sampling frame contained email addresses of GP Practice Managers within the localities of 10 of the 17 PCTs in existence at the time of the study, with the remaining PCTs agreeing to use their existing networks to disseminate the survey invitation.

In October 2012, five GP practices were randomly selected from the sampling frame and invited to pilot the questionnaire. Two of these practices, consisting of 20 registered GPs participated in the pilot and the feedback received was used to improve the questionnaire.

The final questionnaire was produced and hosted online using SelectSurvey.net (ClassApps, USA). No sample size calculation was undertaken as all eligible practices were invited to complete the survey via email during November 2012. One email reminder was sent

Table 1 Clinical scenarios presented to survey participants

Scenario A: Treatment failure in a young woman
A 20 year old lady re-attends surgery and complains that the loin pain and frequent urination symptoms reported to you the previous week had worsened despite finishing a complete course of trimethoprim (no sample was taken previously).

Scenario B: Probable uncomplicated UTI
A 43 year old woman complains of pain passing urine and frequency. She feels well otherwise and has not previously been treated for a UTI.

Scenario C: Probable UTI in an adult male
A 51 year-old man attends your surgery complaining of pain passing urine and perineal tenderness. On examination you find suprapubic tenderness and a temperature of 38.5 C is measured.

Scenario D: Possible asymptomatic UTI in pregnancy
During a routine antenatal clinic an 18 year old girl who is 20 weeks pregnant produces a cloudy urine sample. She reports no symptoms or discomfort. The urine dipstick tests positive for nitrite but negative for leukocytes and protein.

Scenario E: Catheterised asymptomatic elderly female
You visit an 82 year old female in a nursing home. She is catheterised, afebrile and has no symptoms but the staff inform you that the urine is cloudy.

out to practices in January 2013 and the survey closed in February 2013.

Statistical analysis

The survey data was collated using Microsoft Excel (Microsoft Redmond, WA). Categorical variables were summarised as counts and proportions with differences between male and female GPs tested using a two-proportion Z test with $p < 0.05$ considered statistically significant. All statistical analyses were performed using STATA v12 (StataCorp, USA). All free text comments were analysed by thematic analysis.

Results

The response rate was 11.3 % (409/3635 GPs) equivalent to a practice response rate of 26 % (248/950). The age group distribution of respondents were 10 % aged under 35 years, 31 % aged 35–45 years, 44 % were aged 46–55 years and 16 % were over 55 years old. Fifty-four percent of the GPs were female (222/409) and a majority (62 %) of responders were qualified for 20 or more years. The age and sex of the responders was broadly comparable with the demographic profile of all GPs in the West Midlands.

Use of prescribing formularies

Eighty-six percent (314/366) of respondents reported that they use antibiotic prescribing formularies to guide prescribing decisions. The majority of these respondents (73 %; 269/366) stated that they used a formulary provided by their PCT; with 45 (12 %) reporting using more than one formulary (Table 2).

Thirty-four percent (123/366) had reviewed compliance with existing policy for the management of UTI in the last 12 months prior to the survey.

Table 2 Reported source of antibiotic prescribing formularies/prescribing guidance used by survey respondents ($N = 352$)

Source of antibiotic formulary	Number using source[b]
Primary Care Trust[a]	269
British National Formulary	46
Local area prescribing committee	17
Practice formulary	13
Local NHS Microbiology department	6
NHS Hospital/Trust	4
Health Protection Agency (now part of Public Health England)	3
NICE	1

[a]On April 2013, PCTs were replaced by Clinical Commissioning Groups
[b]Note some respondents mentioned more than one source

Influence of laboratory antimicrobial susceptibility results on antibiotic prescribing

Two hundred and fifty (70 %) respondents indicated that susceptibility results 'always' or 'frequently' influenced their antibiotic prescribing decisions for UTI. There was a significant difference (79 vs. 68 %; $p = 0.021$) between female and male GPs in the use of laboratory results to guide prescribing following treatment failure (Table 3). Only 6/362 (2 %) GPs reported that laboratory results infrequently or never influenced their prescribing in the case of reported resistance to initial therapy.

Factors influencing GPs decision to send urine specimens for diagnostic microbiology

Half (183/366) of the respondents reported that their practice had a policy to guide urine sampling for microbiological examination.

There was considerable variation among respondents regarding the approximate proportion of clinical consultations for suspected UTI that resulted in a urine specimen being sent for diagnostic microbiology (median 50 %, IQR 30 to 75 %).

Clinical scenarios

In scenarios A, C and D (Table 4) the majority of GPs would submit a urine specimen for diagnostic microbiology (98, 98 and 97 % respectively), which is in-line with Public Health England (PHE) national guidance [16]. In scenario B, 40 % of GPs indicated that they would submit a urine specimen for microbiological testing, even though PHE guidance recommends samples should not be sent for examination routinely for uncomplicated UTI in female adults <65 years of age. There was a difference in urine sampling between genders for the catheterised asymptomatic elderly female scenario (scenario E) with 32 % of male GPs indicating they would submit a sample, compared to 43 % of female GPs ($p = 0.034$), whereas PHE guidance recommends that urine specimens should only be sent for examination in catheterized patients when features of systemic infection are observed.

The majority of GPs follow PHE guidance [16] by prescribing an antibiotic empirically for probable treatment failure (scenario A, 80 %), suspected uncomplicated UTI (scenario B, 78 %) and probable UTI in a male adult (scenario C, 98 %) (Table 4).

There was significant variation between male and female GPs for prescribing antibiotics in the suspected UTI in pregnancy scenario (scenario D) where 43 % of female GPs would prescribe compared to 30 % of male GPs ($p = 0.0123$).

One hundred and four (104/409, 25 %) GPs entered additional free text comments.

Table 3 Influence of laboratory results on antibiotic prescribing decision (number that would prescribe/number of respondents)

	Male				Female			
	Always	Frequently	Infrequently	Never	Always	Frequently	Infrequently	Never
General prescribing	22 % (37/167)	46 % (77/167)	25 % (41/167)	7 % (11/167)	21 % (40/190)	51 % (97/190)	22 % (42/190)	6 % (12/190)
In the case of a treatment failure	68 % (114/168)	29 % (49/168)	2 % (3/168)	1 % (1/168)	79 % (154/195)	19 % (38/195)	1 % (2/195)	1 % (1/195)
When resistance is reported to initial prescribed agent	81 % (136/168)	16 % (27/168)	2 % (4/168)	1 % (1/168)	86 % (168/195)	13 % (26/195)	1 % (1/195)	0 % (0/195)

The main themes emerging from the analyses was the use of urinary dipstick test to investigate UTI in some of the scenarios presented, particularly scenario A (55/104, 53 %); the need to gather additional clinical information (15/104,14 %); inclination to send urine specimens by default (14/104, 13 %), and influence of the timing of the consultation in determining whether to take a specimen due to specimen transport issues (8/104, 8 %).

Discussion

We consider this to be the first study examining the role of specific organisational and behavioral factors in the observed variation of urine sampling for diagnostic microbiology, and antibiotic prescribing for patients with UTIs among GPs serving a region of England. We found that the existence of a practice policy to guide sampling for diagnostic microbiology varied considerably across the region, as did the proportion of GPs that would submit a specimen and/or prescribe an antibiotic in a number of clinical scenarios. Understanding GPs knowledge and attitude towards the management of UTI within a region will aid interpretation of local AMR surveillance data, help guide appropriate use of regional laboratory resources and inform targeted interventions to promote antimicrobial stewardship.

A commonly cited issue in interpreting routinely reported AMR data from community settings is sampling bias, which may lead to observed levels of resistance that

Table 4 Count and percentage of GPs requesting urine samples and prescribing antibiotics for each clinical scenario

Clinical scenarios	Number (%) of GPs requesting a specimen	Number (%) of GPs that would prescribe an antibiotic
A. Treatment failure in a young women	344/352 (98 %)	284/353 (80 %)
B. Probable uncomplicated UTI	144/359 (40 %)	270/345 (78 %)
C. Probable UTI in an adult male	348/354 (98 %)	344/352 (98 %)
D. Possible asymptomatic UTI in pregnancy	341/353 (97 %)	129/352 (37 %)
E. Catheterised asymptomatic elderly female	134/354 (38 %)	5/348 (1 %)

overestimate the burden of AMR in the general population. Only half of the GPs who responded reported having a practice policy to guide clinical sampling for diagnostic microbiology. There was considerable variation in the estimated proportion of clinical consultations for suspected UTI in which a urine specimen is sent for diagnostic microbiology. However we found that the response was broadly consistent for the scenarios involving: treatment failure, probable UTI in an adult male and possible UTI in pregnancy, and therefore using clinical scenarios may provide a more reliable insight into GP sampling practice than relying on a general view of GPs prescribing habits [4].

We found 40 % of GPs would submit a sample for diagnosis of the most commonly encountered presentation of uncomplicated UTIs, although PHE guidance recommends not sending urine samples for this presentation [16, 17]. This is a similar finding to a study in Wales in 2006 that found 56 % of randomly selected GPs would submit a urine specimen for probable uncomplicated UTI [4]. Also PHE guidance for management of UTIs in catheterised patients recommends that a urine sample should only be sent if there are signs of systemic infection [16], however 38 % of respondents would send a urine specimen in the catheterised asymptomatic elderly female scenario (Table 4). These results indicate non-compliance with guidance for certain clinical scenarios and a degree of inappropriate microbiological testing. A German study in 2005 concluded that most patients in their study were not treated according to current guidelines and for half the patients the decision to prescribe an antibiotic or the antibiotic prescribed was inappropriate [18].

It is plausible that this non-compliance with the guidance may be driven by ambiguity in the advice provided by existing national guidance. The National Institute for Health and Care Excellence (NICE) Clinical Knowledge Summaries advise that a urine sample should be sent to the laboratory for all women with suspected UTI associated with visible or non-visible haematuria [17]; however PHE guidance advises that urine samples should not be routinely submitted from women <65 of age, and if there are signs of UTI, including haematuria, then only empirical treatment should be given [16]. We recommend that these guidelines are reviewed so unambiguous evidence based guidance is made available to GPs.

Whilst acknowledging the importance of autonomy in clinical decision making, there is value in developing and utilising standardised, evidence based sampling policies to ensure that diagnostic and treatment decisions are both clinically effective and cost-effective [5]. Increasingly limited healthcare resources make a compelling case for standardising sampling policies, but this will only be achieved with consensus between microbiologists, community clinicians and policy makers.

The majority of respondents in our survey used local prescribing formularies produced by their PCTs. As PCTs were abolished at the end of March 2013 and replaced with Clinical Commissioning Groups (CCGs), we are unsure whether these formularies have been updated and are still being utilised. We recommend that CCGs work with their GP practices to review and update existing formularies.

A small proportion of respondents (14 %) indicated that they do not use a prescribing formulary to guide treatment decisions. We cannot tell from our survey if the non-utilisation of a formulary by these GPs results in inappropriate prescribing but we recommend that this issue be routinely assessed through the regular auditing and feedback of individual prescribing patterns and implementation of other interventions to address inappropriate prescribing as part of a wider antimicrobial stewardship programme.

The symptoms of UTI are often distressing to the patient, requiring immediate empirical therapy [19]. In our clinical scenarios most GPs would prescribe an antibiotic empirically for scenarios A, B and C (Table 4), which is in-line with national PHE guidance [16]; although it was surprising to find that a fifth of GP respondents would not prescribe an antibiotic in the treatment failure scenario (scenario A) given the presence of worsening symptoms.

Just over a third of our survey respondents indicated that they would prescribe an antibiotic for a suspected asymptomatic UTI in pregnancy (scenario D); even though national guidance recommends that treatment should only be considered after bacteriuria is confirmed by culture [16].

We found the gender of the GP was a factor in the responses to some of the survey questions, with a greater proportion of female GPs reporting being influenced by laboratory results, taking specimens and prescribing in scenarios D and E.

A possible explanation may be differences in patient empathy with particular patients groups or difference in the desire to meet patient expectations [20]. A large English study in 2009 found a higher proportion of male

GPs prescribing antibiotics in the community, and suggested male GPs perceive a greater pressure from patients to prescribe [8]. We therefore suggest that further behavioural studies are required to better understand variation in prescribing between genders and help inform the design of interventions aimed at changing prescribing habits.

There were some limitations to our study. The low response rate raises the possibility of non-response bias and its potential effect on the external validity of our study. We believe any effect on our estimates and the generalisability of our findings is low given that the demographic profile of our respondents is similar to that of all GPs in the West Midlands. In the free text comments, 3 GP respondents indicated that they may delay prescribing in some of the clinical scenarios; however the 'yes' or 'no' response options to these questions prevented the capture of this information.

Our analyses and interpretation of the free text comments may not be representative of the cohort of respondents as the number of comments was relatively small. However emerging themes from the analysis of these comments suggests that some GPs may be more inclined to send urine specimens by default. This needs to be explored further using alternative qualitative research methods such as focus groups.

For our next steps we intend to survey CCGs to determine whether antibiotic prescribing formularies developed by the PCTs are still being used and updated since the abolition of PCTs. We are also currently exploring the use of mobile device technologies to deliver timely localised AMR surveillance data and national prescribing guidance directly to clinicians in community settings and healthcare commissioners to support the management of UTI.

Conclusion

The delivery of clinical care of consistent high quality will benefit from the implementation of antimicrobial stewardship programmes in community settings that include prescribing formularies based on local AMR surveillance and unambiguous national guidance on the management of infections. These, and policies to guide clinical specimen sampling will also facilitate the cost-effective use of available laboratory, and other finite healthcare resources.

Abbreviations
AMR: antimicrobial resistance; CCG: Clinical Commissioning Groups; GP: general practitioner; NICE: National Institute for Health and Care Excellence; PCT: Primary Care Trust; PHE: Public Health England; UTI: urinary tract infection.

Acknowledgement
We would like to thank Shakeel Suleman for statistical input.

Funding
This work was supported by Public Health England and the University of Birmingham.

Authors' contributions
DI contributed to the acquisition and synthesis of the data and drafted the original manuscript, which was then amended with suggestions by all authors. OE, PMH and SG contributed to the conception and design of the work. DI and OE contributed to the analysis of the data. All authors contributed to the interpretation of data, and agreed to be accountable for all aspects of this work. All authors read and approved the final manuscript.

Competing interests
PMH has received honoraria for developing and delivering educational presentations for Eumedica, Pfizer, Merck, Novartis, MagusCommunications, Wyeth; funded research from Pfizer, Eumedica; Consultancy for Pfizer, Novartis, Basilea, Novacta, Novolytics, Merck, Wyeth, Optimer. He is a director of ModusMedica a medical education company. All other authors declare that they have no competing interests.

Consent for publication
Not applicable.

Author details
[1]Field Epidemiology Service, Public Health England, 5 St Philips Place, Birmingham, UK. [2]Public Health Laboratory, Public Health England, Heart of England NHS Foundation Trust, Birmingham, UK. [3]Institute of Microbiology and Infection, Biosciences, University of Birmingham, Birmingham, UK.

Reference List
1. CDC. Antibiotic Resistance Threats in the United States, 2013. http://www.cdc.gov/drugresistance/threat-report-2013/pdf/ar-threats-2013-508.pdf. Accessed 16 Dec 2015.
2. Department of Health. UK five year antimicrobial resistance strategy 2013 to 2018. https://www.gov.uk/government/uploads/system/uploads/attachment_data/file/244058/20130902_UK_5_year_AMR_strategy.pdf. Accessed 16 Dec 2015.
3. Ironmonger D, Edeghere O, Gossain S, Bains A, Hawkey PM. Am Web: a novel interactive web tool for antimicrobial resistance surveillance, applicable to both community and hospital patients. J Antimicrob Chemother. 2013;68:2406–13.
4. Hillier S, Bell J, Heginbothom M, Roberts Z, Dunstan F, Howard A, et al. When do general practitioners request urine specimens for microbiology analysis? The applicability of antibiotic resistance surveillance based on routinely collected data. J Antimicrob Chemother. 2006;58:1303–6.
5. McNulty CA, Bowen J, Clark G, Charlett A, Cartwright K. How should general practitioners investigate suspected urinary tract infection? variations in laboratory-confirmed bacteriuria in south west England. Commun Dis Public Health. 2004;7:220–6.
6. Petersen I, Hayward AC. Antibacterial prescribing in primary care. J Antimicrob Chemother. 2007;60 Suppl 1:i43–7.
7. Shapiro DJ, Hicks LA, Pavia AT, Hersh AL. Antibiotic prescribing for adults in ambulatory care in the USA, 2007–09. J Antimicrob Chemother. 2014;69:234–40.
8. Wang KY, Seed P, Schofield P, Ibrahim S, Ashworth M. Which practices are high antibiotic prescribers? a cross-sectional analysis. Br J Gen Pract. 2009;59:e315–20.
9. Public Health England. Antimicrobial surveillance programme antimicrobial utilisation and resistance (ESPAUR) report 2015. 10-10-2014. https://www.gov.uk/government/uploads/system/uploads/attachment_data/file/477962/ESPAUR_Report_2015.pdf. Accessed 16 Dec 2015.
10. Bell BG, Schellevis F, Stobberingh E, Goossens H, Pringle M. A systematic review and meta-analysis of the effects of antibiotic consumption on antibiotic resistance. BMC Infect Dis. 2014;14:13.
11. Costelloe C, Metcalfe C, Lovering A, Mant D, Hay AD. Effect of antibiotic prescribing in primary care on antimicrobial resistance in individual patients: systematic review and meta-analysis. BMJ. 2010;340:c2096.
12. Howard AJ, Magee JT, Fitzgerald KA, Dunstan FD. Factors associated with antibiotic resistance in coliform organisms from community urinary tract infection in Wales. J Antimicrob Chemother. 2001;47:305–13.
13. Vellinga A, Tansey S, Hanahoe B, Bennett K, Murphy AW, Cormican M. Trimethoprim and ciprofloxacin resistance and prescribing in urinary tract infection associated with Escherichia coli: a multilevel model. J Antimicrob Chemother. 2012;67:2523–30.
14. Hawker JI, Smith S, Smith GE, Morbey R, Johnson AP, Fleming DM, et al. Trends in antibiotic prescribing in primary care for clinical syndromes subject to national recommendations to reduce antibiotic resistance, UK 1995–2011: analysis of a large database of primary care consultations. J Antimicrob Chemother. 2014;69:3423–30.
15. Health and Social Care Information Centre. General and Personal Medical Services, England - 2002–2012. http://www.hscic.gov.uk/catalogue/PUB09536. Accessed 16 Dec 2015.
16. Public Health England. Urinary tract infection: diagnosis guide for primary care. https://www.gov.uk/government/publications/urinary-tract-infection-diagnosis. Accessed 16 Dec 2015.
17. NICE guidelines. Clinical Knowledge Summaries. Urinary tract infection (lower) - women. 2015. http://cks.nice.org.uk/urinary-tract-infection-lower-women#!scenario:1. Accessed 16 Dec 2016.
18. Hummers-Pradier E, Ohse AM, Koch M, Heizmann WR, Kochen MM. Management of urinary tract infections in female general practice patients. Fam Pract. 2005;22:71–7.
19. Gupta K, Hooton TM, Stamm WE. Increasing antimicrobial resistance and the management of uncomplicated community-acquired urinary tract infections. Ann Intern Med. 2001;135:41–50.
20. Coenen S, Michiels B, Renard D, Denekens J, Van RP. Antibiotic prescribing for acute cough: the effect of perceived patient demand. Br J Gen Pract. 2006;56:183–90.

Detection of CTX-M-15 beta-lactamases in Enterobacteriaceae causing hospital- and community-acquired urinary tract infections as early as 2004, in Dar es Salaam, Tanzania

Joel Manyahi[1,2*], Sabrina J. Moyo[1,2], Marit Gjerde Tellevik[3], Faustine Ndugulile[2], Willy Urassa[2], Bjørn Blomberg[1,3] and Nina Langeland[1,3]

Abstract

Background: The spread of Extended Spectrum β-lactamases (ESBLs) among *Enterobacteriaceae* and other Gram-Negative pathogens in the community and hospitals represents a major challenge to combat infections. We conducted a study to assess the prevalence and genetic makeup of ESBL-type resistance in bacterial isolates causing community- and hospital-acquired urinary tract infections.

Methods: A total of 172 isolates of *Enterobacteriaceae* were collected in Dar es Salaam, Tanzania, from patients who met criteria of community and hospital-acquired urinary tract infections. We used E-test ESBL strips to test for ESBL-phenotype and PCR and sequencing for detection of ESBL genes.

Results: Overall 23.8% (41/172) of all isolates were ESBL-producers. ESBL-producers were more frequently isolated from hospital-acquired infections (32%, 27/84 than from community-acquired infections (16%, 14/88, $p < 0.05$). ESBL-producers showed high rate of resistance to ciprofloxacin (85.5%), doxycycline (90.2%), gentamicin (80.5%), nalidixic acid (84.5%), and trimethoprim-sulfamethoxazole (85.4%). Furthermore, 95% of ESBL-producers were multi-drug resistant compared to 69% of non-ESBL-producers ($p < 0.05$). The distribution of ESBL genes were as follows: 29/32 (90.6%) $bla_{CTX-M-15}$, two bla_{SHV-12}, and one had both $bla_{CTX-M-15}$ and bla_{SHV-12}. Of 29 isolates carrying $bla_{CTX-M-15}$, 69% (20/29) and 31% (9/29) were hospital and community, respectively. Bla_{SHV-12} genotypes were only detected in hospital-acquired infections.

Conclusion: $bla_{CTX-M-15}$ is a predominant gene conferring ESBL-production in *Enterobacteriaceae* causing both hospital- and community-acquired infections in Tanzania.

Keywords: ESBL, Urinary tract infections, Tanzania

Background

Extended Spectrum β-lactamases (ESBLs) have been observed in virtually all species of the family *Enterobacteriaceae*. Spread of ESBL-producing strains from general wards to intensive care units (ICU) and into the community can contribute to the further propagation of these resistant strains [1].

ESBLs are responsible for resistance against beta-lactam antibiotics such as penicillins, cephalosporins, monobactams and sometimes also carbapenems [2]. Organisms carrying ESBL enzymes often display co-resistance to other antibiotics including aminoglycosides, quinolones, trimethoprim-sulfamethoxazole and tetracycline [3, 4]. Spread of ESBL-producing bacterial isolates in the community has made empirical treatment of infections more difficult, and narrows the treatment options to expensive antibiotics like colistin and carbapenems.

* Correspondence: manyahijoel@yahoo.com
[1]Department of Clinical Science, University of Bergen, Bergen, Norway
[2]Department of Microbiology and Immunology, Muhimbili University of Health and Allied Sciences, Dar es Salaam, Tanzania
Full list of author information is available at the end of the article

Recent studies in Africa and Europe have found substantial increase in ESBL-producing Gram-negative bacteria causing community urinary tract infections, particularly harboring the $bla_{CTX-M-15}$ allele [5–7]. Previously, studies in Tanzania have detected a substantial amount of ESBL-producing bacteria among the inpatients in intensive care and pediatric units in Tanzania [8, 9]. However, little is known regarding the frequency of ESBL-producers and ESBL genes in community-acquired (CA) and hospital-acquired (HA) urinary tract infections in Tanzania. A more recent study found a predominance of the $bla_{CTX-M-15}$ genotype from human feces in a community setting [10].

Previous studies performed at Muhimbili National Hospital documented the presence of ESBL-producers, predominantly of the $bla_{CTX-M-15}$ genotype, in hospital-acquired infections [8, 9]. Therefore, we decided to examine bacterial isolates collected prospectively for a period of six months in 2004 at Muhimbili National Hospital in Dar es Salaam, aiming at investigating whether ESBL-producers were present in the community setting, when hospital-acquired $bla_{CTX-M-15}$ -producers were first reported in Tanzania. We also aimed to compare the ESBL genotypes circulating in the community to those found in the hospital setting.

Methods
Study setting and patient population
The study was conducted at Muhimbili National Hospital (MNH, Dar es Salaam, Tanzania. MNH is a tertiary health care facility that serves a population of about 4 million residents. The Department of Microbiology, MNH, receives samples from inpatients in the hospital wards, from the outpatient clinics and private health facilities in the city. Included in the study were samples from inpatients and outpatients with urinary tract infections seen at MNH between June 2004 and January 2005. Hospital-acquired infections were defined as those occurring in inpatients admitted at MNH for at least 72 h. Community-acquired infections were defined as those occurring in patients attending outpatient clinics at MNH. A UTI was defined as a positive urine culture of $\geq 10^5$ CFU/ml of pure bacterial growth.

Clinical isolates
A total of 172 isolates of *Enterobacteriaceae* were collected, 84 and 88 isolates from hospital and community patients, respectively. All isolates were identified to the species level using established conventional procedures, the API 20E system (bioMérieux SA, Marcy l'Etoile, France) or the Vitek 2 system (BioMérieux, Inc., Durham, N.C).

Antimicrobial susceptibility testing
All isolates were tested for antimicrobial susceptibility using the disk diffusion method according to the Clinical & Laboratory Standards Institute's guidelines [11]. The antimicrobials tested included amoxicillin/clavulanic acid (20/10µg), gentamicin (10µg), chloramphenicol (30µg), trimethoprim/sulfamethoxazole (1.25/23.75µg), doxycycline (30µg), nitrofurantoin(30µg), nalidixic acid (30µg), imipenem (10µg), ciprofloxacin (5µg), cefotaxime (30µg), ceftriaxone(30µg) and ceftazidime (30µg). Multidrug-resistant (MDR) bacteria were those bacteria which showed resistance to three or more classes of antimicrobial agents [12], classes including β-lactam/β-lactamase inhibitors, cephalosporins (ceftriaxone, ceftazidime, cefotaxime), aminoglycosides, fluoroquinolones (ciprofloxacin), tetracycline, cabepenems, Nitrofurantoin and trimethoprim-sulfamethoxazole. For ESBL isolates classes defining MDR excluded Penicillins and cephalosporins.

ESBL detection
All isolates with reduced susceptibilities to ceftazidime (zone of inhibition < 22mm), ceftriaxone (zone inhibition <25 mm) and cefotaxime (zone inhibition <27 mm) disks according to CLSI guidelines [11], were tested for an ESBL using E-test ESBL strips as previously described [8] and PCR. Isolates with reduced susceptibilities to cephalosporin were confirmed ESBL by either using E-tests ESBL strips or PCR.

Detection and identification of ESBL genotypes
All strain with reduced susceptibility to cephalosporin were examined for the presence of the bla_{TEM}, bla_{SHV} and bla_{CTX-M} genes by PCR, using genomic DNA isolated by boiling. For bla_{TEM} amplification the primers described by Dubois et al. were used [13]. The cycling conditions were 95°C for 15 min, followed by 30 cycles of denaturation at 95°C for 1 min, annealing at 55°C for 1 min, elongation at 72°C for 1 min, followed by a final extension of 72°C for 10 min.

For bla_{SHV} amplification the primers SHV-1F (5′ – CGG CCT TCA CTC AAG GAT G – 3′) and SHV-1R (5′ – CGG STT AGC GTT GCC AGT – 3′) were used. The cycling conditions were the same as for those of blaTEM, but with an annealing temperature of 60°C. In PCR amplification targeting the blaCTX-M gene the primer pairs described by Pagani et al. [14] were used. The cycling conditions for these two primer pairs were initial activation at 95°C for 15 min, followed by 30 cycles of denaturation at 95°C for 30 s, annealing at 50°C for 40 s, elongation at 72°C for 1 min, followed by a final extension at 72°C for 10 min, and initial activation at 95°C for 15 min, followed by 30 cycles of denaturation at 95°C for 50 s, annealing at 50°C for 40 s, elongation at 72°C for 1 min, followed by a final extension at 72°C for 10 min. HotStarTaq Master Mix Kit (Qiagen, Hilden, Germany) and 1 μM of each primer were used for all PCR amplifications.

The PCR products were purified using either QIAquick PCR Purification Kit (Qiagen, Hilden, Germany) or ExoSAP- IT (GE Healthcare). Both strands were sequenced using the same primers as for PCRs, and sometimes internal sequencing primers were added as described by Arpin et al., Bermudes et al. and Rasheed et al. [15–17]. The BigDye® Terminator v3.1 Cycle Sequencing Kit (Applied Biosystems, Foster City, CA) were used for sequencing, followed by analysis by capillary electrophoresis with an ABI Prism 3700 DNA Analyzer (Applied Biosystems). Point mutations were accepted if present in both the forward and reverse sequences.

Data analysis
Data were analysed using SPSS software version 20.0 (IBM SPSS statistics 20.0, SPSS Inc., Chicago, IL, USA). Chi-square test was used to determine associations between categorical variables, $p < 0.05$ was considered statistically significant.

Results
Prevalence of ESBL isolates
During the study period a total of 172 bacterial isolates from hospital- and community-acquired urinary tract infections were consecutively collected. The most frequent bacteria isolated were *Escherichia coli* (64%), followed by *Klebsiella pneumoniae* (15.7%) and other *Enterobacteriaceae* accounted for 20.3%. Of the 172 bacterial isolates, 23.8% (41/172) were ESBL-producers (Table 1). ESBL-producing isolates were more frequent from the hospital setting 32% (27/84) than from the community setting (16%, (14/88); $p < 0.05$). The proportion of ESBL positive *E. coli* isolates was significantly higher in hospital-

acquired infections (20.3%, 11/54) compared to community-acquired infections (7.1% (4/56); $p < 0.05$). In *K. pneumoniae* isolates, ESBL-production was equally frequent in hospital- and community-acquired infections (33.3% each). The proportion of *Enterobacter cloacae* isolates producing ESBL was significantly higher in the hospital setting (71% (5/7)) than in the community setting (25% (1/4); $p > 0.05$).

Antimicrobial susceptibility pattern
Overall, ESBL-producing isolates showed significantly higher rates of resistance towards ciprofloxacin (85.5%), doxycycline (90.2%), gentamicin (80.5%), nalidixic acid (84.5%) and trimethoprim-sulfamethoxazole (85.4%) ($p < 0.05$) compared to non-ESBL producers. All ESBL and non-ESBL-producers were susceptible to imipenem (Table 2). Multi-drug resistant was high (95%) of ESBL-producers compared to 69% of non-ESBL-producing bacteria ($p < 0.05$).

When comparing rates of resistance between HA and CA ESBL, we found that hospital-acquired *E. coli* and *K. pneumoniae* were more frequently resistant to ciprofloxacin, gentamicin and nalidixic acid than those isolated from community-acquired infections (Table 3).

Non-ESBL-producing *E. coli* and *K. pneumoniae* from hospital- and community-acquired infections were less frequently resistant to gentamicin, nalidixic acid and ciprofloxacin. However, non-ESBL-producing *E. coli* from outpatients showed moderately high rates of resistance to trimethoprim-sulfamethoxazole, nitrofurantoin and doxycycline compared to isolates from inpatients. Higher rates of resistance to amoxicillin-clavulanic acid and trimethoprim-sulfonamide were observed in hospital-acquired as compared to community-acquired isolates of non-ESBL-producing *K. pneumoniae*. (Susceptibility profile for other isolates see Additional file 1: Table S1).

Table 1 Distribution of ESBL positive and ESBL negative bacteria isolated from hospital- and community-acquired urinary tract infections

Bacteria spp.	Hospitalized patients			Community patients			Total
	ESBL (+)	ESBL (−)	Subtotal	ESBL (+)	ESBL (−)	Subtotal	
E. coli	11	43	54(64.3)	4	52	56(64)	110(64)
K. pneumoniae	4	8	12(14.3)	5	10	15(17)	27(15.7)
E. cloacae	5	2	7(8.3)	1	3	4(4.5)	11(6.4)
C. freundii	3	2	5(6)	1	3	4(4.5)	9(5.2)
M. morganii	1	1	2(2.3)	1	4	5(5.6)	7(4.1)
P. mirabilis	3	1	4(4.8)	2	1	3(3.3)	7(4.1)
P. rettgeri	0	0	0	0	1	1(1.1)	1(0.6)
Total	27	57	84(100)	14	74	88	172(100)

HA hospital acquired, *CA* community-acquired

Table 2 Antimicrobial resistance pattern for ESBL and Non- ESBL bacteria isolates, (% of resistance isolates within each group)

Antibiotic	E. coli		K. pneumoniae		E. cloacae		C. freundii		P. mirabilis		M. morganii		P. rettgeri
	ESBL(+) (n = 15)	ESBL (−) (n = 95)	ESBL (+) (n = 9)	ESBL (−) (n = 18)	ESBL (+) (n = 6)	ESBL (−) (n = 5)	ESBL (+) (n = 4)	ESBL (−) (n = 5)	ESBL (+) (n = 5)	ESBL (−) (n = 2)	ESBL (+) (n = 2)	ESBL (−) (n = 5)	ESBL (−) (n = 1)
AMC	NA	14.7	NA	44.4	NA	80	NA	50	NA	0	NA	20	100
CTX	NA	0.0	NA	0	NA	0	NA	0	NA	0	NA	0	0
CTZ	NA	0.0	NA	0	NA	0	NA	0	NA	0	NA	0	0
CRO	NA	1.1	NA	0	NA	0	NA	0	NA	0	NA	0	0
IMP	0	0	0	0	0	0	0	0	0	0	0	0	0
CHL	26.7	37.9	88.9	50	83.3	20	75	0	100	0	100	60	100
CIP	86.7	27.4	66.7	22.2	83.3	0	50	0	100	0	100	60	0
DO	100	73.7	66.7	44.4	83.3	60	100	40	100	100	100	80	100
CN	80	18	88.9	22.2	50	0	75	0	100	0	100	20	0
NAL	86.7	37.9	66.7	27.8	75	20	100	0	100	0	100	80	100
NIT	33.3	10.5	77.8	33.3	83.3	60	75	20	100	100	100	100	100
SXT	93.3	72.6	66.7	72.2	83.3	20	75	20	100	0	100	80	0

AMC Amoxicillin-clavulanic acid, CTX cefotaxime, CTZ ceftazidime, CRO ceftriaxone, IMP imipenem, CHL chloramphenicol, CIP ciprofloxacin, DO doxycycline, CN gentamicin, NAL nalidixic acid, NIT nitrofurantoin, SXT trimethoprim-sulfamethoxazole
NA Not applicable

Molecular characterization of ESBL producing bacteria

An ESBL genotype could be identified for 32 of the all ESBL confirmed isolates (Table 4). Among these, 90.6% (29/32) were $bla_{CTX-M-15}$ positive, 6.25% (2/32) were bla_{SHV-12} positive and one isolate was found to carry both $bla_{CTX-M-15}$ and bla_{SHV-12}. None of the isolate carried bla_{TEM}. Of the 29 isolates carrying $bla_{CTX-M-15}$, 69% (20/29) were hospital isolates and 31% (9/29) from community settings. (All three isolates harboring bla_{SHV-12} were from hospital setting (E. coli, E. cloacae and Citrobacter freundii). All isolates carrying $bla_{CTX-M-15}$ displayed high rates of resistance to non β-lactam agents, including ciprofloxacin (88%), gentamicin (81.5%) and trimethoprim-sulfamethoxazole (89%).

Discussion

In recent years there has been an alarming increase in community acquired infections with ESBL-producing bacteria [5, 12, 18]. Spread of these strains in the community is a major concern to patient healthcare, since

Table 3 Antimicrobial resistance pattern of E. coli and K. pneumoniae isolates from Hospital-acquired and Community-acquired urinary tract infections (% of resistance isolates within each group)

Antibiotic	E. coli (n = 110)				K. pneumoniae (n = 27)			
	Hospital acquired		Community acquired		Hospital acquired		Community acquired	
	ESBL (+) (n = 11)	ESBL (−) (n = 43)	ESBL (+) (n = 4)	ESBL (−) (n = 52)	ESBL (+) (n = 4)	ESBL (−) (n = 8)	ESBL (+) (n = 5)	ESBL (−) (n = 10)
AMC	NA	11.6	NA	17.3	NA	62.5	NA	30.0
CTX	NA	0	NA	0	NA	0	NA	0
CTZ	NA	0	NA	0	NA	0	NA	0
CRO	NA	0	NA	0	NA	0	NA	0
IMP	0	0	0	0	0	0	0	0
CHL	27.3	41.9	25.0	34.6	75.0	62.5	100	40.0
CIP	90.9	32.6	75.0	23.1	100	25.0	40.0	20.0
DOX	100	69.8	100	76.9	75.0	62.5	60.0	30.0
CN	90.9	16.3	50.0	21.2	100	37.5	80.0	10.0
NAL	90.0	41.9	75.0	34.6	100	25.0	40.0	30.0
NIT	27.3	27.3	50.0	50.0	100	100	60.0	60.0
SXT	90.9	62.8	100	80.8	75.0	87.5	60.0	60.0

(+) = positive; (−) = negative
AMC Amoxicillin-clavulanic acid, CTX cefotaxime, CTZ ceftazidime, CRO ceftriaxone, IMP imipenem, CHL chloramphenicol, CIP ciprofloxacin, DO doxycycline, CN gentamicin, NAL nalidixic acid, NIT nitrofurantoin, SXT trimethoprim-sulfamethoxazole

Table 4 ESBL genotypes in bacteria isolated from hospital-acquired and community-acquired urinary tract infections

Bacteria spp.	CTX-M-15			SHV-12			CTX-M-15/SHV-12	
	HA	CA	Subtotal	HA	CA	Subtotal	HA	CA
E. coli	10	4	14	0	0	0	1	0
K. pneumoniae	4	3	7	0	0	0	0	0
E. cloacae	3	1	4	1	0	1	0	0
C. freundii	2	0	2	1	0	1	0	0
M. morganii	1	1	2	0	0	0	0	0
Total	20	9	29	2	0	0	1	0

HA Hospital acquired, *CA* community acquired

most display multidrug resistance, limiting outpatient treatment options. The resultant increasing use of broad-spectrum antibiotics to treat infections caused by ESBL-producers is expected to lead to further emergence of antimicrobial resistance. However, little data exist on molecular characterization of ESBL isolates causing community-acquired urinary tract infections in Tanzania and Africa. The current study shows that ESBL-producing isolates caused both community and hospital-acquired urinary tract infections in 2004, when CTX-M-15 was first reported in Tanzania.

The overall frequency of ESBL-producing *Enterobacteriaceae* among urinary tract pathogens in this study was 23.8%. The frequency of ESBL-producing pathogens was significantly higher in hospital-acquired compared to community-acquired uropathogens. Our finding is in agreement with other studies [19–22] reporting higher frequency of ESBL-producers in hospital-acquired urinary tract infections compared to community-acquired infections. A possible explanation for this could be that hospital-acquired infections were more likely associated with prolonged hospitalization, comorbidities, previous antibiotic use and urinary catheterization which are well-known risk factors for acquisition of ESBL-producing pathogens [19]. However, the finding of ESBL-producing isolates in community urinary infections is worrisome because of the limited treatment options, considering most of these isolates display multidrug resistance.

Similar to other studies in Africa [4, 10, 22], we found that ESBL-producing isolates from both hospital and community settings displayed high rates of resistance to ciprofloxacin, trimethoprim-sulfamethoxazole, gentamicin, nalidixic acid and doxycycline. Resistance to commonly prescribed oral antimicrobials in these resource-limited settings, specifically to ciprofloxacin and trimethoprim-sulfamethoxazole, limits outpatient therapeutic options. Considering that most of the outpatients present with uncomplicated urinary tract infections, opting to injectable and expensive antimicrobials increases health-care burdens. We also found non-ESBL-producing *E. coli* from community-acquired

urinary tract infections had moderate to high rates of resistance to trimethoprim-sulfamethoxazole, doxycycline and nitrofurantoin. This could be expected, since oral antimicrobials are inexpensive and easily available over the counter, and self-treatment is common in Africa; these are well known factors driving emergence of antimicrobial resistance bacteria.

Among 41 ESBL defined isolates, 78% were found to carry ESBL genes. Our finding of a predominance of CTX-M-15 is in line to previous and recent studies from hospital and community urinary tract infections [6, 7, 18, 23], and our finding concurs with those of studies from the same setting, which found CTX-M-15 as the dominant ESBL genotype [8–10, 24]. CTX-M types ESBLs, in particular CTX-M-15, are known for their rapid dissemination world-wide among the members of *Enterobacteriaceae* [6, 12, 23, 25, 26]. It has also been suggested that the widespread use of ceftriaxone and cefotaxime could be a reason of emergence and spread of CTX-M enzymes [27].

Our study had some limitations; one our isolates were collected in 2004 and may not imply the current situation. However, our findings shed lights on community spread of ESBL-producers and suggest existence in Tanzania at least since 2004. Second being a laboratory-based study, clinical information was not obtained, and we could not analyze risk factors for ESBL infections. Furthermore, epidemiological typing to assess clonality of the isolates was not performed, and this could have added value to the understanding of the epidemiological spread of ESBL genes.

Conclusion

In conclusion, we report the presence of *Enterobacteriaceae* harboring CTX-M-15 type ESBL causing community-acquired urinary tract infections in Tanzania as early as 2004. Furthermore, both ESBL and non-ESBL-producing isolates displayed high rates of multidrug resistance. Further investigation needs to be performed to understand the transmission dynamics of CTX-M type of ESBL resistance.

Acknowledgement
We would like to acknowledge members of Department of Microbiology and Immunology, Muhimbili National Hospital, Dar es Salaam, Tanzania, the Department of Microbiology, Haukeland University Hospital, Bergen, Norway and the Department of Clinical Science, University of Bergen, Bergen, Norway, for their technical and financial support during the molecular study.

Authors' contributions
JM, SM, MGT, FN, WU, BB, NL conceived and designed the study. FN collected study data. FN and MGT performed the experiments. JM drafted the manuscript. All authors read and approved the manuscript.

Competing interests
The authors declare that they have no competing interests.

Consent for publication
Not applicable.

Author details
[1]Department of Clinical Science, University of Bergen, Bergen, Norway. [2]Department of Microbiology and Immunology, Muhimbili University of Health and Allied Sciences, Dar es Salaam, Tanzania. [3]National Centre for Tropical Infectious Diseases, Department of Medicine, Haukeland University Hospital, Bergen, Norway.

References
1. Bosi C, Davin-Regli A, Bornet C, Mallea M, Pages JM, Bollet C. Most Enterobacter aerogenes strains in France belong to a prevalent clone. J Clin Microbiol. 1999;37:2165–9.
2. Paterson DL, Bonomo RA. Extended-spectrum beta-lactamases: a clinical update. Clin Microbiol Rev. 2005;18:657–86.
3. Canton R, Coque TM. The CTX-M beta-lactamase pandemic. Curr Opin Microbiol. 2006;9:466–75.
4. Meier S, Weber R, Zbinden R, Ruef C, Hasse B. Extended-spectrum beta-lactamase-producing Gram-negative pathogens in community-acquired urinary tract infections: an increasing challenge for antimicrobial therapy. Infection. 2011;39:333–40.
5. Hammami S, Saidani M, Ferjeni S, Aissa I, Slim A, Boutiba-Ben Boubaker I. Characterization of extended spectrum beta-lactamase-producing Escherichia coli in community-acquired urinary tract infections in Tunisia. Microb Drug Resist. 2013;19:231–6.
6. Ibrahimagic A, Bedenic B, Kamberovic F, Uzunovic S. High prevalence of CTX-M-15 and first report of CTX-M-3, CTX-M-22, CTX-M-28 and plasmid-mediated AmpC beta-lactamase producing Enterobacteriaceae causing urinary tract infections in Bosnia and Herzegovina in hospital and community settings. J Infect Chemother. 2015;21:363–9.
7. Barguigua A, El Otmani F, Talmi M, Zerouali K, Timinouni M. Prevalence and types of extended spectrum beta-lactamases among urinary Escherichia coli isolates in Moroccan community. Microb Pathog. 2013;61–62:16–22.
8. Blomberg B, Jureen R, Manji KP, Tamim BS, Mwakagile DS, Urassa WK, et al. High rate of fatal cases of pediatric septicemia caused by gram-negative bacteria with extended-spectrum beta-lactamases in Dar es Salaam, Tanzania. J Clin Microbiol. 2005;43:745–9.
9. Ndugulile F, Jureen R, Harthug S, Urassa W, Langeland N. Extended spectrum beta-lactamases among Gram-negative bacteria of nosocomial origin from an intensive care unit of a tertiary health facility in Tanzania. BMC Infect Dis. 2005;5:86.
10. Mshana SE, Falgenhauer L, Mirambo MM, Mushi MF, Moremi N, Julius R, et al. Predictors of blaCTX-M-15 in varieties of Escherichia coli genotypes from humans in community settings in Mwanza, Tanzania. BMC Infect Dis. 2016;16:187.
11. CLSI. Perfomance standards for antimicrobial susceptibility testing; fifteenth information supplement vol. CLSI document M100-S15. Clinical and Laboratory Standards Institute: Wayne; 2005.
12. Woodford N, Ward ME, Kaufmann ME, Turton J, Fagan EJ, James D, et al. Community and hospital spread of Escherichia coli producing CTX-M extended-spectrum beta-lactamases in the UK. J Antimicrob Chemother. 2004;54:735–43.
13. Dubois V, Poirel L, Marie C, Arpin C, Nordmann P, Quentin C. Molecular characterization of a novel class 1 integron containing bla(GES-1) and a fused product of aac3-Ib/aac6'-Ib' gene cassettes in Pseudomonas aeruginosa. Antimicrob Agents Chemother. 2002;46:638–45.
14. Pagani L, Luzzaro F, Ronza P, Rossi A, Micheletti P, Porta F, et al. Outbreak of extended-spectrum beta-lactamase producing Serratia marcescens in an intensive care unit. FEMS Immunol Med Microbiol. 1994;10:39–46.
15. Arpin C, Labia R, Andre C, Frigo C, El Harrif Z, Quentin C. SHV-16, a beta-lactamase with a pentapeptide duplication in the omega loop. Antimicrob Agents Chemother. 2001;45:2480–5.
16. Bermudes H, Jude F, Chaibi EB, Arpin C, Bebear C, Labia R, et al. Molecular characterization of TEM-59 (IRT-17), a novel inhibitor-resistant TEM-derived beta-lactamase in a clinical isolate of Klebsiella oxytoca. Antimicrob Agents Chemother. 1999;43:1657–61.
17. Rasheed JK, Jay C, Metchock B, Berkowitz F, Weigel L, Crellin J, et al. Evolution of extended-spectrum beta-lactam resistance (SHV-8) in a strain of Escherichia coli during multiple episodes of bacteremia. Antimicrob Agents Chemother. 1997;41(3):647–53.
18. Kariuki S, Revathi G, Corkill J, Kiiru J, Mwituria J, Mirza N, et al. Escherichia coli from community-acquired urinary tract infections resistant to fluoroquinolones and extended-spectrum beta-lactams. J Infect Dev Ctries. 2007;1:257–62.
19. Kader AA, Angamuthu K. Extended-spectrum beta-lactamases in urinary isolates of Escherichia coli, Klebsiella pneumoniae and other gram-negative bacteria in a hospital in Eastern Province, Saudi Arabia. Saudi Med J. 2005; 26:956–9.
20. Latifpour M, Gholipour A, Damavandi MS. Prevalence of Extended-Spectrum Beta-Lactamase-Producing Klebsiella pneumoniae Isolates in Nosocomial and Community-Acquired Urinary Tract Infections. Jundishapur J Microbiol. 2016;9:e31179.
21. Khanfar HS, Bindayna KM, Senok AC, Botta GA. Extended spectrum beta-lactamases (ESBL) in Escherichia coli and Klebsiella pneumoniae: trends in the hospital and community settings. J Infect Dev Ctries. 2009;3:295–9.
22. Moyo SJ, Aboud S, Kasubi M, Lyamuya EF, Maselle SY. Antimicrobial resistance among producers and non-producers of extended spectrum beta-lactamases in urinary isolates at a tertiary Hospital in Tanzania. BMC Res Notes. 2010;3:348.
23. Fam N, Leflon-Guibout V, Fouad S, Aboul-Fadl L, Marcon E, Desouky D, et al. CTX-M-15-producing Escherichia coli clinical isolates in Cairo (Egypt), including isolates of clonal complex ST10 and clones ST131, ST73, and ST405 in both community and hospital settings. Microb Drug Resist. 2011;17:67–73.
24. Mshana SE, Imirzalioglu C, Hain T, Domann E, Lyamuya EF, Chakraborty T. Multiple ST clonal complexes, with a predominance of ST131, of Escherichia coli harbouring blaCTX-M-15 in a tertiary hospital in Tanzania. Clin Microbiol Infect. 2011;17(8):1279–82.
25. Blanco VM, Maya JJ, Correa A, Perenguez M, Munoz JS, Motoa G, et al. [Prevalence and risk factors for extended-spectrum beta-lactamase-producing Escherichia coli causing community-onset urinary tract infections in Colombia]. Enferm Infecc Microbiol Clin. 2016;34(9):559–65.
26. Rossolini GM, D'Andrea MM, Mugnaioli C. The spread of CTX-M-type extended-spectrum beta-lactamases. Clin Microbiol Infect. 2008;14 Suppl 1:33–41.
27. Wang H, Kelkar S, Wu W, Chen M, Quinn JP. Clinical isolates of Enterobacteriaceae producing extended-spectrum beta-lactamases: prevalence of CTX-M-3 at a hospital in China. Antimicrob Agents Chemother. 2003;47(2):790–3.

Urinary tract infection among fistula patients admitted at Hamlin fistula hospital, Addis Ababa, Ethiopia

Matifan Dereje[1*], Yimtubezinesh Woldeamanuel[2], Daneil Asrat[2] and Fekade Ayenachew[3]

Abstract

Background: Urinary Tract Infection (UTI) causes a serious health problem and affects millions of people worldwide. Patients with obstetric fistula usually suffer from incontinence of urine and stool, which can predispose them to frequent infections of the urinary tract. Therefore the aim of this study was to determine the etiologic agents, drug resistance pattern of the isolates and associated risk factor for urinary tract infection among fistula patients in Addis Ababa fistula hospital, Ethiopia.

Methods: Across sectional study was conducted from February to May 2015 at Hamlin Fistula Hospital, Addis Ababa, Ethiopia. Socio-demographic characteristics and other UTI related risk factors were collected from study participants using structured questionnaires. The mid-stream urine was collected and cultured on Cysteine lactose electrolyte deficient agar and blood agar. Antimicrobial susceptibility was done by using disc diffusion method and interpreted according to Clinical and Laboratory Standards Institute (CLSI). Data was entered and analyzed by using SPSS version 20.

Results: Out of 210 fistula patients investigated 169(80.5%) of the patient were younger than 25 years. Significant bacteriuria was observed in 122/210(58.1%) and 68(55.7%) of the isolates were from symptomatic cases. E.coli 65(53.7%) were the most common bacterial pathogen isolated followed by Proteus spp. 31(25.4%). Statistical Significant difference was observed with history of previous UTI ($P = 0.031$) and history of catheterization ($P = 0.001$). Gram negative bacteria isolates showed high level of resistance (>50%) to gentamicin and ciprofloxacin, while all gram positive bacteria isolated were showed low level of resistance (20–40%) to most of antibiotic tested.

Conclusions: The overall prevalence of urinary tract infection among fistula patient is 58.1%. This study showed that the predominant pathogen of UTI were E.coli followed by Proteus spp. It also showed that amoxicillin-clavulanic acid was a drug of choice for urinary tract bacterial pathogens.

Keywords: UTI, Fistula patients, Hamlin Fistula Hospital, Addis Ababa, Ethiopia

Background

Urinary Tract Infections (UTIs) is an infection caused by the presence and growth of pathogens anywhere in the urinary tract including a kidney, ureter, bladder, and urethra. It is one of the most common bacterial infections in women, and 50% to 60% of adult women experience a UTI during their lifetime [1].

Patients with obstetric fistula (OF) can have frequent bladder infections, incontinence of urine and stool. Many of these patients might live with these conditions for several years. This may further predispose them to health related problems like urinary tract infections [2].

Obstetric fistula (or vaginal fistula) is a severe medical condition in which a fistula (hole) develops between the rectum and vagina (recto-vaginal fistula (RVF)) or between the bladder and vagina (vesico-vaginal fistula (VVF)) after severe or failed childbirth, when adequate medical care is not available [3]. Vesico-vaginal and recto-vaginal fistulas are debilitating complications of

---

* Correspondence: matiy2016@yahoo.com
[1]Department of medicine, Collages of medicine and health sciences, Ambo University, Ambo, Ethiopia
Full list of author information is available at the end of the article

obstructed labor, which primarily affect women and girls in developing countries [4].

Other causes include poorly performed abortion, sexual abuse and rape, other surgical trauma, gynecological cancers or other related radiotherapy treatments and, perhaps the most important, limited or no access to obstetrical care or emergency services [5].

It has been cited as one of the most dramatic and physically, psychologically, and socially damaging, yet preventable, complications of labor.

The most common symptom of recto-vaginal fistula is passage of bowl contents through the vagina. It may also cause inflammation of vagina, which result in burning, itching and discharge; or inflammation of bladder which cause frequent and sometimes painful urination. There are also some physical complications like damage to the cervix or pelvic bones, neurological conditions, leakage of urine and/or feces into the vagina, urogenital infections, ammonia dermatitis, genital lacerations, kidney infections and amenorrhea [3].

Women with obstetric fistula also face other significant physical and social challenges, including infertility, social isolation and unemployment [6].

In general, obstetric fistula treatment needs prolonged hospitalization and bladder catheterization which may contribute for the development of urinary tract infections in women who have OF.

Although it is difficult to determine precise rates, according to the World Health Organization (WHO) and the United Nations Population Fund Agency (UNFPA), estimated 50,000 to 100,000 women develop obstetric fistulas each year admitted at Hamlin fistula hospital, Addis Ababa, Ethiopia [7].

Methods
Study design, area and period
A cross sectional study was conducted from February to May 2015 at Hamlin Fistula Hospital, Addis Ababa, Ethiopia. The hospital is located in Addis Ababa at Lideta subcity

In Ethiopia, it is estimated that 9 000 women annually develop a fistula, where only 1200 of them are treated [8]. However, data on impact of UTI on obstetric fistula patients and distribution and antimicrobial drug susceptibility patterns among urinary pathogen isolated from such patients are scarce. Therefore, the aim of this study was to determine the prevalence of UTI, antimicrobial susceptibility pattern of bacterial isolates and the associated risk factors among obstetric fistula patients.

Study population
During the period from February to May, a total of 210 fistula patients admitted to the Hamlin Fistula Hospital were screened for significant bacteriuria. The study populations were all fistula patients who were treated during the study period. All consenting fistula patients selected as study participant were included in the study. After obtaining informed consent, study participants were interviewed about their socio-demographic characteristics, presence and duration of their clinical manifestations and information on related risk factors by using a structured questionnaire.

Culture and identifications
About 10 to 20 ml clean-catch mid-stream urine was collected from fistula patients. The sample was inoculated onto cysteine lactose electrolyte deficient agar (CLED) media and blood agar with calibrated loop of 0.001 ml [9]. The inoculated media was incubated overnight (18–24 h) at 37 °C. After overnight incubation, the bacterial growth on the respective media was observed, and total colony count was done and checked for significant bacteriuria [10].

A significant bacteriuria was considered if urine culture yields $\geq 10^5$ CFU/mL midstream urine. All positive urine cultures showing significant bacteriuria was sub cultured and further identified by their characteristics appearance on their respective media (colony morphology) and confirmed by the pattern of biochemical reactions (indole production, citrate utilization, motility test, urease test, oxidase test, coagulase and catalase tests) using the standard procedures [10, 11].

Antimicrobial susceptibility testing
Disk diffusion method was employed for antibiotic susceptibility testing as recommended by CLSI [12]. Mueller-Hinton agar (Oxoid) was used for susceptibility testing. Antibiotics discs (Oxoid Ltd) used were: Ceftriaxone (CRO) (30 µg), Chloramphenicol (C) (30 µg), Gentamicin (CN) (10 µg), Ciprofloxacin (CIP) (10 µg),) Nitrofurantion (F) (300 µg), and amoxicillin– clavulanic acid (AMC) (30 µg).

Briefly pure bacterial culture was transferred into a tube containing 5 ml sterile normal saline (0.85% NaCl) and mixed gently until it forms a homogenous suspension. The turbidity of the suspension was adjusted to the optical density of McFarland 0.5. A standard inoculum adjusted to 0.5 McFarland was swabbed on to Muller-Hinton agar (Oxoid) and antibiotic discs were dispensed after drying the plate for 3–5 min and incubated at 37 °C for 24 h. Diameter of the zone of inhibition around the disc was measured to the nearest millimeter using a metal caliper and the isolate was classified as sensitive, intermediate and resistant according to [12].

Quality control
E. coli (ATCC 25922), S. aureus (ATCC25923) and P. aeruginosa (ATTC 27853) were used as reference

strains for culture and sensitivity testing throughout the study [12].

Statistical analysis

Data was entered and analyzed using SPSS version 20 software. Odds ratio was used to screen the possible potential risk factors and to compare the proportion of bacterial isolates with patients' demographic information and comparison of antimicrobial resistances. *P*-value <0.05 was considered statistically significant.

Results

The data collected in this study consisted of 210 fistula patients admitted to Hamlin Fistula Hospital for surgical repair. All were investigated for presence or absence of urinary bacterial pathogen during the study period between February and May, 2015. The age range of study participants was 12 to 42 years (mean age of 21 years). Majority of the study participants 118 (56.2%) were in the age group of 21–25 years and 196(93.3%) were from rural settings. Overall 134(63.8%) of the study participant had less than 500 ETB personal monthly incomes. A high proportion 77(36.7%) of the study participants are divorced and 99 (47.1%) had a previous history of catheterizations (Table 1).

Significant bacteriuria was observed in 122 (58.1%) of 210 fistula patients screened for urinary tract infections (Table 3). The overall prevalence of bacterial isolates of the current study was 58.1% and 68(55.7%) of the isolates were from symptomatic cases (Table 2).

Of the total of 117 (55.7%) symptomatic cases 68 (58.1%) of them were positive for significant bacteriuria while from the total of 93(44.3%) asymptomatic cases 54(58.1%) were positive for significant bacteriuria. The odds of developing UTI for both symptomatic and asymptomatic patients are the same, OR 95% CI (1002(0.577–1.74), which indicate there is no association between clinical sign and significant bacteria isolates. In general no statistically significant differences were observed in the isolation frequency of each pathogen in the two groups (*p* > 0.05) as shown in Table 2.

Of the 122 isolates only 5(4.1%) of them were gram positive bacteria while nearly all 117 (95.9%) were gram negative bacteria. *E. coli* 65(53.7%) were the commonest bacterial pathogen isolated and followed by *Proteus* spp.31 (25.4%). *Klebsiella spp.* and *Pseudomonas spp.* accounted for 14(11.5%) and 4(3.27%) respectively. Others found in small number included *Serratia spp.*3 (2.46%), *Coagulase negative Staphylococcus* 3 (2.46%) and *S. aureus* 2(1.64%). *Serretia spp., coagulase negative staphylococcus and S. aureus* were only isolated from symptomatic fistula patients (Table 3).

Table 1 Socio demographic characteristics of 210 Fistula patients investigated for UTIs at Hamlin Fistula hospital, Addis Ababa, Ethiopia

Variables	Frequency	Percent (%)
Age (years)		
10–15	2	1.0
16–20	49	23.3
21–25	118	56.2
26–30	25	11.9
31–40	9	4.3
36–40	6	2.9
>40	1	0.5
Residence		
Rural	196	93.3
Urban	14	6.7
Educational status		
Illiterate	163	77.6
Primary school	44	21.0
Above primary school	3	1.4
Occupations		
Merchant	34	16.2
Farmer	62	29.5
Student	17	8.1
House Wife	67	31.9
Daily Laborer	23	11.0
Others	7	3.3
Marital status		
Single	72	34.3
Married	61	29.0
Divorced	77	36.7
Personal income (ETB)		
Less than 500	134	63.8
500–1000	51	24.3
1001–1500	17	8.1
Above 1500	8	3.8
Previous history of catheterization		
Yes	99	47.1
No	111	52.9
Previous history of UTI		
Yes	85	40.5
No	125	59.5

ETB Ethiopian birr

Risk factors associated with urinary tract infections

Significant bacteriuria was strongly associated with history of previous UTI and history of catheterizations (*p* < 0.05) as shown in Table 4. Statistical significance difference was observed in relation to previous history of

Table 2 Significant bacteriuria among symptomatic and asymptomatic fistula patient's investigated for UTIs in Hamlin Fistula Hospital, Addis Ababa, Ethiopia

Fistula patients with UTI	Significant bacteriuria		Total	OR(95% CI)	P value
	Yes	No			
Symptomatic No. (%)	68(58.1)	49(41.9)	117(55.7)	1.002(0.577–1.74)	0.994
Asymptomatic No. (%)	54(58.1)	39(41.9)	93(44.3)		
Total No. (%)	122(58.1)	88(41.9)	210(100)		

catheterization and UTI with OR (95%CI) 2.739(1.547, 4.849), P value = 0.001 and OR (95%CI) 1.879(1.060, 3.331), P value = 0.031 respectively.

The average duration of hospital stay among fistula patient screened for UTI was 30 days with range of 1 to 60 days. From admitted patient 38(18.1%) was screened for UTI within two days of admission while 22(18%) of them were with significant bacterial isolates. Of the total 210 study participants 122(58.1%) study participants were diagnosed with significant bacteriuria. The majority these patients 100/122 (82%) stayed in hospital for more than 3 days. There is no statistical significance difference observed in relation to duration of hospital stay with the OR (95%CI) (0.990(0.486, 2.017) and P value > 0.05. Educational status, marital status, occupation and other independent variables used were not show statistical significance difference with P value >0.05 as shown in Table 5.

Antimicrobial susceptibility testing
Gram negative bacteria
The resistance pattern of gram negative bacteria ($n = 117$) against 6 antimicrobial agents are shown in Table 6. Gram negative bacteria isolates showed low level of resistance to most of antimicrobial tested, 21.4% to amoxicillin -clavulanic acid and ceftriaxone and 33.3% to both nitrofurantoin and chloramphenicol. Intermediate level of resistance (3.4– 7.7%) was observed to most of antimicrobial tested

except amoxicillin -clavulanic acid. High level of resistance (>50%) was observed to gentamicin and ciprofloxacin. Among the isolates *Klebsiella spp.*shows low rate of resistance to ceftriaxone (14.3%) and nitrofurantoin (7.5%), while the same rate of intermediate resistance level (7.5%) to gentamicin, nitrofurantoin and ceftriaxone were observed. The isolate also shows high rate of resistance to ciprofloxacin (78.6%).

Pseudomonas spp. shows low rate of resistance (20%) to both ciprofloxacin and chloramphenicol and high rate of resistance (80%) to nitrofurantoin, while it was not showed any resistance level to both gentamicin and ceftriaxone.

E.coli was the commonest bacterial pathogen isolated which showed low resistance rate (21.6%, 24.6%, and 32.2%) to amoxicillin- clavulanic acid, ceftriaxone and chloramphenicol, respectively. The isolates also shows high rate of resistance to ciprofloxacin (56.9%) and gentamicin(53.8%). *Proteus spp.*and *Serratia spp.* were also other bacterial isolates which showed the high level of resistance to gentamicin (61.3% and 66.6%) respectively, while they were showed low resistance rate to ceftriaxone (19.4%, 33.3%).

Gram positive bacteria
The resistance pattern of gram positive bacteria ($n = 5$) against 6 antimicrobial agents are shown in Table 7. All gram positive bacteria isolated were 100% sensitive to Amoxicillin-clavulanic acid and ciprofloxacin. Low level of resistance (20–40%) was observed to all the rest of antibiotic tested.

Table 3 Frequency and types of bacterial species isolated from asymptomatic and symptomatic UTI among fistula patients at Hamlin Fistula Hospital, Addis Ababa, Ethiopia

Bacteria species isolated	Symptomatic UTI No. (%)	Asymptomatic UTI No. (%)	Total No. (%)
E. coli	31(45.5)	34(62.9)	65(53.3)
Klebsiella spp.	9(13.2)	5(9.2)	14(11.5)
Pseudomonas spp.	2(2.9)	2(3.7)	4(3.3)
Proteus spp.	18(26.4)	13(24.7)	31(25.4)
Serratia spp.	3(4.4)	0(0.0)	3(2.45)
CONS	3(4.4)	0(0.0)	3(2.45)
S.aureus	2(2.9)	0(0.0)	0(0.0)
Total	68(55.7)	54(44.3)	122(100)

CONS cougulase negative staphylococcus

Table 4 Risk factors associated with significant bacteria isolated from obstetric fistula patients at Hamlin fistula hospital, Addis Ababa, Ethiopia

Variables	Significant bacteria isolated		OR(95%CI), P-value
	Yes N. (%)	No N. (%)	
Previous history of catheterization			
yes	70(57.4)	29(33.3)	2.739(1.547, 4.849),0.001
No	52(42.6)	59(67.7)	
Previous history of UTI			
yes	57(46.7)	28(31.8)	1.879(1.060, 3.331), 0.031
No	65(53.3)	60(68.2)	

Table 5 Significant bacteriuria in relation to socio-demographic characteristics of obstetric fistula patients at Hamlin Fistula Hospital, Addis Ababa, Ethiopia

Variables	Significant bacteriuria		Total No. (%)	P-value
	Yes No. (%)	No No. (%)		
Age (years)				
10–15	2(100)	0(00)	2(1.0)	
16–20	24(40.7)	25(59.3)	49(23.3)	
21–25	72(61)	46(39)	118(56.2)	0.765
26–30	15(60)	10(40)	25(11.9)	
31–35	6(66.6)	3(33.3)	9(4.3)	
36–40	2(33.3)	4(66.6)	6(2.9)	
Above 40	1(100)	0(00)	1(.5)	
Marital status				
Single	40(55.5)	32(44.5)	72(34.3)	0.856
Married	38(62.9)	23(37.1)	61(29.0)	
Divorced	44(57.1)	33(42.9)	77(36.7)	
Educational status				
Illiterate	97(59.5)	66(40.5)	163(77.6)	0.534
Primary School	23(52.7)	21(46.3)	44(21.0)	
Greater	1(33.3)	2(66.6)	3(1.4)	
Occupations				
Merchant	17(50)	17(50)	34(16.2)	0.52
Farmer	33(53.2)	29(46.8)	61(29.5)	
Student	7(41.2)	10(58.8)	17(8.1)	
House Wife	45(67.1)	22(32.9)	77(31.9)	
Daily Laborer	16(69.6)	7(30.4)	23(11.0)	
Others	4(57.1)	3(42.9)	7(3.3)	
Personal income(ETB)				
Less 500	78(58.2)	56(41.8)	134(63.8)	0.955
500–1000	29(56.8)	22(53.2)	51(24.3)	
1001–1500	11(64.7)	6(35.3)	17(8.1)	
Above 1500	4(50)	4(50)	8(3.8)	
Residence				
Rural	112(91.8)	84(95.4)	196(93.3)	0.31
Urban	10(8.2)	4(4.6)	14(6.7)	
Duration of hospital stay				
Less than 3 days	22(18)	16(18.2)	38(18.1)	0.978
Equal or above 3 days	100(82)	72(81.8)	172(81.9)	

ETB Ethiopian birr

Discussion

A variety of enteropathogenic bacteria are known to cause UTI worldwide. UTIs are among the most common bacterial infections in humans, both in the community and hospital settings. It is a serious health problem affecting millions of people each year and is the leading cause of gram-negative bacteremia [13]. Patients with obstetric fistula (OF) can have frequent bladder infections, incontinence of urine and stool. Many of these patients might live with these conditions for several years. This may further predispose them to health related problems like urinary tract infections [2]. However, there is a lack of concrete evidences that show the magnitude of UTI and antimicrobial sensitivity patterns in obstetric fistula patients throughout the world and it is difficult to compare all the current findings with previous reports.

This study finding showed that low socioeconomic status was one of the factors that were not significantly associated with increased UTI (*P* value = 0.955) as indicated in Table 5. This report was the same with other report from Thailand which report insignificant association between UTI and socio economic status [14]. Another study on pregnant women in North West Ethiopia showed that pregnant women who had monthly income of less than 500 Ethiopian birr have (18.9%) more likely to have bacteriuria than those who had high socioeconomic income level [15]. Also other study in Egypt on UTI showed the presence of association between low income level and UTI [16]. This could be due to the relation of low socioeconomic status with nutrition and immunity especially in fistula patients.

This study finding also showed that educational status was one of the factors that was not significantly associated with increased UTI (*P* value =0.534) as indicated in Table 5. The frequency of UTI (59.5%) was higher among illiterate fistula patients when compared with others. This study was the same as other studies which indicate absence of association between level of education and UTI among pregnant women in Pakistan [17] and in Tanzania [18].

In general, the overall prevalence of UTI in the present study was 58.1%, which is almost similar with other report from India (60%) [19]. But the present finding of UTI was lower than other studies from Libya (65.7%) [20] and Nigeria (76.1%) [21].

Lower report was also reported from other African country Tanzania [18] and Nigeria (47.5%) [22]. The prevalence of present study was also higher than other reports from Ethiopia; North West Ethiopia [23]; (52.8%) [24], Addis Ababa [25] and Dessie [26].

In this study, the most commonly isolated organisms were *Escherichia coli* (53.7%), *Proteus* spp.(25.4%) and, *Klebsiella spp.*(11.5%). Similar isolate with different frequency was found on study done in Libya, *Escherichia coli* (33.98%), *Proteus* spp. (21.48%) and *Klebsiella pneumoniae*(10.3%) [20].

According to previous study done in West Ethiopia *Citrobacter* (24.5%) [24] was the most dominant bacterial isolated while in this study *Citrobacter* was not isolated

Table 6 Antimicrobial resistance pattern of gram negative bacteria isolated from fistula patient at Hamlin Fistula Hospital, Addis Ababa, Ethiopia

Bacterial isolates		Antimicrobial Tested					
		AMC	CIP	CN	F	C	CRO
E. coli (n = 65)	S	51(78.4)	28(43.1)	25(48.5)	36(55.4)	41(63.1)	45(69.2)
	I	0(0.0)	0(0.0)	5(7.7)	3(4.6)	3(4.6)	4(6.1)
	R	14(21.6)	37(56.9)	35(53.8)	26(40)	21(32.2)	16(24.6)
Klebsiella spp. (n = 14)	S	14(100)	3(21.4)	6(42.8)	12(85.7)	10(71.4)	11(78.6)
	I	0(0.0)	0(0.0)	1(7.1)	1(7.5)	0(0.0)	1(7.5)
	R	0(0.0)	11(78.6)	7(50)	1(7.5)	4(28.6)	2(14.3)
Pseudomonas spp. (n = 4)	S	1(20)	3(80)	4(100)	1(20)	3(80)	4(100)
	I	0(0.0)	0(0.0)	0(0.0)	0(0.0)	0(0.0)	0(0.0)
	R	3(80)	1(20)	0(0.0)	3(80)	1(20)	0(0.0)
Proteus spp. (n = 31)	S	25(80.6)	13(41.9)	12(48.7)	20(64.5)	17(54.8)	21(67.7)
	I	0(0.0)	4(12.9)	0(0.0)	2(6.5)	1(3.2)	4(12.9)
	R	6(19.4)	14(45.9)	19(61.3)	9(29)	13(41.9)	6(19.4)
Serratia spp. (n = 3)	S	1(33.3)	0(0.0)	1(33.3)	3(100)	3(100)	2(66.6)
	I	0(0.0)	1(33.3)	0(0.0)	0(0.0)	0(0.0)	0(0.0)
	R	2(66.6)	2(66.6)	2(66.6)	0(0.0)	0(0.0)	1(33.3)
Total (n = 117)	S	92(78.6)	47(40.2)	48(41)	72(61.5)	74(63.2)	83(70.9)
	I	0(0.0)	5(4.3)	6(5.1)	6(5.1)	4(3.4)	9(7.7)
	R	25(21.4)	65(55.5)	63(53.8)	39(33.3)	39(33.3)	25(21.4)

CRO Ceftriaxone, *C* Chloramphenicol, *CN* Gentamicin, *F* Nitrofurantoin, *CIP* Ciprofloxacin, *AMC* Amoxicillin- clavulanic acid

and *Escherichia coli (53.7%)* was the most dominant isolated similar to other many studies *(39%, 44.9%, 31.7%)* respectively [19, 27, 28].

In the present study, the prevalence of symptomatic and asymptomatic bacteriuria were the same (58.1%), with the OR (95%CI) of 1.002(0.577-1.74) and *P* value of 0.978, which indicate there is no statistically significant differences observed in the isolation frequency of each pathogen in the two groups ($p > 0.05$) (Table 5). This study was the same as previous study done in North

Table 7 Antimicrobial resistance pattern of gram positive bacteria isolated from fistula patients at Hamlin Fistula Hospital, Addis Ababa, Ethiopia

Bacterial isolates		Antimicrobial tested					
		AMC	CIP	CN	F	C	CRO
CONs (n = 3)	S	3(100)	3(100)	1(33.3)	2(66.6)	2(66.6)	2(66.6)
	I	0(0.0)	0(0.0)	0(0.0)	0(0.0)	0(0.0)	0(0.0)
	R	0(0.0)	0(0.0)	2(66.6)	1(33.3)	1(33.3)	1(33.3)
S.aureus (n = 2)	S	2(100)	2(100)	2(100)	2(100)	2(100)	2(100)
	I	0(0.0)	0(0.0)	0(0.0)	0(0.0)	0(0.0)	0(0.0)
	R	0(0.0)	0(0.0)	0(0.0)	0(0.0)	0(0.0)	0(0.0)
Total (n = 5)	S	5(100)	5(100)	3(60)	4(80)	4(80)	4(80)
	I	0(0.0)	0(0.0)	0(0.0)	0(0.0)	0(0.0)	0(0.0)
	R	0(0.0)	0(0.0)	2(40)	1(20)	1(20)	1(20)

West Ethiopia where no statistically significant differences were observed [28].

The finding of this study also revealed that past history of UTI had strong association with UTI with the OR (95%CI) 1.879 (1.060, 3.331) and *P* value = 0.031 as indicated in Table 4. Similar finding were reported from North West Ethiopia [15, 28]. Another study in Tanzania also reported that past history of UTI was a risk factor for UTI during pregnancy [18]. But absence of association was reported from Thailand [14].

This finding also revealed that history of catheterization had strong association with UTI with the OR (95%CI) 2.739(1.547, 4.849) and *P* value = 0.001, which is almost similar with other reports where catheterization is the most important risk factor for the development of catheter associated bacteriuria [29].

In this report, gram negative bacteria isolated showed high level of resistance to ciprofloxacin and gentamicin (>50%) and intermediate level of resistance (3.4– 7.7%) was observed to most of antimicrobial tested except amoxicillin-clavulanic acid.

This is in contrast to previous study done in Ethiopia, where gentamicin considered as appropriate antimicrobial for empirical treatment of urinary tract infections [26]. According to percent study all gram negative bacteria isolate were sensitive (61.5%–78.6%) to amoxicillin-clavulanic acid, nitrofurantoin, ceftriaxone and chloramphenicol. The same result were also reported from other previous study in Ethiopia were amoxicillin–clavulanic acid was appropriate drug of choice for UTI [30]. Low level of resistance (20–40%) was observed to all gram positive isolates against ceftriaxone, chloramphenicol, gentamicin and nitrofurantoin. This study also reveals 100% sensitivity to Amoxicillin-clavulanic acid and ciprofloxacin for all gram positive bacteria isolates. The same result was reported from other previous Ethiopian studies where low level of resistance (8.6%–34.3) was reported with the same antibiotic tested with the current studies [28].

In conclusion overall prevalence of urinary tract infection among fistula patient was 58.1%. The prevalence of significant bacteriuria among both asymptomatic and symptomatic fistula patients was almost the same. This study showed that the predominant pathogen of UTI were *E.coli*. Significant bacteriuria was significantly associated with history of previous UTI and history of catheterization. This study also showed that amoxicillin-clavulanic acid was a drug of choice for both gram negative and gram positive bacteria while ciprofloxacin and ceftriaxone were found effective against gram negative and positive bacteria isolated respectively.

Conclusions

The overall prevalence of urinary tract infection among fistula patients was 58.1%. Significant bacteriuria was significantly associated with history of previous UTI and history of catheterization. This study also showed that the predominant pathogen of UTI were *E.coli* and agumantin and ciprofloxacin were the drug of choice for gram positive bacteria while CAF and ceftraxone were found effective against gram negative bacteria isolated.

Abbreviations

CLED: Cysteine lactose electrolyte deficient agar; CLSI: Clinical and Laboratory Standards Institute; RVF: Recto vaginal fistula; UNFPA: United nations population fund agency; UNFPA: United nations population fund agency; UTI: Urinary tract infection; VUR: Vesicoureteral reflux; VVF: Vesico vaginal fistula; WHO: World health organization

Acknowledgements

We are thankful to all Addis Ababa Hamlin fistula hospital laboratory staff for their excellent technical support. We are grateful to all the participant fistula patients for their kind cooperation and Addis Ababa University for their financial support.

Authors' contributions

MD carried out the experiment work, analyzed the data, and wrote the manuscript. DA and YW helped to revise and edited the manuscript. All authors have read and approved the final manuscript.

Competing interests

The authors declare that they have no competing interests

Consent for publication

Not applicable

Author details

[1]Department of medicine, Collages of medicine and health sciences, Ambo University, Ambo, Ethiopia. [2]Department of Microbiology, Immunology & Parasitology, School of Medicine, Addis Ababa University, Addis Ababa, Ethiopia. [3]Addis Ababa Hamlin Fistula Hospital, Addis Ababa, Ethiopia.

References

1. Czaja CA, Hooton TM. Update on acute uncomplicated urinary tract infection in women. PostgradMed. 2006;119:39–45.
2. Hilton P. Vesicovaginal fistulas in developing countries. Int J Gynaecol Obstet. 2003;82:285–95.
3. Miller S, Lester F, Webster M, Cowan B. Obstetric fistula: a preventable tragedy. J Mid Wifery Women's Health. 2005;50:286–94.
4. Rovner ES. Urinary fistulae. In: Clinical manual of urology. 3rd ed. 2001. p. 323–36.
5. Menefee SA, Wall LL. Incontinence, prolapse, and disorders of the pelvic floor. In: Berek IJ, editor. Novak's Gynecology. 13th ed. Philadelphia: Lippincott Williams &Wilkins; 2011. p. 645–710.
6. McFadden E, Taleski SJ, Bocking A, Rachel F, Mabeya H. Retrospective review of predisposing factors and surgical outcomes in obstetric fistula patients at a single teaching hospital in Western Kenya. J Obstet Gynaecol Can. 2011;33(1):30–5.
7. United Nations Population Fund and Engender Health. Obstetric fistula needs assessment report: findings from nine African countries. New York: United Nations Population Fund and Engender Health; 2011.
8. UNFPA and Engender Health. Obstetric fistula needs assessment report finding from nine African countries. In Women's Health and Education centers.2009; 1–5
9. Graham JC, Galloway A. The laboratory diagnosis of urinary tract infection. JClin Pathol. 2001;54:911–9.
10. Cheesbourgh M. Medical laboratory manual for tropical countries. 2nd ed. 2006.
11. Vandepitte J, Verhaegen J, Engbaek K, Rohner P, Piot C. Basic laboratory proceduresin clinical bacteriology. 2nd ed. 2003.
12. Clinical and Laboratory Standards Institute. Performance standards for antimicrobial susceptibility testing Seventeenth information supplement. Wayne Pennsylvania: CLSI document M100-S17; 2007.
13. El-Naggar W, Hassan R, Barwa R, Shokralla S and Elgaml A. (2010) Molecular diagnosis of gram negative bacteria in urinary tract infections. Egyptian Journal of Medical Microbiology.2010;19(1):93.
14. Kovavisarach E, Vichaipruck M. Risk factors related to asymptomatic bacteriuria in pregnant women. J Med Assoc Thai. 2009;92:606–10.
15. Emiru T, Beyene G, Tsegaye W, Melaku S. Associated risk factors of urinary tract infection among pregnant women at Felege Hiwot Referral Hospital, Bahir Dar, North West Ethiopia. BMC Res Notes. 2013;25(6):292.
16. Dimetry SR, El-Tokhy HM, Abdo NM. Urinary tract infection and adverse outcome of pregnancy. J Egypt Public Health Assoc. 2007;82:203–18.
17. Sheikh MA, Khan MS, Khatoon A. Incidence of urinary tract infection during pregnancy. Eas Mediterr Health. 2000;6:265–71.
18. Masinde A, Gumodoka B, Kilonzo A, Mshana SE. Prevalence of urinary tract infection among pregnant women at Bugando medical centre, Mwanza. Tanzania J Health Res. 2009;11:154–61.
19. Alka Nerurkar, Priti Solanky, Shanta S,Nai k. Bacterial pathogens in urinary tract infection and antibiotic susceptibility pattern. JPBMS. 2012;21(21):2.
20. Khamees SS. Urinary tract infection: causative agents, the relation between bacteriuria and pyuria. World Applied Sci J. 2012;20(5):683–6.
21. Adeoye I, Oladeinde O, Uneke J, Adeoye J. An assessment of asymptomatic bacteriuria among women with vesico-vaginal fistula in South-Eastern Nigeria. Nepal J Epidemiol. 2011;1(2):64–9.
22. Okonko IO, Ijandipe LA, Ilusanya AO, Donbraye-Emmanuel OB, Ejembi J, Udeze AO, Egun OC, Fowotade A, Nkang AO. Detection of urinary tract infection among pregnant women in oluyoro catholic hospital, Ibadan, south-western Nigeria. J Microbiol. 2010;6(1):16–24.
23. Ferede G, Yismaw G, Wondimeneh Y, Sisay Z. The prevalence and antimicrobial susceptibility pattern of bacterial uropathogens isolated from pregnant women. Eur J Exp Bio. 2012;2(5):1497–502.

24. Wondimeneh Y, Muluye D, Alemu A, Atinafu A, Yitayew G, Gebrecherkos T, Alemu AG, Damtie D, Ferede G. Urinary tract infection among obstetric fistula patients at Gondar University Hospital, Northwest Ethiopia. BMC Women's Health. 2014;14:12.

25. Assefa A, Asrat D, Woldeamanuel Y, GHiwot Y, Abdella A, Melesse T. Bacterial profile and drug susceptibility pattern of urinary tract infection in pregnant women at Tikur Anbessa specialized hospital Addis Ababa, Ethiopia. Ethiopia Med J. 2008;46:227–35.

26. Kibret M, Abera B. Prevalence and antibiogram of bacterial isolates from urinary tract infections at dessie health research laboratory. Ethiopia Asian Pac J TropBiomed. 2014;4(2):164–8.

27. Foxman B, Manning SD, Tallman P. Uropathogenic Escherichia coli are more likely than comensal E. coli to be shared between heterosexual sex partners. Am J Epidemiol. 2002;156(12):1133–40.

28. Yismaw G, Asrat D, Woldeamanuel Y, Chandrashekhar G. Urinary tract infection: bacteria etiologies, drug resistance profile and associated risk factors in diabetic patients attending Gondar university hospital. European J Exp Biol. 2012;2(4):889–98.

29. Loeb M, Hunt D, Halloran K. Stop orders to reduce inappropriate urinary Catheterization in hospitalized patients: a randomized, controlled trial. J Gen Intern Med. 2008;23:816–20.

30. Teshager L, Asrat D, Gebre-selassie S, Tamiru S. Catheterized and non-catheterized Urinary tract infections among patients attended at Jimma university teaching hospital. Ethiop Med J. 2008;46(1):55–62.

Cost-effectiveness of ceftolozane/tazobactam compared with piperacillin/tazobactam as empiric therapy based on the in-vitro surveillance of bacterial isolates in the United States for the treatment of complicated urinary tract infections

Teresa L Kauf[1], Vimalanand S. Prabhu[2,6]* (iD), Goran Medic[3], Rebekah H. Borse[2], Benjamin Miller[4], Jennifer Gaultney[3], Shuvayu S. Sen[2] and Anirban Basu[5]

Abstract

Background: A challenge in the empiric treatment of complicated urinary tract infection (cUTI) is identifying the initial appropriate antibiotic therapy (IAAT), which is associated with reduced length of stay and mortality compared with initial inappropriate antibiotic therapy (IIAT). We evaluated the cost-effectiveness of ceftolozane/tazobactam compared with piperacillin/tazobactam (one of the standard of care antibiotics), for the treatment of hospitalized patients with cUTI.

Methods: A decision-analytic Monte Carlo simulation model was developed to compare the costs and effectiveness of empiric treatment with either ceftolozane/tazobactam or piperacillin/tazobactam in hospitalized adult patients with cUTI infected with Gram-negative pathogens in the US. The model applies the baseline prevalence of resistance as reported by national in-vitro surveillance data.

Results: In a cohort of 1000 patients, treatment with ceftolozane/tazobactam resulted in higher total costs compared with piperacillin/tazobactam ($36,413 /patient vs. $36,028/patient, respectively), greater quality-adjusted life years (QALYs) (9.19/patient vs. 9.13/patient, respectively) and an incremental cost-effectiveness ratio (ICER) of $6128/QALY. Ceftolozane/tazobactam remained cost-effective at a willingness to pay of $100,000 per QALY compared to piperacillin/tazobactam over a range of input parameter values during one-way and probabilistic sensitivity analysis.

Conclusions: Model results show that ceftolozane/tazobactam is likely to be cost-effective compared with piperacillin/tazobactam for the empiric treatment of hospitalized cUTI patients in the United States.

Keywords: Cost-benefit analysis, Ceftolozane, Piperacillin, Tazobactam, Urinary tract infections, United States, Drug resistance

* Correspondence: vimalanand.prabhu@merck.com
[2]Merck & Co., Inc., Kenilworth, NJ, USA
[6]Merck & Co., Inc., 2000 Galloping Hill Rd., Kenilworth, NJ 07033, USA
Full list of author information is available at the end of the article

Background

Gram-negative pathogens are a major cause of hospital-treated infections, accounting for 38% of all healthcare associated infections in the US [1–3]. Complicated urinary tract infections (cUTI), which are defined as UTIs associated with factors that compromise the urinary tract or host defense, are commonly caused by Gram-negative pathogens [4]. In the US, the prevalence of cUTI has been estimated at 24.2 per 1000 hospital discharges. Accounting for 70–80% of cUTIs [5], catheter-associated cUTIs make up a large group of cUTIs predominantly caused by Gram-negative pathogens [3, 6–8], including resistant pathogens, and reflect 28% of device-associated and procedure–associated infections [2, 9].

cUTI is often treated empirically as organism identification and susceptibility is not available at diagnosis. Patients with resistant pathogens are more likely to receive initially inappropriate antibiotic therapy (IIAT), defined as microbiological documentation of an infecting pathogen that was not effectively treated at the time of identification, instead of initially appropriate antibiotic therapy (IAAT) [10, 11]. Antibiotic resistance is associated with significant adverse impact on clinical outcomes, and increased consumption of health-care resources, leading to higher costs [12]. In a retrospective, matched-cohort analysis of patients admitted to the hospital with UTI in the US, patients with infections caused by extended-spectrum β-lactamase (ESBL) producing bacteria experienced IIAT 61.8% of the time as compared to 5.5% for patients with ESBL negative infections. Further, patients experienced two additional days in the hospital and an all-cause mortality rate of 9.1% with ESBL positive infections compared to 1.8% in ESBL negative infections. The increased length of stay and increased mortality in patients receiving IIAT vs. IAAT is also seen in other bacterial infections where antibiotics are administered for initial empiric therapy [13].

The goal of empiric therapy, therefore, is to increase the chances of IAAT. Thus, the antibacterial spectrum of the empiric antibiotic agent should cover the most relevant pathogens. Clinicians making decisions about empiric therapy for patients with cUTI not only consider the pathogens most likely colonizing the site of infection and knowledge of any prior bacteria known to colonize a given patient, but also local resistance patterns or antibiograms [14]. Local in-vitro antibiotic susceptibility data available through institutional antibiograms are more likely to reflect the current local resistance patterns compared with efficacy data from clinical trials alone as clinical trials are conducted internationally in geographically diverse populations. The application of local surveillance data for up-to-date clinical practice guidelines has been shown to be essential in patient care of cUTI given the evolving bacterial susceptibility [15].

Given the clinical and economic burden associated with IIAT, it is necessary to consider not only the clinical benefits but also the economic benefits that an empiric therapy could provide as a result of better coverage and improved susceptibility. There is a growing need to evaluate new and effective therapies that can offer a higher probability of appropriate empiric coverage compared to current antibacterial drugs.

In this study, we assess the cost-effectiveness of ceftolozane/tazobactam compared with piperacillin/tazobactam as empiric therapy in the treatment of hospitalized US patients aged 18 years or older with cUTI. Piperacillin/tazobactam is commonly used for empiric therapy of cUTI when resistance is suspected, as recommended in treatment guidelines [16, 17]. Ceftolazone/tazobactam is a novel cephalosporin/β-lactamase inhibitor combination available for treatment of adult cUTI patients. Ceftolozane/tazobactam has demonstrated broad activity against Gram-negative pathogens, including ESBL-producing Enterobacteriaceae and multi-drug resistant *Pseudomonas aeruginosa* [18].

Methods

Model structure

A patient-level decision analytic Monte Carlo micro-simulation model was developed to estimate the quality-adjusted life expectancy and costs of persons diagnosed with cUTI in order to conduct a cost-utility analysis of ceftolozane/tazobactam compared with piperacillin/tazobactam in the target patient population. The model tracks index patients through different phases of cUTI from diagnosis until death. A graphical representation of the model structure with all treatment pathways is provided in Fig. 1. The model incorporates treatment switching algorithms that depend upon patient level data regarding the underlying pathogen and its susceptibility to various antibiotics. As a result, an individual patient simulation that captures patient level information and history is a more appropriate model as opposed to a Markov model with transition probabilities that do not depend on history.

Hospitalized patients enter the model at the time of cUTI diagnosis, which is assumed to be concurrent with collecting the urine culture and initiation of empiric antimicrobial therapy. Each patient in the model receives empiric antibiotic treatment with either ceftolozane/tazobactam or piperacillin/tazobactam. Patients continue empiric treatment until culture results are available (assumed to occur after 3 days). Culture results include organism identification and susceptibility for ceftolozane/tazobactam, piperacillin/tazobactam, and other drugs that patients could be given, consistent with standard treatments. Once culture results are known, patients are switched to the least expensive therapy to which the

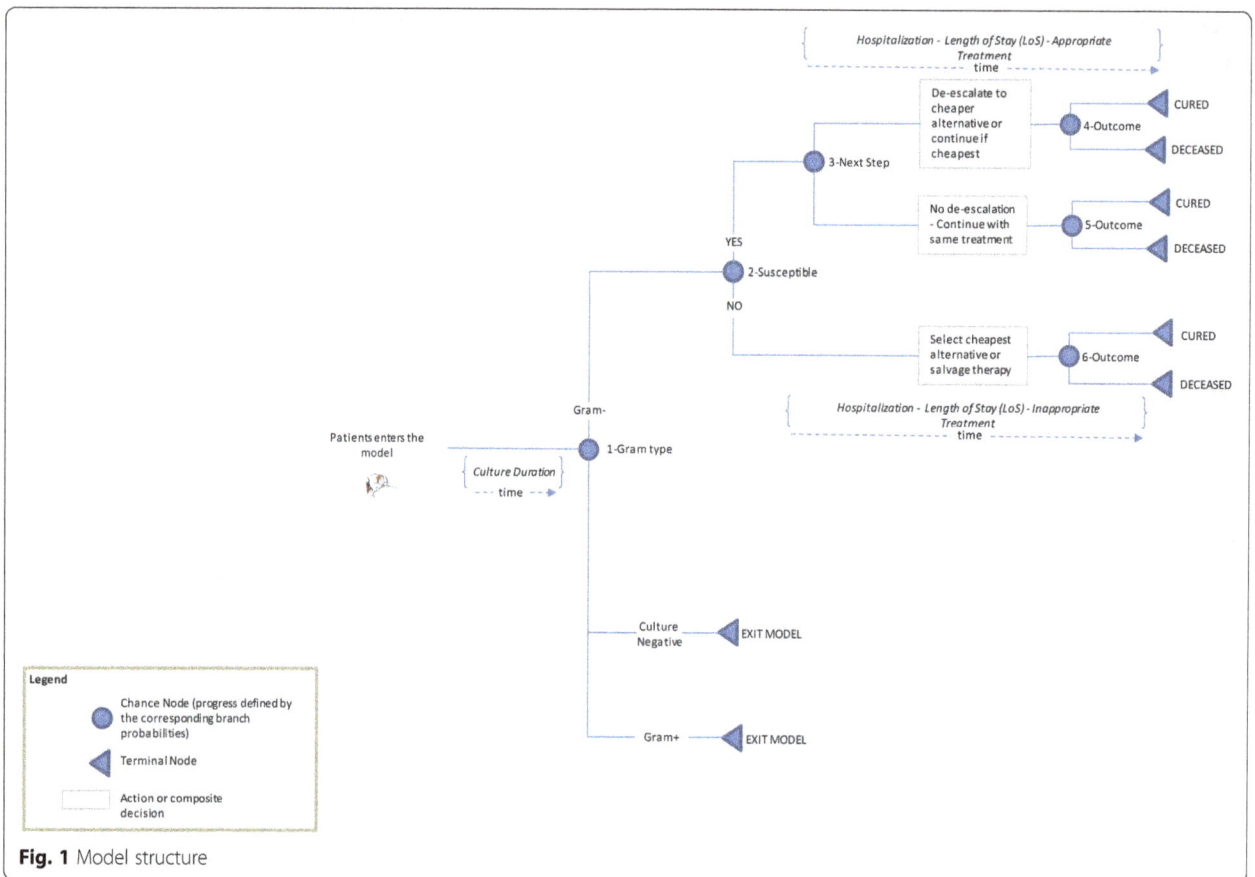

Fig. 1 Model structure

causative pathogen is susceptible. Patients may be maintained on the same drug (initial drug is appropriate and cheapest), de-escalated to a cheaper drug (initial drug is appropriate, but another drug that is cheaper and to which the pathogen is susceptible is available), or escalated (initial therapy is inappropriate, another drug to which the pathogen is susceptible is available, with patient escalated to the cheapest drug to which the pathogen is susceptible). If the pathogen is not susceptible to any of the drugs for which culture results were obtained, patients are switched to salvage therapy, assumed in this analysis as the combination of meropenem and colistin. Patients with Gram-positive infections exit the model after 3 days of initial therapy (Fig. 1). As the underlying pathogen is unknown at diagnosis, patients suspected of a Gram-negative infection but infected with a Gram-positive pathogen may be inadvertently prescribed drugs for the treatment of a Gram-negative infection. While empiric therapy with these drugs adds to the cost, it does not have any impact on the resolution of symptoms. As both ceftolozane/tazobactam and piperacillin/tazobactam are not indicated for Gram-positive pathogens, we assume that disease progression, after determination of culture results, and therefore the subsequent costs and outcomes, are similar across both arms. Drug acquisition

costs until culture results become available are included; however, we did not include any other costs as they are likely to be same for both arms.

The patient-level simulation begins with the random selection of an isolate from the Program to Assess Ceftolozane/Tazobactam Susceptibility (PACTS) surveillance dataset [19], such that each isolate represents a single patient. Isolates were sampled so that the resulting pathogen distribution reflects that of cUTI, as determined by an analysis of Premier hospital discharge data. Details regarding PACTS and Premier data are provided in Additional File 1.

Each patient enters the decision tree, and relevant costs are accumulated as they progress through one of the treatment pathways. This process is repeated for a large number of patients, and corresponding results are used to produce point estimates and confidence intervals for total costs per comparator. The analysis was performed on a cohort of 1000 patients, with the patients for each comparator arm being identical. The appropriateness of initial antibiotic therapy influences each patient's length of hospital stay. Once the patient finishes the entire duration of antibiotic therapy, mortality rate is dependent on whether the patient received IAAT or IIAT.

For patients who survive, we assume that they experience an average length of life based on their life expectancy and incur health care expenditure comparable to the average of a person their age [20].

Interventions

The empiric treatment comparators considered in the model are ceftolozane/tazobactam and piperacillin/tazobactam. The following drugs were considered for switching (escalation/de-escalation) upon pathogen confirmation: aztreonam, cefepime, ceftazidime, ceftriaxone, ciprofloxacin, doripenem, imipenem, levofloxacin, meropenem and tigecycline.

Time horizon, discounting and payer perspective

A lifetime horizon is applied to capture the utility and costs of healthy survivors. Costs and outcomes are discounted at 3% [21]. A US healthcare perspective is taken to evaluate costs.

Clinical inputs

Susceptibility data from the PACTS dataset were used to evaluate the appropriateness of the treatments in the model (Additional file 1). Five-percent of patients were Gram positive based on the Phase-III trial results [22]. The other key clinical inputs are summarized in Table 1.

Mortality rates and length of stay were based on MacVane et al. (2014) [23]. Duration of empiric therapy was assumed to be 3 days. US life-tables were used for the prediction of life expectancy (according to gender) [24].

Economic inputs

Hospitalization costs per day were derived from the 2013 Healthcare Cost and Utilization Project (HCUP), based on primary diagnoses of urinary tract infection (ICD-9 code 590.10, 590.11, 590.2, 590.3, 590.80, 590.81, 590.9, 597, and 599) and catheter/device-associated infections (ICD-9 codes 996.64 and 996.65) [25]. The average cost per hospital day for cUTI patients, inflated to 2015 using the Gross Domestic Product (GDP) price index, was $1746.27.

Daily drug costs were based on wholesale average cost at labeled doses [26]. Salvage therapy costs were based on combination therapy with meropenem and colistin.

For healthy survivors, lifetime health care expenditure was calculated using average annual age-adjusted values [20] inflated to 2015 values using the Gross Domestic Product (GDP) price index (Table 1) [27].

A utility value of 0.85 (assumption) was applied to cured patients for the remainder of their lives (Table 1) [28].

Analysis

The model compared ceftolozane/tazobactam with piperacillin/tazobactam from the perspective of the US hospital payer. The population was restricted to the US PACTS dataset for all available isolates from years 2011 to 2013. The susceptibility evaluation used Clinical and Laboratory Standards Institute (CLSI) breakpoints. A susceptibility breakpoint of 2 mg/L for all pathogens was assumed for ceftolozane/tazobactam, except for *Pseudomonas* spp. where a susceptibility breakpoint of 4 mg/L was used [29].

To compare the two treatment strategies, the following outcomes were estimated from the model: proportions of patients appropriately and inappropriately treated (sensitive/resistant to empiric therapy), cost per QALY saved, drug costs, hospitalization costs, proportion of cases by pathogen, total costs (undiscounted), and total QALYs (undiscounted and discounted). Differences in these outcomes of interest were estimated, along with the incremental cost-effectiveness ratio (ICER) calculated as total incremental cost per incremental QALY gained.

In order to evaluate uncertainty, one-way sensitivity analyses (OWSA) and probabilistic sensitivity analysis (PSA) were performed.

The model assessed the sensitivity of the model results to all the input data for which uncertainty has been defined one parameter at a time by means of OWSA. Beta distributions for utilities, gamma distributions for resource use and costs, reported statistical measures of uncertainty, where available, and otherwise within a range of ±10%. The ten parameters with the greatest impact were summarized in a tornado diagram.

For the PSA, new model input parameter values were repeatedly sampled from the defined distributions and the corresponding model output was calculated. The output values of 10,000 parameter samples were calculated to reflect the uncertainty in model output given the uncertainty of the input parameters.

For each treatment strategy, the probability of cost-effectiveness was expressed with cost-effectiveness acceptability curves, calculated as the number of iterations out of the total number of iterations for which the net monetary benefit (NMB) was greatest for a given treatment strategy out of all strategies. The NMB was calculated as the QALYs multiplied by a willingness to pay (WTP) ratio minus the costs, where a WTP of $100,000 was the amount decision makers were assumed to be willing to pay per additional QALY gained [30].

Scenario analyses

Appropriate use of carbapenems is important as they are often used as the last line of defence against increasingly difficult-to treat Gram-negative pathogens. In the base case, the de-escalation algorithm ensures that patients continue treatment on the least expensive antibiotic to which an isolate is susceptible following the empiric therapy period.

Table 1 Model inputs

Mortality rates	Mean	Lower bound	Upper bound	Distribution for PSA	Source
Mortality rate with appropriate empiric treatment	0.018	0.016	0.020	Beta	MacVane et al. [23]
Mortality rate with inappropriate empiric antibiotic	0.072	0.065	0.079	Beta	MacVane et al. [23]
Duration of therapy	Mean	Lower bound	Upper bound	Distribution for PSA	Source
Duration of empiric therapy	3 days	3 days	3 days	Gamma	MacVane et al. [23]
Total LOS for IAAT (inc. empiric therapy)	4 days	3 days	6 days	Gamma	MacVane et al. [23]
Additional LOS associated with IIAT	2 days	1 days	2 days	Gamma	MacVane et al. [23]
Quality of life adjustment	Mean	Lower bound	Upper bound	Distribution for PSA	Source
Health utility for survivors	0.85	0.70	1.00	Beta	Assumption
Hospital costs	Mean	Lower bound	Upper bound	Distribution for PSA	Source
Hospital cost per day (average USD 2015)	$1746.27	$1397.01	$2095.52	Gamma	AHQR [35]
Discounting	Mean	Lower bound	Upper bound	Distribution for PSA	Source
Benefits discount rate (per annum)	3%	3%	3%	Gamma	AMCP [21]
Drug name	Cost per day (USD 2015)				Source
Ceftolozane/tazobactam	$249.00				Analy$ource database [1]
Aztreonam	$84.24				
Cefepime	$23.04				
Ceftazidime	$19.80				
Ceftriaxone	$6.40				
Ciprofloxacin	$5.26				
Doripenem	$125.22				
Imipenem	$73.12				
Levofloxacin	$6.24				
Meropenem	$81.51				
Piperacillin/tazobactam	$43.08				
Tigecycline	$238.44				
Salvage[a]	$164.31				
Lifetime health care expenditure	Annual cost				Source
<25 years	$477				Basu [20]
25 to 34 years	$790				Basu [20]
35 to 44 years	$947				Basu [20]
45 to 54 years	$1422				Basu [20]
55 to 64 years	$2106				Basu [20]
65 to 74 years	$2758				Basu [20]
75 years and above	$3100				Basu [20]

LOS Length of stay, IAAT Initial appropriate antibiotic therapy, IIAT Initial inappropriate antibiotic therapy
[a]Salvage therapy consists of meropenem + colistin for cost purposes

However, an alternative algorithm, the carbapenem-sparing option, was designed to evaluate the impact of the de-escalation algorithm on the cost-effectiveness results. In this scenario, a carbapenem therapy (doripenem, imipenem or meropenem) is selected only if there is no other treatment alternative to which the pathogen is susceptible. Even if a carbapenem was the cheapest agent available to which the pathogen was susceptible, it would not be used if another non-carbapenem (e.g., a cephalosporin) was available.

Two additional scenarios were designed to evaluate the impact of risk factors associated with infection due to resistant pathogens, as identified in the literature [31, 32]. Information regarding the risk factors for infection due to resistant pathogens in cUTI was available for patients in the PACTS dataset, including (a) nosocomial infection, (b) age ≥ 65 years, and (c) admission to the intensive care unit (ICU). Scenario analyses were performed firstly using only nosocomial isolates and secondly using only nosocomial isolates for high risk patients aged ≥65 years, requiring an ICU stay or experiencing a catheter-associated infection.

Lastly, an additional scenario was also performed where lifetime health care expenditure for healthy survivors was excluded.

Results
Base case results
The average age of the cohort was 75.1 years. Distribution of the major Gram-negative pathogens was as follows: 58% *Escherichia coli*, 18% *Klebsiella pneumoniae*, 10% *Psuedomonas aeruginosa*, and 8% *Proteus mirabilis*.

The key results from the model are summarized in Table 2. In the base case, ceftolozane/tazobactam resulted in higher total costs than piperacillin/tazobactam ($36,413/patient vs. $36,028/patient, respectively), a greater number of discounted QALYs (9.19/patient vs. 9.13/patient, respectively) and 249 hospitalization days saved.

In patients receiving ceftolozane/tazobactam, 7.8% of pathogens were resistant compared with 20.2% of pathogens in those receiving piperacillin/tazobactam Table 3. There were 22.2 deaths (2.2%) in patients treated with ceftolozane/tazobactam compared with 28.9 (2.9%) in those treated with piperacillin/tazobactam. Amongst those who died, a larger proportion was resistant to initial therapy with piperacillin/tazobactam compared with ceftolozane/tazobactam.

When examining results for QALYs in more detail, ceftolozane/tazobactam generated a total of 0.06 discounted additional QALYs per patient compared with piperacillin/tazobactam. The average QALYs gained by patients treated with ceftolozane/tazobactam and piperacillin/tazobactam was 9.19 versus 9.13 (discounted), respectively.

Per patient lifetime health care expenditure and per patient drug costs were higher for ceftolozane/tazobactam compared with piperacillin/tazobactam ($28,651 vs. $28,444 and $766 vs. $155, respectively) Table 4. These were partly offset by hospital costs, with a lower average hospital cost per patient for patients treated with ceftolozane/tazobactam compared with those treated with piperacillin/tazobactam ($6996 vs. $7429, respectively). The resultant total cost per patient was higher for ceftolozane/tazobactam compared with piperacillin/tazobactam ($36,413 vs. $36,028, respectively).

For ceftolozane/tazobactam, 99.8% of patients who received IAAT were de-escalated after 3 days (following culture results), which was higher compared with piperacillin/tazobactam at 97.0%. In patients who received IIAT, an equal percentage of patients for each comparator (1.6%) required salvage therapy with meropenem + colistin.

Sensitivity analyses
The results of the one-way sensitivity analysis are presented in a tornado graph (Fig. 2). Varying the average cost per

Table 2 Summary of results

	Ceftolozane/tazobactam	Piperacillin/tazobactam	Incremental Ceftolozane/tazobactam - Piperacillin/tazobactam
Total costs per patient (USD 2015)	$36,413	$36,028	$385
Total QALYs (undiscounted) per patient	11.82	11.74	0.08
Total QALYs (discounted) per patient	9.19	9.13	0.06
Incremental Cost Effectiveness Ratio (Cost per discounted QALY gained)			$6128
Hospitalization days saved per patient			0.25

QALY Quality-adjusted life year

hospital day resulted in the largest impact on the resultant ICER. Other input parameters influencing the model results included: the health utility value applied to survivors, susceptibilities, mortality rate associated with IIAT and IAAT, and the additional length of stay associated with IIAT.

The PSA shows that in all instances, ceftolozane/tazobactam is more effective and more costly than piperacillin/tazobactam (Fig. 3); however, ceftolozane/tazobactam has a 100% probability of being cost-effective at a willingness-to-pay threshold of $100,000/QALY gained.

Scenario analyses
Table 5 provides the results of the scenario analyses. In all scenarios, ceftolozane/tazobactam resulted in higher total costs and a greater number of discounted QALYs than piperacillin/tazobactam. The carbapenem-sparing scenario and the scenario using only nosocomial isolates in high risk patients (aged ≥65 years, ICU stay, or catheter-associated infection) both resulted in ICERs that were very similar to the base case ($6020/QALY and $6037/QALY, respectively). Whilst the ICERs for the scenario using only nosocomial isolates (25% of the patients from the US PACTS dataset) and the scenario where lifetime health care expenditure was excluded were lower than in the base case ($3825/QALY and $2842/QALY, respectively).

Discussion
The objective of this analysis was to evaluate the use of ceftolozane/tazobactam compared with piperacillin/tazobactam in the empiric treatment of adult US patients with cUTI at risk of infection due to a resistant Gram-negative pathogen. Model results suggest that

Table 3 Appropriateness of empiric therapy

	Ceftolozane/tazobactam	Piperacillin/tazobactam
Resistant to initial therapy (%)	7.8	20.2
Susceptible to initial therapy (%)	92.2	79.8

Table 4 Cost results (USD 2015)

	Ceftolozane/ tazobactam	Piperacillin/ tazobactam	Incremental Ceftolozane/tazobactam - Piperacillin/tazobactam
Hospital costs per patient	$6996	$7429	-$433
Drug costs per patient	$766	$155	$612
Lifetime health care expenditure per patient	$28,651	$28,444	$207

the use of ceftolozane/tazobactam as empiric treatment is cost-effective compared with piperacillin/tazobactam. Ceftolozane/tazobactam was associated with a higher proportion of patients with IAAT, resulting in reduced hospitalizations and increased QALYs.

The present study is the first economic evaluation of ceftolozane/tazobactam compared to the standard of care in the treatment of cUTI. The benefits of using ceftolozane/ tazobactam as empiric therapy in this study are predominantly due to the proportion of the isolates that are susceptible to this therapy, as compared to the reference therapy. Therefore, the source and reliability of the susceptibility data are important. A strength of this study is the use of real-world surveillance data for the US from the PACTS surveillance database rather than clinical trial data. A similar approach to ours was used in the study by Sader et al. 2007 where they used the SENTRY Antimicrobial Surveillance Program, a large multinational data source on pathogen prevalence and antimicrobial susceptibility, to estimate the effectiveness of tigecycline in complicated skin and skin structure infections [33]. The findings of Sader et al. 2007 demonstrated the variation in prevalence of bacterial pathogens, highlighting the need to take into account local data on both frequency and susceptibility patterns [33]. Therefore, it is important to note that antimicrobial resistance varies by location, which could impact the cost-effectiveness of ceftolozane/tazobactam compared to piperacillin/tazobactam. For example, a recent study by Lin et al. 2015 compared the costs and effectiveness of ceftriaxone, ertapenem,

and levofloxacin in treatment of community-acquired complicated urinary tract infections from a single center perspective [34]. Future studies evaluating the cost-effectiveness of ceftolozane/tazobactam applying local surveillance data are warranted.

A few limitations to the study deserve mention. Firstly, the PACTS dataset does not contain enough information to specifically target (a) cUTI patients and (b) all patients in the PACTS dataset at risk for resistant infection. Therefore, the true proportion of resistant pathogens in the target cohort and, consequently, the cost-consequence analysis of ceftolozane/tazobactam may have been underestimated. Secondly, the model does not account for further treatment changes after any initial de-escalation/escalation, with patients assumed to be fully cured or deceased at the end of hospitalization. Recurrence and/or re-admission were not incorporated in this model. Additionally, the model excludes bacterial resistance over time and costs of antibiotic preparation and administration, monitoring, and adverse events. These costs were assumed to be similar across treatments and/or minor. Similarly, dose adjustments were not considered.

The PACTS database includes monomicrobial infections; however, infections can be polymicrobial. Underlying polymicrobial susceptibility data are required to accurately model polymicrobial infections. We used the Premier database, which is a polymicrobial database, to define the distribution for our underlying pathogens. The sum of pathogens from the Premier study exceeded 100% as patients could have polymicrobial infections. As the model only considers monomicrobial infection, the Premier distributions had to be normalized to 100%. While our model is a first step in that direction and defines a way to model monomicrobial infections, more data are needed on polymicrobial infections to accurately model such infections.

The costs reported in this analysis may be overestimated since the isolates in PACTS may under-

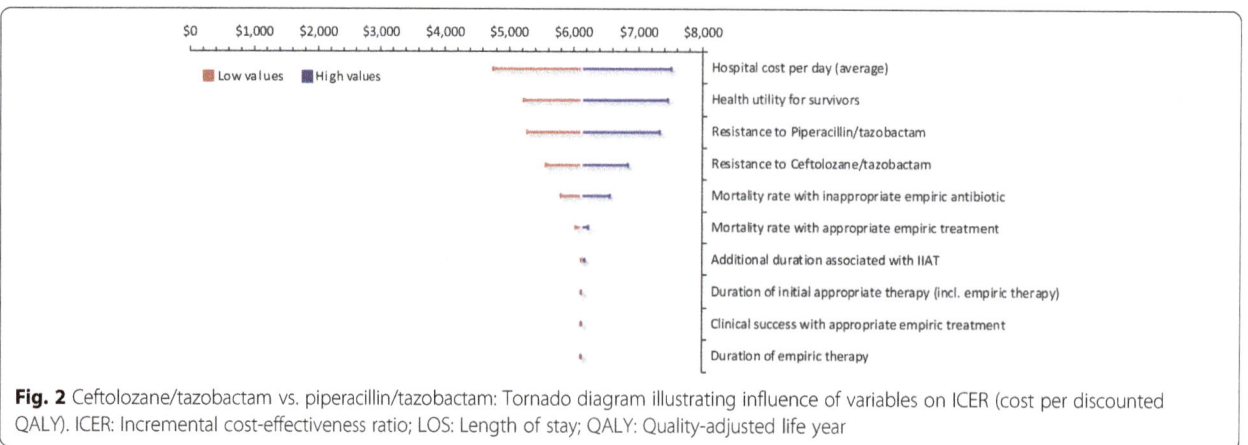

Fig. 2 Ceftolozane/tazobactam vs. piperacillin/tazobactam: Tornado diagram illustrating influence of variables on ICER (cost per discounted QALY). ICER: Incremental cost-effectiveness ratio; LOS: Length of stay; QALY: Quality-adjusted life year

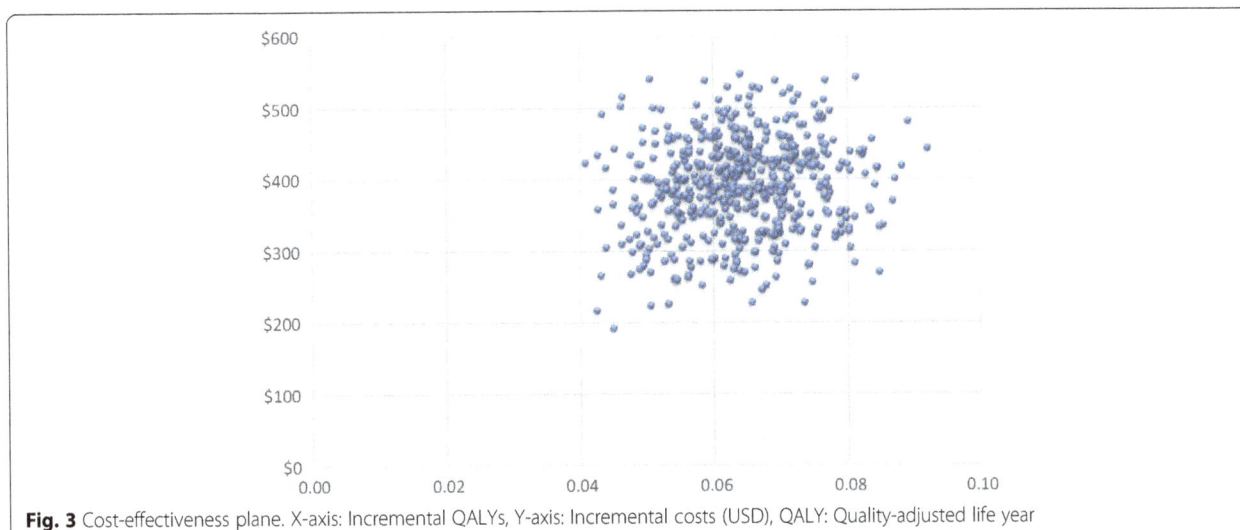

Fig. 3 Cost-effectiveness plane. X-axis: Incremental QALYs, Y-axis: Incremental costs (USD), QALY: Quality-adjusted life year

represent pathogen resistance in the target population of cUTI patients at risk of resistant infection. Costs are a function of several model parameters including duration of empiric therapy, susceptibility among comparators, and particularly the increase in length of stay (LOS) due to IIAT. Furthermore, the differences in costs are derived solely from differences in

antimicrobial activity between ceftolozane/tazobactam and piperacillin/tazobactam.

The results of our analysis were largely unchanged in both the high risk scenarios and the carbapenem-sparing scenario, with ceftolozane/tazobactam remaining similarly cost-effective. Due to increasing antibacterial resistance and scarcity of new classes of antibacterial drugs to treat Gram-

Table 5 Scenario analysis results

	Ceftolozane/ tazobactam	Piperacillin/ tazobactam	Incremental Ceftolozane/tazobactam - Piperacillin/tazobactam
Results for carbapenem-sparing scenario where non-carbapenem drugs are given precedence			
Total costs per patient (USD 2015)	$36,416	$36,038	$378
Total QALYs (discounted) per patient	9.19	9.13	0.06
Incremental Cost Effectiveness Ratio (Cost per discounted QALY gained)			$6020
Results using only nosocomial isolates	Ceftolozane/ tazobactam	Piperacillin/ tazobactam	Incremental Ceftolozane/tazobactam - Piperacillin/tazobactam
Total costs per patient (USD 2015)	$42,737	$42,358	$378
Total QALYs (discounted) per patient	12.37	12.27	0.10
Incremental Cost Effectiveness Ratio (Cost per discounted QALY gained)	-	-	$3825
Results for high risk patients (aged 65 years, requiring an ICU stay or catheter-associate infection) using nosocomial isolates	Ceftolozane/ tazobactam	Piperacillin/ tazobactam	Incremental Ceftolozane/tazobactam - Piperacillin/tazobactam
Total costs per patient (USD 2015)	$37,947	$37,557	$390
Total QALYs (discounted) per patient	10.10	10.03	0.07
Incremental Cost Effectiveness Ratio (Cost per discounted QALY gained)	-	-	$6037
Results when lifetime health care expenditure for health survivors is excluded	Ceftolozane/ tazobactam	Piperacillin/ tazobactam	Incremental Ceftolozane/tazobactam - Piperacillin/tazobactam
Total costs per patient (USD 2015)	$7762	$7583	$179
Total QALYs (discounted) per patient	9.19	9.13	0.06
Incremental Cost Effectiveness Ratio (Cost per discounted QALY gained)	-	-	$2842

QALY Quality-adjusted life year

negative bacteria, it is necessary to preserve the efficacy of existing drugs to cure common and life-threatening infections [12].

The exclusion of lifetime health care expenditures in our base case analysis approximately halved the incremental costs, resulting in a lower ICER. For our analysis, ceftolozane/tazobactam remained cost-effective; however, inclusion of lifetime healthcare expenditure may have a potential impact on comparisons which are borderline cost-effective or cost-saving.

Conclusion
Model-based analysis indicate that ceftolozane/tazobactam is cost-effective compared with piperacillin/tazobactam for the empiric treatment of cUTI in hospitalized patients.

Abbreviations
CLSI: Clinical and Laboratory Standards Institute; cUTI: Complicated urinary tract infection; ESBL: Extended-spectrum β-lactamase; GDP: Gross Domestic Product; HCUP: Healthcare Cost and Utilization Project; IAAT: Initial appropriate antibiotic therapy; ICD-9: International Classification of Diseases, Ninth Edition; ICER: Incremental cost-effectivness ratio; IIAT: Initial inappropriate antibiotic therapy; LOS: Length of stay; NMB: Net monetary benefit; OWSA: One-way sensitivity analyses; PACTS: Program to Assess Ceftolozane/Tazobactam Susceptibility; PSA: Probabilistic sensitivity analysis; QALYs: Quality-adjusted life years; US: United States

Acknowledgements
The authors would like to thank Jason Foo of Mapi B.V. for providing medical writing assistance.

Funding
This study was funded by Merck & Co., Inc.

Authors' contributions
VP, GM, RB, TK, BM, SS and AB were involved in the conception and design. VP, GM, JG, RB, TK, BM and SS were involved in data collection. VP, GM, JG, TK, BM, SS and AB were involved in data interpretation. VP, JG and TK were involved in writing the manuscript. All authors read and approved the final manuscript.

Competing interests
TK was an employee at Merck & Co., Inc. at the time the study was conducted. VP, RB and SS are employees of Merck & Co., Inc. and hold Merck stocks and stock options. GM, BM and AB have no potential conflicts of interest to declare. JG has served as a consultant to Merck and has received research funding from Merck. GM, BM and AB have no potential conflicts of interest to declare.

Consent for publication
Not applicable.

Author details
[1]Shire International GmbH, Zug, Switzerland. [2]Merck & Co., Inc., Kenilworth, NJ, USA. [3]MAPI Group, Houten, The Netherlands. [4]Shire, Lexington, MA, USA. [5]University of Washington, Seattle, WA, USA. [6]Merck & Co., Inc., 2000 Galloping Hill Rd., Kenilworth, NJ 07033, USA.

References
1. Allegranzi B, Bagheri Nejad S, Combescure C, Graafmans W, Attar H, Donaldson L, Pittet D: Burden of endemic health-care-associated infection in developing countries: systematic review and meta-analysis. Lancet (London, England) 2011, 377(9761):228–241.
2. Sievert DM, Ricks P, Edwards JR, Schneider A, Patel J, Srinivasan A, Kallen A, Limbago B, Fridkin S, National Healthcare Safety Network T, et al. Antimicrobial-resistant pathogens associated with healthcare-associated infections: summary of data reported to the National Healthcare Safety Network at the Centers for Disease Control and Prevention, 2009-2010. Infection control and hospital epidemiology: the official journal of the Society of Hospital Epidemiologists of America. 2013;34(1):1–14.
3. European Centre for Disease Prevention and Control (ECDC): Antimicrobial resistance surveillance in Europe 2011. Annual report of the European Antimicrobial Resistance Surveillance Network (EARS-Net) 2012.
4. Flores-Mireles AL, Walker JN, Caparon M, Hultgren SJ. Urinary tract infections: epidemiology, mechanisms of infection and treatment options. Nat Rev Microbiol. 2015;13(5):269–84.
5. Lo E, Nicolle LE, Coffin SE, Gould C, Maragakis LL, Meddings J, Pegues DA, Pettis AM, Saint S, Yokoe DS. Strategies to prevent catheter-associated urinary tract infections in acute care hospitals: 2014 update. Infection control and hospital epidemiology: the official journal of the Society of Hospital Epidemiologists of America. 2014;35(Suppl 2):S32–47.
6. Food and Drug Administration (FDA). Center for Drug Evaluation and Research (CDER). Guidance for industry. Complicated urinary tract infections: Developing drugs for treatment. 2012.
7. Davis N, Flood H: The pathogenesis of urinary tract infections; 2011.
8. Nicolle LE, Louie TJ, Dubois J, Martel A, Harding GK, Sinave CP. Treatment of complicated urinary tract infections with lomefloxacin compared with that with trimethoprim-sulfamethoxazole. Antimicrob Agents Chemother. 1994;38(6):1368–73.
9. Hidron AI, Edwards JR, Patel J, Horan TC, Sievert DM, Pollock DA, Fridkin SK, National Healthcare Safety Network T, Participating National Healthcare Safety Network F. NHSN annual update: antimicrobial-resistant pathogens associated with healthcare-associated infections: annual summary of data reported to the National Healthcare Safety Network at the Centers for Disease Control and Prevention, 2006-2007. Infect Control Hosp Epidemiol. 2008;29(11):996–1011.
10. Kollef MH, Sherman G, Ward S, Fraser VJ. Inadequate antimicrobial treatment of infections: a risk factor for hospital mortality among critically ill patients. Chest. 1999;115(2):462–74.
11. Falagas ME, Barefoot L, Griffith J, Ruthazar R, Snydman DR. Risk factors leading to clinical failure in the treatment of intra-abdominal or skin/soft tissue infections. Eur J Clin Microbiol Infect Dis. 1996;15(12):913–21.
12. WHO: Antimicrobial resistance: Global report on surveillance. In 2014. >http://www.who.int/drugresistance/documents/surveillancereport/en/. Accessed 21 Jan 2016.
13. Edelsberg J, Berger A, Schell S, Mallick R, Kuznik A, Oster G. Economic consequences of failure of initial antibiotic therapy in hospitalized adults with complicated intra-abdominal infections. Surg Infect. 2008;9(3):335–47.
14. Leekha S, Terrell CL, Edson RS. General principles of antimicrobial therapy. Mayo Clin Proc. 2011;86(2):156–67.
15. Koningstein M, van der Bij AK, de Kraker ME, Monen JC, Muilwijk J, de Greeff SC, Geerlings SE, van Hall MA, Group I-AS. Recommendations for the empirical treatment of complicated urinary tract infections using surveillance data on antimicrobial resistance in the Netherlands. PLoS One. 2014;9(1):e86634.
16. Grabe M, Bjerklund-Johansen TE, Botto H, Cek M, Naber KG, Tenke P, Wagenlehner F. Guidelines on urological infections. In: European Association of Urology. 2010;
17. Hsueh PR, Hoban DJ, Carmeli Y, Chen SY, Desikan S, Alejandria M, Ko WC, Binh TQ. Consensus review of the epidemiology and appropriate antimicrobial therapy of complicated urinary tract infections in Asia-Pacific region. J Inf Secur. 2011;63(2):114–23.
18. Zhanel GG, Chung P, Adam H, Zelenitsky S, Denisuik A, Schweizer F, Lagace-Wiens PR, Rubinstein E, Gin AS, Walkty A, et al. Ceftolozane/tazobactam: a novel cephalosporin/beta-lactamase inhibitor combination with activity against multidrug-resistant gram-negative bacilli. Drugs. 2014;74(1):31–51.
19. Sader HS, Farrell DJ, Flamm RK, Jones RN. Ceftolozane/tazobactam activity tested against aerobic Gram-negative organisms isolated from intra-abdominal and urinary tract infections in European and United States hospitals (2012). J Infect. 2014;69(3):266-77.

20. Basu A: Estimating costs and valuations of non-health benefits in cost-effectiveness analysis, in chapter 8, second panel on cost-effectiveness analysis in health and medicine: Oxford university press; forthcoming 2016.

21. AMCP. The AMCP Format For Formulary Submissions Version 3.1. In; 2012. http://www.amcp.org/practice-resources/amcp-format-formulary-submisions.pdf. Accessed 21 Jan 2016.

22. Wagenlehner FM, Umeh O, Steenbergen J, Yuan G, Darouiche RO: Ceftolozane-tazobactam compared with levofloxacin in the treatment of complicated urinary-tract infections, including pyelonephritis: a randomised, double-blind, phase 3 trial (ASPECT-cUTI). Lancet (London) 2015, 385(9981):1949–1956.

23. MacVane SH, Tuttle LO, Nicolau DP. Impact of extended-spectrum beta-lactamase-producing organisms on clinical and economic outcomes in patients with urinary tract infection. J Hosp Med. 2014;9(4):232–8.

24. United States Life Tables http://www.cdc.gov/nchs/products/life_tables.htm. Accessed 21 Jan 2016.

25. 2012 Healthcare Cost and Utilization Project (HCUP). https://hcupnet.ahrq.gov/. Accessed 10 Nov 2014.

26. AnalySource Suite of Drug Pricing Services https://www.analysource.com. Accessed 21 Jan 2016.

27. Using appropriate price indices for analyses of health care expenditures or income across multiple years. http://meps.ahrq.gov/about_meps/Price_Index.shtml. Accessed 21 Jan 2016.

28. Jansen JP, Kumar R, Carmeli Y. Cost-effectiveness evaluation of ertapenem versus piperacillin/tazobactam in the treatment of complicated intraabdominal infections accounting for antibiotic resistance. Value in health: the journal of the International Society for Pharmacoeconomics and Outcomes Research. 2009;12(2):234–44.

29. Zerbaxa U.S. Prescribing Information [http://www.merck.com/product/usa/pi_circulars/z/zerbaxa/zerbaxa_pi.pdf]. Accessed 21 Jan 2016.

30. Framework Summary [http://icer-review.org/wp-content/uploads/2016/02/Value-Assessment-Framework-One-Pager.pdf].

31. Marchaim D, Gottesman T, Schwartz O, Korem M, Maor Y, Rahav G, Karplus R, Lazarovitch T, Braun E, Sprecher H, et al. National multicenter study of predictors and outcomes of bacteremia upon hospital admission caused by Enterobacteriacee producing extended-spectrum beta-lactamases. Antimicrob Agents Chemother. 2010;54(12):5099–104.

32. Aloush V, Navon-Venezia S, Seigman-Igra Y, Cabili S, Carmeli Y. Multidrug-resistant Pseudomonas Aeruginosa: risk factors and clinical impact. Antimicrob Agents Chemother. 2006;50(1):43–8.

33. Sader HS, Mallick R, Kuznik A, Fritsche TR, Jones RN. Use of in vitro susceptibility and pathogen prevalence data to model the expected clinical success rates of tigecycline and other commonly used antimicrobials for empirical treatment of complicated skin and skin-structure infections. Int J Antimicrob Agents. 2007;30(6):514–20.

34. Lin HA, Yang YS, Wang JX, Lin HC, Lin Y, Chiu CH, Yeh KM, Lin JC, Chang FY. Comparison of the effectiveness and antibiotic cost among ceftriaxone, ertapenem, and levofloxacin in treatment of community-acquired complicated urinary tract infections. J Microbiol Immunol Infect. 2015;

35. 2013 Healthcare Cost and Utilization Project (HCUP). [http://hcupnet.ahrq.gov/].

Outcomes of high-dose levofloxacin therapy remain bound to the levofloxacin minimum inhibitory concentration in complicated urinary tract infections

Eliana S. Armstrong[*], Janelle A. Mikulca, Daniel J. Cloutier[*], Caleb A. Bliss and Judith N. Steenbergen

Abstract

Background: Fluoroquinolones are a guideline-recommended therapy for complicated urinary tract infections, including pyelonephritis. Elevated drug concentrations of fluoroquinolones in the urine and therapy with high-dose levofloxacin are believed to overcome resistance and effectively treat infections caused by resistant bacteria. The ASPECT-cUTI phase 3 clinical trial (ClinicalTrials.gov, NCT01345929 and NCT01345955, both registered April 28, 2011) provided an opportunity to test this hypothesis by examining the clinical and microbiological outcomes of high-dose levofloxacin treatment by levofloxacin minimum inhibitory concentration.

Methods: Patients were randomly assigned 1:1 to ceftolozane/tazobactam (1.5 g intravenous every 8 h) or levofloxacin (750 mg intravenous once daily) for 7 days of therapy. The ASPECT-cUTI study provided data on 370 patients with at least one isolate of Enterobacteriaceae at baseline who were treated with levofloxacin. Outcomes were assessed at the test-of-cure (5–9 days after treatment) and late follow-up (21–42 days after treatment) visits in the microbiologically evaluable population ($N = 327$).

Results: Test-of-cure clinical cure rates above 90% were observed at minimum inhibitory concentrations ≤4 μg/mL. Microbiological eradication rates were consistently >90% at levofloxacin minimum inhibitory concentrations ≤0.06 μg/mL. Lack of eradication of causative pathogens at the test-of-cure visit increased the likelihood of relapse by the late follow-up visit.

Conclusions: Results from this study do not support levofloxacin therapy for complicated urinary tract infections caused by organisms with levofloxacin minimum inhibitory concentrations ≥4 μg/mL.

Keywords: Ceftolozane/tazobactam, cUTI, Fluoroquinolones, Levofloxacin, Resistance

Background

Complicated urinary tract infection (cUTI) is associated with significant morbidity and increased health care costs, particularly as resistance to first-line antimicrobial agents has become widespread [1, 2]. Hospitalization for cUTIs caused by Gram-negative bacteria (typically Enterobacteriaceae such as *Escherichia coli*) in the United States increased by approximately 50% from 2000 to 2009, whereas the incidence of infections caused by extended-spectrum β-lactamase (ESBL)–positive organisms increased by approximately 300% in the same time period [3].

Fluoroquinolones such as levofloxacin have historically been an attractive therapy for cUTI (including pyelonephritis) because of their high drug concentrations in the urine and their demonstrated clinical efficacy [4]. However, their future usefulness is threatened by alarmingly high rates of fluoroquinolone resistance, often occurring in combination with other resistance mechanisms including ESBL production. A surveillance study of 24 US hospitals found that less than 70% of non-ESBL–producing isolates of *E. coli* were susceptible to ciprofloxacin or

* Correspondence: eliana.s.armstrong@gmail.com;
danieljcloutier44@gmail.com
Merck & Co., Inc., 2000 Galloping Hill Road, Kenilworth, NJ 07033, USA

levofloxacin, and this number fell to less than 10% for ESBL-producing strains [5]. The challenge of fluoroquinolone resistance is even greater in other regions of the world [6]. Resistance to fluoroquinolones can occur through a combination of point mutations in the target gyrase and topoisomerase genes, plasmid-mediated mechanisms (eg, qnr), and upregulated efflux of the drug [7, 8]. The spread of these resistance mechanisms has been facilitated by their strong association with the worldwide pandemic clone of E. coli, ST-131 [9].

In the clinical management of cUTI, it remains common practice to treat patients empirically, at least during the 2- to 3-day time period required to obtain standard culture results [10, 11]. As resistance increases, recommendations either to avoid empiric use of fluoroquinolones or to use these antibacterials judiciously based on local surveillance data are becoming more prevalent [12, 13]. Guidance directed toward uncomplicated urinary tract infections, published by the Infectious Diseases Society of America and the European Society for Clinical Microbiology and Infectious Diseases, supports a 3-day course of fluoroquinolone therapy, but only in regions where the resistance rate is lower than 10% [14].

Previous clinical studies have concluded that high urinary tract concentrations of fluoroquinolones are sufficient to allow successful outcomes for nonsusceptible isolates. One large post hoc analysis examined a population in whom the level of fluoroquinolone resistance was relatively low (<10%) [15]. Patients received levofloxacin (750 mg intravenously) or ciprofloxacin (either 400 mg intravenously or 500 mg orally) for 10 days. Forty-two fluoroquinolone-resistant isolates (levofloxacin minimum inhibitory concentration [MIC] ≥ 8 µg/mL and ciprofloxacin MIC ≥ 4 µg/mL) were reported. Six isolates had levofloxacin or ciprofloxacin MICs ranging from 8 to 32 µg/mL and were eradicated with treatment, and 13 isolates with fluoroquinolone MICs >32 µg/mL persisted. The outcomes of the remaining 23 isolates were not presented. A smaller study of a 500-mg dose of levofloxacin conducted in a setting of higher levofloxacin resistance calculated a 90% probability of microbiological eradication of Gram-negative bacilli at an MIC of 2 µg/mL. Eradication was evaluated only 2 days after therapy, however, a time when levofloxacin may still be present in the urine and suppressing the growth of organisms that could result in a different microbiological outcome after the drug has cleared [16]. In vitro urinary bactericidal titer experiments demonstrated that the concentration of levofloxacin in urine following a 750-mg dose was bactericidal to E. coli isolates with MICs ≤ 32 µg/mL [17].

In this exploratory analysis, we examined the clinical and microbiological outcomes of treatment with high-dose, extended-duration levofloxacin (750 mg for 7 days)

by levofloxacin MIC in a large sample of patients with cUTI caused by Enterobacteriaceae in the ASPECT-cUTI phase 3 clinical trial.

Methods
Study population
ASPECT-cUTI (ClinicalTrials.gov, NCT01345929 and NCT01345955) was a large, global, phase 3 program that evaluated the efficacy and safety of ceftolozane/tazobactam versus levofloxacin for the treatment of adult hospital patients with cUTI, including pyelonephritis [18]. The trials were approved by appropriate regulatory agencies and local institutional review boards (IRB) and were conducted in accordance with International Conference on Harmonisation/Good Clinical Practice guidelines and the principles of the Declaration of Helsinki. All patients provided written informed consent. Patients with cUTI (defined in [18]) were randomly assigned 1:1 to ceftolozane/tazobactam (1.5 g intravenous every 8 h) or levofloxacin (750 mg intravenous once daily) for 7 days of therapy. Patients were included in the microbiological modified intent-to-treat (mMITT) population if they received any amount of study drug and had at least one but not more than two causative uropathogen(s) growing at $\geq 10^5$ CFU/mL from a study-qualifying pretreatment baseline urine specimen. The microbiologically evaluable (ME) population was the subset of the mMITT population who adhered to study procedures and had interpretable urine culture results at the test-of-cure (TOC) visit (5–9 days after the last dose of study drug).

The ASPECT-cUTI study provided data on 370 patients in the mMITT population and 327 patients in the ME population who had ≤ 1 isolate of Enterobacteriaceae at baseline and were treated with levofloxacin. A total of 333 Enterobacteriaceae were isolated from 327 patients in the ME population. Susceptibility data were available for 313 of these isolates.

Levofloxacin efficacy analysis
An exploratory analysis of levofloxacin-treated patients with an Enterobacteriaceae isolate and characterized levofloxacin susceptibility from the screening visit in ASPECT-cUTI was conducted to evaluate the microbiological and clinical outcomes at the TOC and late follow-up (LFU) visits (21–42 days after the last dose of study drug). The ME population was selected for analysis to exclude patients with indeterminate outcomes. Clinical cure at the TOC visit was defined as complete resolution, substantial improvement (ie, reduction in severity of all baseline signs and symptoms), or return to premorbid signs and symptoms without the need for additional antibiotic therapy. Microbiological eradication was defined as a TOC urine culture with $< 10^4$ CFU/mL of the baseline uropathogen. The per-pathogen microbiological and clinical outcomes at the

TOC visit were stratified by levofloxacin MIC of each baseline infecting organism. Clinical outcomes for patients who were classified as clinical cures at the TOC visit and who returned for the LFU visit were classified as sustained, indeterminate, or relapsed based on the sustained resolution or relapse in clinical signs and symptoms of cUTI that were absent at the TOC visit. Relative proportions of each of these categories were examined for patients whose infections were microbiologically eradicated versus those who had persisting positive cultures at the TOC visit.

Susceptibility testing
Susceptibility and quality control testing of study isolates was performed by ICON Laboratories (Farmingdale, NY) in accordance with Clinical and Laboratory Standards Institute (CLSI) guidelines. Quality control testing was performed concurrent with testing of clinical study isolates. Interpretation of susceptibility test results and acceptable quality control ranges were based on CLSI document M100-S22 [19]. Study isolates initially characterized as levofloxacin-resistant (MIC >4 µg/mL) [19] were retested to determine the levofloxacin MIC end point up to 256 µg/mL.

Statistical analysis
Descriptive statistics were used to summarize the demographics, baseline characteristics, clinical outcomes, microbiological outcomes, and genotypes of patients, and 95% confidence intervals (CIs) were calculated by the Wilson score methodology to compare the relapse rates at LFU. Statistical analyses were performed using SAS version 9.1 (SAS Institute Inc., Cary, NC).

Results
Demographics and baseline clinical characteristics of 370 levofloxacin-treated patients with ≥1 isolate each of Enterobacteriaceae identified at baseline in the mMITT population are shown in Table 1. Most patients had pyelonephritis (82.7%) and most were enrolled in Europe (74.9%); 24.3% were 65 years of age or older.

Clinical and microbiological outcomes of levofloxacin treatment stratified by levofloxacin MICs are listed in Table 2. High rates of clinical cure (90–100%) were observed at levofloxacin MICs ≤4 µg/mL. Rates of microbiological eradication were also consistently high (>90%) at levofloxacin MICs ≤0.06 µg/mL. However, at levofloxacin MICs >0.06 µg/mL, a trend toward decreasing eradication rates was observed.

A higher percentage of patients with persistent infection at the TOC visit experienced relapse by the LFU visit than did patients whose infections were eradicated at the TOC visit (18.5% vs 1.3%; difference, 17.2%; 95% CI, 8.7–29.6%) (Table 3).

Table 1 Characteristics of levofloxacin-treated patients with ≥1 isolate of Enterobacteriaceae identified at baseline (mMITT population)

Characteristic	Levofloxacin N = 370
Age, years	
Mean (SD)	48.0 (20.26)
Range, n (%)	18–87
≥ 65–< 75	47 (12.7)
≥ 75	43 (11.6)
Sex, n (%)	
Male	82 (22.2)
Female	288 (77.8)
Race, n (%)	
White	317 (85.7)
Black or African American	6 (1.6)
Asian	30 (8.1)
Other	17 (4.6)
Region, n (%)	
Eastern Europe	277 (74.9)
Western Europe	0
North America	9 (2.4)
South America	39 (10.5)
Rest of world	45 (12.2)
Diagnosis, n (%)	
Pyelonephritis	306 (82.7)
cLUTI	64 (17.3)
Creatinine clearance, mL/min, n (%)	
Normal (≥80)	250 (67.6)
Mild impairment (≥50–< 80)	92 (24.9)
Moderate impairment (≥30–< 50)	27 (7.3)
Severe impairment (<30)	1 (0.3)

cLUTI complicated lower urinary tract infection, *mMITT* microbiological modified intent-to-treat, *SD* standard deviation

Discussion and conclusions
In several recent and ongoing clinical trials in cUTI, levofloxacin has been used as the comparator against such agents as doripenem [20], plazomicin (NCT01096849), ceftolozane/tazobactam [18], and eravacycline (NCT01978938). A recent meta-analysis examined multiple cUTI trials before ASPECT-cUTI and identified microbiological eradication rates at the TOC visit in the microbiological intent-to-treat population of 81% for doripenem, 79% for levofloxacin, and 80.5% for imipenem-cilastatin, confirming that levofloxacin has a place in the armamentarium for cUTI [21]. In an era of increasing and evolving antibiotic resistance, however, decisions about clinical usefulness must be made at the local hospital and individual patient level [22].

Table 2 Microbiological eradication and clinical cure following levofloxacin treatment stratified by MIC (Enterobacteriaceae isolates, ME population)

Baseline levofloxacin MIC, μg/mL	Microbiological eradication, n/N (%)	Clinical cure, n/N (%)
≤0.015	9/10 (90.0)	10/10 (100)
0.03	120/126 (95.2)	124/126 (98.4)
0.06	38/40 (95.0)	37/40 (92.5)
0.125	9/11 (81.8)	10/11 (90.9)
0.25	6/8 (75.0)	8/8 (100)
0.5	14/17 (82.4)	17/17 (100)
1	5/6 (83.3)	6/6 (100)
2	1/1 (100)	0/1 (0)[a]
4	3/9 (33.3)	9/9 (100)
8	11/17 (64.7)	15/17 (88.2)
16	20/44 (45.5)	36/44 (81.8)
32	4/13 (30.8)	11/13 (84.6)
64	1/6 (16.7)	4/6 (66.7)
128	0/1 (0)	0/1 (0)

ME microbiologically evaluable, *MIC* minimum inhibitory concentration, *n* number of isolates assigned to an outcome of eradication or clinical cure, *N* number of isolates at each levofloxacin MIC

Four E. coli isolates were not retested to determine MIC end points and were excluded from this analysis. Five patients had 2 Enterobacteriaceae isolates identified at baseline. Four patients had a clinical response of cure, and 1 patient had a clinical response of failure. Clinical response for these patients was counted once for each isolate at its respective MIC

[a] This isolate was present in combination with a second isolate that had a levofloxacin MIC of 16 μg/mL; the patient's clinical response was failure

High-dose levofloxacin treatment (750 mg once daily for 7 days) in ASPECT-cUTI resulted in clinical cure for the more than 90% of patients with Enterobacteriaceae infections who had MICs ≤4 μg/mL. Nevertheless, persistence of the baseline pathogen became more frequent as the MIC increased, with an eradication rate of <90% observed at an MIC of only 0.125 μg/mL. A similar decrease in the microbiological eradication rate with levofloxacin treatment above a levofloxacin MIC of 0.06 μg/mL was observed during the phase 3 doripenem studies, though the total numbers of patients treated was smaller [20].

The clinical significance of failure to eradicate the causative pathogen while resolving clinical symptoms is unknown, but multiple studies have shown that fluoroquinolone resistance is strongly correlated with persistence of symptoms [23] and recurrence of infection [24]. The results presented in this study show that, as expected, an increase in levofloxacin MIC was correlated with a decrease in microbiological eradication rate with levofloxacin treatment. Clinical cure without microbiological eradication of the causative pathogen was more likely (difference, 17.2%; 95% CI, 8.7–29.6%) to result in a relapse of cUTI at the LFU visit. The levofloxacin-resistant isolates from this study had high levofloxacin MICs that were associated with common and highly conserved fluoroquinolone resistance mechanisms, most typically point mutations in gyrA and parC (data not shown).

Pharmacokinetic/pharmacodynamic (PK/PD) targets for fluoroquinolone treatment in cUTI have been studied in depth. Typically, AUC/MIC ratios of 100 or C_{max}/MIC ratios of 10 are associated with good clinical outcomes [25], though 90% microbiological eradication of Gram-negative cUTI pathogens has been reported at targets as low as 31.46 and 2.74, respectively [16]. Data on the pharmacokinetics of levofloxacin in either serum or urine were not obtained during ASPECT-cUTI; therefore, direct analysis of these outcomes as they relate to the levofloxacin concentration is not possible. Administration of single 750-mg doses of levofloxacin to 10 healthy adults was reported to produce AUC and C_{max} values of 93 ± 15 μg·h/mL and 7.6 ± 1.2 μg/mL in serum and 7328 ± 3237 μg·h/mL and 620 ± 324 μg/mL in urine, respectively [17]. Conservatively applying the lower bound of the PK ranges and the higher PK/PD targets predicts that levofloxacin MICs of 0.5 μg/mL should be treatable in serum. In urine, the value is between 16 and 32 μg/mL, depending on whether the C_{max} or the AUC parameter is used. However, elevated MIC treatment targets based on urinary concentrations are not supported by the outcomes in this study, which is the first to examine a population with high levels of levofloxacin resistance using a stringent criterion for microbiological eradication.

In summary, these clinical data demonstrate that high-dose, extended-duration levofloxacin treatment (750 mg for

Table 3 Impact of microbiological outcome at TOC on clinical outcome at LFU (ME population)

Microbiological outcome at TOC visit	Clinical outcome at LFU visit			% Difference in relapse between persisted and eradicated (95% CI)
	Sustained	Indeterminate	Relapse	
Eradicated, n/N (%)	225/229 (98.3)	1/229 (0.4)	3/229 (1.3)	17.2 (8.7–29.6)
Persisted, n/N (%)	42/54 (77.8)	2/54 (3.7)	10/54 (18.5)	

CI confidence interval, *LFU* late follow-up, *ME* microbiologically evaluable, *TOC* test-of-cure

Four patients had 2 Enterobacteriaceae isolates identified at baseline and a clinical response of cure at the TOC visit. These patients were counted once for this analysis by assignment to the "persisted at TOC group" if 1 isolate persisted (1 patient) and to the "eradicated at TOC group" if both isolates were eradicated (3 patients). All 4 experienced sustained response at the LFU visit

7 days) of patients with cUTIs was less likely to be successful when the MIC of the infecting organism was ≥4 µg/mL and less likely to be sustainable when the MIC was >0.06 µg/mL.

Abbreviations

CFU: Colony-forming unit; CI: Confidence interval; CLSI: Clinical and Laboratory Standards Institute; cUTI: Complicated urinary tract infection; ESBL: Extended-spectrum β-lactamase; LFU: Late follow-up; ME: Microbiologically evaluable; MIC: Minimum inhibitory concentration; mMITT: Microbiological modified intent-to-treat; PD: Pharmacodynamic; PK: Pharmacokinetic; TOC: Test-of-cure

Acknowledgements

Editorial support for this manuscript was provided by Jean Turner of PAREXEL, Hackensack, NJ, USA, and Sally Mitchell, PhD, and Sarah Utley, PhD, of ApotheCom, Yardley, PA, and was funded by Merck & Co., Inc., Kenilworth, NJ, USA.

Funding

This work was supported by Merck & Co., Inc., Kenilworth, NJ, USA. Employees of the study sponsor, in collaboration with the authors, were involved in the study design, data collection and analysis, decision to publish, and preparation of the manuscript.

Authors' contributions

E.S.A. substantially contributed to the acquisition and analysis of the data, interpretation of results, drafting and critically revising the manuscript for important intellectual content, gave approval of the final version of the manuscript to be published, and agreed to be accountable for the integrity of the data and the accuracy of the work. J.A.M. substantially contributed to the interpretation of the study data, drafting and critically revising the manuscript for important intellectual content, gave approval of the final version of the manuscript to be published, and agreed to be accountable for the integrity of the data and the accuracy of the work. D.J.C. substantially contributed to the conception of the study, analysis of the data, interpretation of results, drafting and critically revising the manuscript for important intellectual content, gave approval of the final version of the manuscript to be published, and agreed to be accountable for the integrity of the data and the accuracy of the work. C.A.B. substantially contributed to the analysis of the data and interpretation of results, drafting and critically revising the manuscript for important intellectual content, gave approval of the final version of the manuscript to be published, and agreed to be accountable for the integrity of the data and the accuracy of the work. J.N.S. substantially contributed to the design and planning of the study, analysis of the data and interpretation of results, and critically revising the manuscript for important intellectual content, gave approval of the final version of the manuscript to be published, and agreed to be accountable for the integrity of the data and the accuracy of the work.

Authors' information

Not applicable.

Competing interests

J.A.M. is a current employee and E.S.A., D.J.C., C.A.B, and J.N.S. are former employees of Merck, Sharp & Dohme Corp., a subsidiary of Merck & Co., Inc., Kenilworth, NJ, USA.
E.S.A. was working under a contract from Pro Unlimited, 7777 Glades Road, Boca Raton, FL 33434, USA, at the time of the study.

Consent for publication

Not applicable.

References

1. Klevens RM, Edwards JR, Gaynes RP. The impact of antimicrobial-resistant, health care-associated infections on mortality in the United States. Clin Infect Dis. 2008;47:927–30.
2. Sader HS, Flamm RK, Jones RN. Frequency of occurrence and antimicrobial susceptibility of Gram-negative bacteremia isolates in patients with urinary tract infection: results from United States and European hospitals (2009–2011). J Chemother. 2014;26:133–8.
3. Zilberberg MD, Shorr AF. Secular trends in Gram-negative resistance among urinary tract infection hospitalizations in the United States, 2000–2009. Infect Control Hosp Epidemiol. 2013;34:940–6.
4. Rafat C, Debrix I, Hertig A. Levofloxacin for the treatment of pyelonephritis. Expert Opin Pharmacother. 2013;14:1241–53.
5. Bouchillon SK, Badal RE, Hoban DJ, Hawser SP. Antimicrobial susceptibility of inpatient urinary tract isolates of Gram-negative bacilli in the United States: results from the study for monitoring antimicrobial resistance trends (SMART) program: 2009–2011. Clin Ther. 2013;35:872–7.
6. Hsueh PR, Hoban DJ, Carmeli Y, Chen SY, Desikan S, Alejandria M, Ko WC, Binh TQ. Consensus review of the epidemiology and appropriate antimicrobial therapy of complicated urinary tract infections in Asia-Pacific region. J Infect. 2011;63:114–23.
7. Hooper DC. Mechanisms of action and resistance of older and newer fluoroquinolones. Clin Infect Dis. 2000;31 suppl 2:S28.
8. Tran JH, Jacoby GA. Mechanism of plasmid-mediated quinolone resistance. Proc Natl Acad Sci U S A. 2002;99:5638–42.
9. Rogers BA, Sidjabat HE, Paterson DL. Escherichia coli O25b-ST131: a pandemic, multiresistant, community-associated strain. J Antimicrob Chemother. 2011;66:1–14.
10. Nicolle LE. Complicated urinary tract infection in adults. Can J Infect Dis Med Microbiol. 2005;16:349–60.
11. Pallett A, Hand K. Complicated urinary tract infections: practical solutions for the treatment of multiresistant Gram-negative bacteria. J Antimicrob Chemother. 2010;65 suppl 3:iii25–33.
12. Bader MS, Hawboldt J, Brooks A. Management of complicated urinary tract infections in the era of antimicrobial resistance. Postgrad Med. 2010;122:7–15.
13. Koningstein M, Van der Bij AK, De Kraker ME, Monen JC, Muilwijk J, De Greeff SC, Geerlings SE, Leverstein-van Hall MA, ISIS-AR Study Group. Recommendations for the empirical treatment of complicated urinary tract infections using surveillance data on antimicrobial resistance in the Netherlands. PLoS One. 2014;9:e86634.
14. Gupta K, Hooton TM, Naber KG, Wullt B, Colgan R, Miller LG, Moran GJ, Nicolle LE, Raz R, Schaeffer AJ, Soper DE. Infectious Diseases Society of America; European Society for Microbiology and Infectious Diseases. International clinical practice guidelines for the treatment of acute uncomplicated cystitis and pyelonephritis in women: a 2010 update by the Infectious Diseases Society of America and the European Society for Microbiology and Infectious Diseases. Clin Infect Dis. 2011;52:e103–20.
15. Peterson J, Kaul S, Khashab M, Fisher A, Kahn JB. Identification and pretherapy susceptibility of pathogens in patients with complicated urinary tract infection or acute pyelonephritis enrolled in a clinical study in the United States from November 2004 through April 2006. Clin Ther. 2007;29:2215–21.
16. Deguchi T, Nakane K, Yasuda M, Shimizu T, Monden K, Arakawa S, Matsumoto T. Microbiological outcome of complicated urinary tract infections treated with levofloxacin: a pharmacokinetic/pharmacodynamic analysis. Int J Antimicrob Agents. 2010;35:573–7.
17. Stein GE, Schooley SL, Nicolau DP. Urinary bactericidal activity of single doses (250, 500, 750 and 1000 mg) of levofloxacin against fluoroquinolone-resistant strains of Escherichia coli. Int J Antimicrob Agents. 2008;32:320–5.
18. Wagenlehner FM, Umeh O, Steenbergen J, Yuan G, Darouiche RO. Ceftolozane-tazobactam compared with levofloxacin in the treatment of complicated urinary-tract infections, including pyelonephritis: a randomised, double-blind, phase 3 trial (ASPECT-cUTI). Lancet. 2015;385:1949–56.
19. Clinical and Laboratory Standards Institute. Performance Standards for Antimicrobial Susceptibility Testing: Twenty-Second Informational Supplement M100-S22. Wayne: Clinical and Laboratory Standards Institute; 2012.

20. Naber KG, Llorens L, Kaniga K, Kotey P, Hedrich D, Redman R. Intravenous doripenem at 500 milligrams versus levofloxacin at 250 milligrams, with an option to switch to oral therapy, for treatment of complicated lower urinary tract infection and pyelonephritis. Antimicrob Agents Chemother. 2009;53:3782–92.

21. Singh KP, Li G, Mitrani-Gold FS, Kurtinecz M, Wetherington J, Tomayko JF, Mundy LM. Systematic review and meta-analysis of antimicrobial treatment effect estimation in complicated urinary tract infection. Antimicrob Agents Chemother. 2013;57:5284–90.

22. Chen YH, Ko WC, Hsueh PR. The role of fluoroquinolones in the management of urinary tract infections in areas with high rates of fluoroquinolone-resistant uropathogens. Eur J Clin Microbiol Infect Dis. 2012;31:1699–704.

23. Can F, Azap OK, Seref C, Ispir P, Arslan H, Ergonul O. Emerging *Escherichia coli* O25b/ST131 clone predicts treatment failure in urinary tract infections. Clin Infect Dis. 2015;60:523–7.

24. Bodro M, Sanclemente G, Lipperheide I, Allali M, Marco F, Bosch J, Cofan F, Ricart MJ, Esforzado N, Oppenheimer F, Moreno A, Cervera C. Impact of antibiotic resistance on the development of recurrent and relapsing symptomatic urinary tract infection in kidney recipients. Am J Transplant. 2015;15:1021–7.

25. Schentag JJ. Clinical pharmacology of the fluoroquinolones: studies in human dynamic/kinetic models. Clin Infect Dis. 2000;31 suppl 2:S40–4.

Management of febrile urinary tract infection among spinal cord injured patients

Aurélien Dinh[1*], Adnène Toumi[2], Constance Blanc[1], Alexis Descatha[1], Frédérique Bouchand[3], Jérôme Salomon[1], Thomas Hanslik[4], Benjamin Bernuz[5], Pierre Denys[5] and Louis Bernard[6]

Abstract

Background: Urinary tract infection (UTI) among patients with neurogenic bladder is a major problem but its management is not well known. We studied the relationship between antibiotic regimen use and the cure rate of those infections among 112 patients with neurogenic bladder.

Methods: We studied a retrospective cohort of febrile UTI among patients with neurogenic bladder. Drug selection was left to the discretion of the treating physicians, in accordance with current guidelines. Patients were divided into 3 groups according to antibiotic treatment duration (<10 days, between 10 and 15 days, and >15 days). We analysed clinical and microbiogical cure rate one month after the end of antibiotic treatment.

Results: The three groups of patients were similar, especially in terms of drug treatment (equal distribution). The cure rates were not significantly different (71.4 %, 54.2 %, and 57.1 %, respectively; $p = 0.34$). Moreover, there was no difference in cure rate between mono and dual therapy (44 % for monotherapy *vs.* 40 % for dual therapy; $p = 0.71$).

Conclusion: This descriptive study supports the efficacy of antimicrobial treatment duration of less than 10 days and the use of monotherapy to treat febrile UTI among patients with neurogenic bladder. A randomized control trial is required to confirm these data.

Keywords: Antibiotic treatment duration, Neurogenic bladder, Urinary tract infection

Background

Urinary tract infection (UTI) is one of the most common infectious diseases, especially among patients with neurogenic bladder. These patients are more likely to develop UTI than the general population [1–3]. Fever during UTI suggests the presence of tissue inflammation, which could lead to severe sepsis [4]. Despite voiding practices maintaining low pressure bladder such as intermittent catheterizations, febrile UTI among patients with neurogenic bladder is still the primary cause of morbidity and hospitalization [1, 5].

Guidelines about the duration of antibiotic treatment for acute pyelonephritis are usually 7 to 14 days, and 21 days for complicated forms such as in patients with neurogenic bladder [6]. Shorter antibiotic treatments are considered helpful to reduce the development of antibiotic resistance and reduce toxicity. No recommendations about the duration of antibiotic treatment currently exist for patients with neurogenic bladder.

We aimed to describe cure rates of febrile UTI, according to different antibiotic treatment regimens, in a cohort of patients with neurogenic bladder who were followed in a specialist rehabilitation center.

Methods

This retrospective study was conducted from January the 1st 2008 to December the 31st 2013 in a University Hospital, with acute care facilities (255 beds, including 43 beds of adult intensive care) and a 108-bed rehabilitation unit (with 40 beds dedicated to spinal cord injured patients). There are about 8400 admissions per year for

* Correspondence: aurelien.dinh@aphp.fr
[1]Infectious Disease Unit, Garches PIFO University Hospital, AP-HP, Versailles Saint Quentin University, Garches, France
Full list of author information is available at the end of the article

complete hospitalization. This study was approved by the Saint-Germain-en-Laye ethical (CPP IDF XI) review committee (N° 06070).

Patients

Hospitalized patients with neurogenic bladder diagnosed with febrile UTI were enrolled in this study if they fulfilled the 3 following criteria: 1) fever > 38 °C; 2) at least one of the following clinical signs lasting less than five days: pyuria, dysuria, frequent urination, urgent urination, perineal or flank pain, clinical autonomic dysreflexia (which is associated with throbbing headaches, profuse sweating, nasal stuffiness, flushing of the skin above the level of the lesion, slow heart rate); 3) a positive urine culture defined as a urine bacterial count $\geq 10^5$ colony-forming units (CFU)/mL [7] ; 4) management as a UTI by the physician on charge, with relevant and appropriate antimicrobial prescription according to usual guidelines, and absence of other possible diagnosis.

Methods

Susceptibility to antibiotics was determined using disk diffusion according to the CA-SFM recommendations [8]. For patients with an indwelling urinary catheter, the urine sample was collected from the port of the catheter.

The following information about antibiotic treatment was collected from medical charts using a standard questionnaire:

- Drug treatment
- Duration: patients were divided into three groups according to the duration of antibiotic treatment. Group 1, less than 10 days of treatment; group 2, between 10 and 15 days of treatment; and group 3, more than 15 days of treatment. Duration was the time during which the patient received microbiologically appropriate antibiotic treatment considering the final result of his urine culture.
- Mono or dual therapy: dual therapy was defined as the simultaneous use of two antibiotics effective against the particular pathogens involved, for at least one day during the course of treatment. Only antibiotics that have shown to be effective against febrile UTI according to international guidelines and with proven efficacy based on susceptibility testing were considered for use in dual therapy and treatment duration [6].

The following information was obtained for each case of febrile UTI at diagnosis: clinical data (including type of neurological deficit and voiding practice), bacteriological data, leukocyte count, C-reactive protein level.

End-point

The cure rate was determined one month after the end of antibiotic treatment from a medical interview [9, 10]. Cure was defined as the complete resolution of symptoms and clinical signs related to UTI without the need for additional or alternative antibiotic therapy. A urine culture was performed at the same time.

Failure was defined as the persistence or progression of symptoms or signs of UTI, or death related to UTI. Patients who could not be evaluated either died due to a condition unrelated to UTI, were lost to follow up, or required another antibiotic treatment during follow up for a concomitant infection outside the urinary tract, were included in the study but not in the outcome analysis. These patients were considered as undetermined.

Statistical analysis

Data analyses were carried out with the SAS 9.3 software (SAS Institute Inc., Cary, NC, USA). Univariate analyses were carried out with chi^2 and Fisher exact tests, including all variables known to be associated with UTI (i.e. statistical or clinically significant): sex, age, type of neurological deficit, type of voiding management, positive blood culture [1, 11, 12].

Statistical significance was defined as $p < 0.05$.

Results

There were 112 cases of febrile UTI among 94 patients with neurogenic bladder. The baseline characteristics of the 94 patients and the outcome of the 112 episodes are listed in Table 1. Of the 94 patients, 83 had a unique episode.

The population was mostly male (80/112) with young adults (mean age: 38.4 years old ± 11.7) and paraplegic patients ($n = 65$; 58 %). The most frequent bladder voiding method was intermittent catheterization ($n = 57$; 51 %). During UTI, patients had a mean temperature of 38.8 °C (±0.6 °C) and mean C reactive protein level was 121 mg/L (±84); 15 % ($n = 17$) of patients had positive blood culture.

The main bacteria involved were *E. coli* ($n = 55$; 49 %), *Pseudomonas aeruginosa* ($n = 19$; 13.5 %) and *Entero-coccus spp.* ($n = 19$; 13.5 %). Twenty nine (26 %) UTIs were polymicrobial, with four involving 3 microorganisms and 25 involving 2. Mean treatment duration was 18.1 days and dual therapy was prescribed in 62 % ($n = 69$) of cases. Global cure rate was 60 % ($n = 67$) and failure 27.5 % ($n = 31$). Fourteen patients (12.5 %) could not be evaluated.

Eleven patients had recurrent febrile UTI: seven patients had two episodes of UTI, three patients had three, and one patient suffered six. Of these patients, three (27 %) had urinary diversion and three others (27 %) used reflex voiding.

Table 1 Characteristics and outcome of 112 febrile urinary tract infection occurring among patients with neurogenic bladder depending on treatment duration

Treatment duration (days)	<10 d	10-15 d	>15 d	Total	P value
Number of febrile UTI[a]	28	35	49	112	
Patient characteristics					
Sex (women/men)	12/16	11/24	9/40	32/80	0.2453
Age: mean year (SD)	49.6 (20.1)	46.5 (24.7)	31 (19.7)	38.4 (11.7)	0.1443
Fever: mean °C (SD)	38.6 (0.33)	38.9 (0.76)	39.07 (0.78)	38.8 (0.6)	0.5469
Neurological deficit N (%)					
Paraplegia	18 (64)	20 (57)	27 (55)	65 (58)	0.2604
Tetraplegia	5 (18)	2 (6)	13 (27)	20 (18)	0.5205
Multiple sclerosis	4 (14)	6 (17)	6 (12)	16(14)	0.9299
Brain injury	1 (4)	7 (20)	3 (6)	11(10)	0.1042
Voiding management N (%)					
Intermittent cathererization	14 (50)	13 (37.1)	30 (62)	57 (51)	0.4564
Indwelling catheter	2 (7)	4 (11)	6 (12)	12 (10)	0.9899
Reflex voiding	7 (25)	8 (23)	7 (14)	22 (19)	0.8349
Urinary diversion	2 (7)	6 (17)	3 (6)	11 (10)	
Others	3 (11)	4 (11)	3 (6)	10 (10)	
Biological variables					
Leukocyte count: median/L (SD)	12. 9 (5.5)	13 (6.9)	12 (5.7)	12.6 (6)	0.4426
CRP mean mg/l (SD)	140 (84)	139 (89)	122(90)	121 (84)	0.9953
Positive blood culture N (%)	3 (10)	5 (14)	9 (18)	17 (15)	0.5246
Microorganism sample N (%)					
E coli	17 (53)	16 (37.2)	22 (33)	55 (49)	
Pseudomonas aeruginosa	6 (18.7)	6 (13.9)	7 (10.6)	19 (13.5)	
Enterococcus	4 (12.5)	7 (16.2)	8 (12)	19 (13.5)	
Klebsiella	2 (6.25)	4 (9.3)	8 (12)	14 (10)	
Proteus	1 (3.12)	3 (7)	4 (6)	8(5.6)	
Others	2 (6.43)	7 (16.4)	17 (26.4))	26 (18.4)	
Antibiotic treatment					
Mean treatment duration (SD)	7.9 (2.3)	13.4 (1.9)	27.3 (9.8)	18.1 (10.7)	0.0250
Mean parenteral treatment duration (median, SD)	8 (8, ±2.2)	6.8 (5, ±5.33)	11.2 (7, ±10.6)	8.2 (6, ±8.3)	
Dual therapy N (%)	17 (61)	18 (52)	34 (70)	69 (62)	0.9669
Antibiotic treatment N (%)					
Third generation cephalosporin	16 (33)	19 (26.3)	32 (32)	67 (30.6)	
Aminoglycosides	12 (25)	18 (25)	21 (21)	51 (23.2)	
Fluoroquinolones	6 (12.5)	14 (19.4)	16 (16)	36 (16.4)	
Penicillin	9 (18.8)	12 (16.7)	14 (14)	35 (16)	
Carbapenem	4 (8.3)	5 (6.9)	11 (11)	20 (9.1)	
Colimycin	1 (2)	2 (2.8)	2 (2)	5 (2.3)	
Cotrimoxazole	0	0	3 (3)	3 (1.4)	
Fosfomycin	0	2 (2.8)	0	2 (1)	
Outcome (1 month)					
Cure N (%)	20 (71.4)	19 (54.2)	28 (57.1)	67 (60.0)	0.3979
Failure N (%) including:	6 (21.6)	10 (28.5)	15 (30.8)	31 (27.5)	

Table 1 Characteristics and outcome of 112 febrile urinary tract infection occurring among patients with neurogenic bladder depending on treatment duration *(Continued)*

Persistence of symptoms	5 (17.8)	9 (25.7)	12 (24.4)	26 (23.2)	
Death related to UTI	1 (3.5)	1 (3)	3 (6.1)	5 (4.4)	
Patients who could not be evaluated N (%)[b]	2 (7.1)	6 (17.1)	6 (12.2)	14 (12.5)	
Requiring another antibiotic treatment for concomitant infection	0	1	4	5	
Lost to follow up	1	1	1	3	
Death unrelated to UTI	1	4	1	6	
Negative urine culture (D30) N (%)	17 (60.7)	15 (42.8)	21 (42.8)	53 (47.3)	0.635

[a]UTI = urinary tract infection
[b]Patients who could not be evaluated: included death unrelated to UTI ($n = 6$); patients lost to follow-up ($n = 3$), and patients requiring another antibiotic treatment for a concomitant infection ($n = 5$)

There was no difference between the variables measured in these patients (sex, age, type of neurogenic deficit, voiding practice) and those measured in patients without recurrent UTI who were included in the study. There was no difference from the general population of the study, except for numerous patients with non-stabilized bladder.

The mean duration of antibiotic treatment for these patients was 17 days (1–60).

All kidney examinations and/or abdominal CT scans were normal: no abscess or obstruction. No surgery or derivation had been performed.

The most commonly prescribed antibiotics, considering only appropriate antimicrobial treatment, were third generation cephalosporins ($n = 67$), aminoglycosides ($n = 51$), and fluoroquinolones ($n = 36$).

Considering the three groups of patients, there was no statistically significant difference in sex ratio, type of neurological deficit, positive blood culture, prescribed antibiotics, and mono or dual therapy. There was no significant difference in the cure rate of the three groups ($p = 0.3979$) (assessed by either a Chi^2 or an exact test). Considering follow up urine culture at day 30, there was no significant difference in bacteriuria rate of the three groups ($p = 0.635$).

Moreover, there was no difference in cure rate between mono and dual therapy (44 % for monotherapy versus 40 % for dual therapy, $p = 0.071$), regardless of the treatment duration.

Discussion

Our study compared the outcomes of febrile UTI among patients with neurogenic bladder according to different appropriate antimicrobial durations, and mono or dual therapy. We did not find any difference between treatment durations of less than 10 days, 10 to 15 days or more than 15 days. Moreover there was no difference between mono and dual antimicrobial therapies.

There are no well-established guidelines for the optimal antibiotic treatment of febrile UTI in patients with neurogenic bladder. Physicians tend to prescribe antibiotics for a long duration, often with dual therapy, depending on voiding difficulties and on the risk of vesico ureteric reflux. However, long term treatment is considered to be associated with a high risk of toxicity; therefore, this practice may be deleterious and could probably lead to the emergence of multidrug resistant bacteria in patients already frequently exposed to antibiotics [13, 14].

The global low cure rate compared to the rate in usual UTI is often associated with neurogenic bladder [1]. The higher cure rate for group 1, which is the shorter antibiotic treatment group, is possibly linked to the absence of randomization. The fast resolution of symptoms of UTI could have led to shorter antimicrobial treatment.

Considering microbiological data as a cure criterion among a population with neurogenic bladder is under debate because of the frequent asymptomatic bacteriuria in this population [14]. The overall rate of negative urine culture was not statistically different in the three groups.

Our study has several limitations. First it is a non-randomized trial and treatment duration was decided on subjective criteria and depended on the physician in charge and the clinical presentation of the UTI. Several patients ($n = 3$) were lost to follow up, treated with antibiotics for another reason ($n = 5$), or died for another reason ($n = 6$), which is a potential bias. Patients had various neurological deficits and voiding practices, leading to a heterogeneous population, and treatment could have different outcome depending on these bladder characteristics. Also, we considered different microorganisms and antimicrobial treatments. Moreover, changes in antibiotic policy over the 6 years could also have affected the analysis.

Although the statistical strength of this study is limited, it nonetheless contains one of the largest cohorts published to date. These patients were treated at a specialist center.

The treatment duration and the use of mono or dual therapy were decided by the physician because this was a non-interventional trial. However, there was no difference in outcome between the three groups of treatment duration.

Our definition of cure which considers only the absence of clinical symptoms is based on the guideline not to treat asymptomatic bacteriuria in patients with neurogenic bladder [2, 3]. This situation is common in this population and the diagnosis of infection is mainly supported by clinical symptoms. Furthermore, the threshold of bacteriuria to diagnose infection in this population is matter of discussion.

Nevertheless, considering microbiological results of urine culture, we found no difference in the three groups of treatment duration ($p = 0.635$).

Treatment duration is a subject of wide debate. Studies suggest that a short length (5 days) of antibiotic treatment should be encouraged for uncomplicated pyelonephritis [15, 16]. Generally shortening antibiotic treatment duration is a leading goal in public health. It is considered as a tool to fight against bacterial resistance and has several other advantages such as the reduction of side effects and cost. Even if we have not measured these components in our study, we are convinced that short antibiotic treatment duration tend towards these advantages.

The only clinical trial to date about UTI in patients with neurogenic bladder revealed that 14 days of ciprofloxacin treatment is associated with a higher cure rate than only three days of this treatment [5]. Three days may not be enough; however, in our study, we find no difference in the outcome of the three treatment groups. These findings support the trend to use short duration antibiotic treatments of less than 14 days.

The use of dual therapy involving aminoglycosides to treat UTI is controversial [17, 18]. Recommendations usually suggest that aminoglycosides should be used only in cases of severe sepsis or for particular bacteria such as *Pseudomonas aeruginosa* or AmpC-producing *Enterobacteriaceae* [6]. Most of these microorganisms are rare in cases of UTI in the general population but more frequent in patients with neurogenic bladder. Furthermore the high frequency of polymicrobial infection can promote the use of a dual therapy.

Aminoglycosides are potentially highly toxic molecules, and their use should be limited to protect renal function. We suggest that the use of aminoglycosides be avoided for UTI among patients with neurogenic bladder, except for cases of AmpC-producing *Enterobacteriaceae* and severe sepsis.

Conclusions

As our study found no difference of outcome between long and short antibiotic treatment duration either with mono or dual therapy, this suggests that a long treatment duration and dual antibiotic therapy could be unnecessary

for the management of febrile UTI in patients with neurogenic bladder.

According to our data, the management of febrile UTI among patients with neurogenic bladder does not seem to require longer treatment duration than for patients without disability. In our center we recommend an appropriate antimicrobial treatment duration of 8 days for patients with neurogenic bladder.

These promising results should be confirmed by additional data and randomized trials.

Abbreviations
UTI: urinary tract infection.

Competing interests
The authors declare that they have no competing interests.

Authors' contributions
AD, PD and LB designed the study. AD, AT, CB, JS, BB and LB supervised data collection and data management. AD, AD, JS, TH, PD and LB analyzed the data. AD, FB, JS, TH, PD and LB prepared the 1st draft of the manuscript. All the authors participated in manuscript preparation and approved the final manuscript for publications.

Acknowledgements
We are grateful to all patients and their relatives for their participation in this study.
We thank Elodie Choisy and Clara Duran for their help.

Funding
No funding was received to support this research project.

Author details
[1]Infectious Disease Unit, Garches PIFO University Hospital, AP-HP, Versailles Saint Quentin University, Garches, France. [2]Infectious Diseases Unit, University Hospital, Monastir, Tunisia. [3]Pharmacy, University Hospital, AP-HP, Versailles Saint Quentin University, Garches, France. [4]Internal Medicine Unit, University Hospital, AP-HP, Versailles Saint Quentin University, Boulogne-Billancourt, France. [5]Physical Medicine and Rehabilitation Department, University Hospital, AP-HP, Versailles Saint Quentin University, Garches, France. [6]Infectious Disease Unit, Bretonneau University Hospital, Tours, France.

References
1. Cardenas DD, Hooton TM. Urinary tract infection in persons with spinal cord injury. Arch Phys Med Rehabil. 1995;76:272–80.
2. Matsumoto T, Takahashi K, Manabe N, Iwatsubo E, Kawakami Y. Urinary tract infection in neurogenic bladder. Int J Antimicrob Agents. 2001;17:293–7.
3. Sauerwein D. Urinary tract infection in patients with neurogenic bladder dysfunction. Int J Antimicrob Agents. 2002;19:592–7.
4. Pinson AG, Philbrick JT, Lindbeck GH, Schorling JB. Fever in the clinical diagnosis of acute pyelonephritis. Am J Emerg Med. 1997;15:148–51.
5. Dow G, Rao P, Harding G, Brunka J, Kennedy J, Alfa M, et al. A Prospective, Randomized Trial of 3 or 14 Days of Ciprofloxacin Treatment for Acute Urinary Tract Infection in Patients with Spinal Cord Injury. Clin Infect Dis. 2004;39:658–64.
6. Gupta K, Hooton TM, Naber KG, Wullt B, Colgan R, Miller LG, et al. International Clinical Practice Guidelines for the Treatment of Acute Uncomplicated Cystitis and Pyelonephritis in Women: A 2010 Update by the Infectious Diseases Society of America and the European Society for Microbiology and Infectious Diseases. Clin Infect Dis. 2011;52:103–20.
7. Esclarín De Ruz A, García Leoni E, Herruzo Cabrera R. Epidemiology and risk factors for urinary tract infection in patients with spinal cord injury. J Urol. 2000;164:1285–9.
8. Société Française de Microbiologie, EUCAST. Comité de l'antibiogramme de la SFM. Recommendations [Internet]. 2015 [cited 2015 Dec 23]. Available

from: http://www.sfm-microbiologie.org/UserFiles/files/casfm/CASFM_
EUCAST_V1_2015.pdf. Accessed 13 Apr 2016.

9.   European Medecines Agency. Guideline on the evaluation of medicinal
     products indicated for treatment of bacterial infections [Internet]. 2011
     [cited 2015 Dec 23]. Available from: http://www.ema.europa.eu/docs/en_
     GB/document_library/Scientific_guideline/2009/09/WC500003417.pdf.
     Accessed 13 Apr 2016.

10. FDA. Complicated Urinary Tract Infections: Developing Drugs for Treatment -
     Guidance for Industry [Internet]. 2015 [cited 2015 Dec 23]. Available from:
     http://www.fda.gov/downloads/Drugs/.../Guidances/ucm070981.pdf.
     Accessed 13 Apr 2016.

11. García Leoni ME, Esclarín De Ruz A. Management of urinary tract infection
     in patients with spinal cord injuries. Clin Microbiol Infect. 2003;9:780–5.

12. The prevention and management of urinary tract infections among people
     with spinal cord injuries. National Institute on Disability and Rehabilitation
     Research Consensus Statement. January 27–29, 1992. J Am Paraplegia Soc.
     1992;15:194–204.

13. Salomon J, Denys P, Merle C, Chartier-Kastler E, Perrone C, Gaillard JL, et al.
     Prevention of urinary tract infection in spinal cord-injured patients: safety
     and efficacy of a weekly oral cyclic antibiotic (WOCA) programme with a
     2 year follow-up - an observational prospective study. J Antimicrob
     Chemother. 2006;57:784–8.

14. Ronco E, Denys P, Bernede-Bauduin C, Laffont I, Martel P, Salomon J, et al.
     Diagnostic Criteria of Urinary Tract Infection in Male Patients With Spinal
     Cord Injury. Neurorehabil Neural Repair. 2010;25:351–8.

15. Sandberg T, Skoog G, Hermansson AB, Kahlmeter G, Kuylenstierna N,
     Lannergård A, et al. Ciprofloxacin for 7 days versus 14 days in women with
     acute pyelonephritis: a randomised, open-label and double-blind, placebo-
     controlled, non-inferiority trial. Lancet. 2012;380:484–90.

16. Talan DA, Stamm WE, Hooton TM, Moran GJ, Burke T, Iravani A, et al. Comparison
     of Ciprofloxacin (7 Days) and Trimethoprim-Sulfamethoxazole (14 Days) for Acute
     Uncomplicated Pyelonephritis in Women. JAMA. 2000;283:1583.

17. Martinez JA, Cobos-Trigueros N, Soriano A, Almela M, Ortega M, Marco F,
     et al. Influence of Empiric Therapy with a Beta-Lactam Alone or Combined
     with an Aminoglycoside on Prognosis of Bacteremia Due to Gram-Negative
     Microorganisms. Antimicrob Agents Chemother. 2010;54:3590–6.

18. Paul M, Grozinsky-Glasberg S, Soares-Weiser K, Leibovici L. Beta lactam antibiotic
     monotherapy versus beta lactam-aminoglycoside antibiotic combination therapy
     for sepsis. Cochrane Database Syst Rev. 2006;1:CD003344.

The influence of antibiotic prophylaxis on bacterial resistance in urinary tract infections in children with spina bifida

Sebastiaan Hermanus Johannes Zegers[1*], Jeanne Dieleman[1], Tjomme van der Bruggen[2], Jan Kimpen[3] and Catharine de Jong-de Vos van Steenwijk[3]

Abstract

Background: Bacterial resistance to antibiotics is an increasingly threatening consequence of antimicrobial exposure for many decades now. In urinary tract infections (UTIs), antibiotic prophylaxis (AP) increases bacterial resistance. We studied the resistance patterns of positive urinary cultures in spina bifida children on clean intermittent catheterization, both continuing and stopping AP.

Methods: In a cohort of 176 spina bifida patients, 88 continued and 88 stopped using AP. During 18 months, a fortnightly catheterized urine sample for bacterial pathogens was cultured. UTIs and significant bacteriuria (SBU) were defined as a positive culture with a single species of bacteria, respectively with and without clinical symptoms and leukocyturia. We compared the percentage of resistance to commonly used antibiotics in the isolated bacteria in both groups.

Results: In a total of 4917 cultures, 713 (14.5%) had a positive monoculture, 54.3% of which were *Escherichia coli*. In the group stopping AP, the resistance percentage to antibiotics in UTI / SBU bacteria was lower than in the group remaining on AP, even when excluding the administered prophylaxis.

Conclusion: Stopping antibiotic prophylaxis for urinary tract infections is associated with reduced bacterial resistance to antibiotics in children with spina bifida.

Background

Due to increasing antibiotic use, bacterial resistance has emerged as an significant healthcare problem. The use of broader antibiotics for infections is driven by local antibiotic susceptibility and is influenced by preventive measures, use of antibiotic prophylaxis and previous antibiotic use.

Prior to the recent AAP Guidelines, there has been a trend to prescribe antibiotic prophylaxis (AP) to prevent recurrence of urinary tract infections (UTIs) and possible subsequent renal parenchymal scarring in otherwise healthy children and children with congenital abnormalities of kidney and urological tract [1]. The time-delay in culture results leads to the prescription of broad-spectrum antibiotics in suspicion of a UTI. Bacterial resistance for an increasing number of antibiotics is therefore seen in UTIs [2–5].

In children with spina bifida, renal insufficiency due to urological impairments and recurrent UTIs has been the major cause of morbidity and mortality [6]. The introduction of clean intermittent bladder catheterization (CIC) in 1972 by Lapides et al. enabled more adequate bladder emptying and a significant decline in UTIs, renal insufficiency and the need for kidney transplantation [7]. However, since the introduction of CIC, many clinicians started prescribing AP to prevent CIC-related UTIs [8–10]. Due to the lack of general guidelines on the use of AP for children with spina bifida applying CIC [11], caretakers were guided by the clinical course in the individual patient to either continue or stop AP.

* Correspondence: b.zegers@mmc.nl
[1]Máxima Medical Center, Post box 77775500 MB Veldhoven, The Netherlands
Full list of author information is available at the end of the article

To study the value of AP in children with spina bifida applying CIC, we conducted the SPIN UTI trial in the Netherlands and Belgium [12]. In this trial 176 patients were randomized to continue or to stop AP. Stopping AP resulted in significantly more non-febrile UTIs (relative risk 1.44, 95% confidence interval 1.13 – 1.83, p 0.003). However, the absolute risk of UTI was low: on average, AP has to be administered for more than two years to prevent one non-febrile, and therefore non-renal scarring UTI. The recommendation from this study was to start AP upon diagnosing spina bifida, and to stop AP as soon as vesico-ureteral reflux is excluded, overactive bladder symptoms are treated with anticholinergics and CIC is properly implemented. Only spina bifida patients with persisting high grade vesico-ureteral reflux and severe overactive bladder despite anticholinergic medication, which results in significantly more UTIs, may benefit from continuation of AP [12].

During the SPIN UTI study, catheterized urine samples of the 176 patients were investigated fortnightly for a period of 18 months by dip stick and subsequent culture only if the dip stick was positive. This resulted in almost 5000 cultures. In case of a positive culture with one strain of bacteria (monoculture), antimicrobial susceptibility was determined. The main aim of the present analysis was to study the difference in antimicrobial susceptibility in positive urine cultures between patients continuing and stopping AP. Our hypothesis was that children stopping prophylaxis would have better susceptibility of bacteria to commonly used antibiotics.

Methods

Patients

All patients with a meningomyelocele (spina bifida) known at the outpatient clinics of Wilhelmina's Children's Hospital in Utrecht, the Netherlands and Gasthuisberg University Hospital in Leuven, Belgium were eligible for inclusion in the study, provided they had been on CIC and AP during the last 6 months. One hundred and seventy-six patients participated in the study. The study period was from February 2005 until March 2009. This study was approved and registered by the ISRCTN, trial number 56278131 (http://bit.ly/2hvP2Uq).

Interventions

Patients were randomly allocated to continue or discontinue AP, using a computer based random concealed allocation scheme. Randomization was stratified for ages under and over 3 years, presence of vesico-ureteral reflux, gender and participating centre. Patients randomized to continuation of AP continued the individually prescribed type and dosage of antibiotics. The dosages and types were allowed to differ between patients according to antimicrobial susceptibility in pre-study

cultures. Patients randomized to stopping of AP were instructed to discontinue the prescribed AP upon study start. The first urine sample was taken two weeks after stopping AP.

Follow-up, outcome measurements, primary outcome definition

During an 18 months follow-up period, fortnightly dip sticks and urine cultures were performed after CIC by the patients themselves, their parents or their primary care takers.

The dip stick for both urinary leukocytes and nitrite (Combur2-LN®, Roche Diagnostics) was rated either as negative (no color change) or as positive (any color change) by the primary care takers. If the dipstick was positive for leukocytes and / or nitrite, a urine culture was performed using a Uricult™ test (Orion Diagnostica, Finland) with MacConkey and CLED media.

In Utrecht, the Netherlands, the Uricult™ was sent to the laboratory of clinical microbiology of the University Medical Centre Utrecht for a 24 hour incubation period at 37 °C (98°F). If rated positive, the Uricult was subcultured on a sheep blood agar for 72 hours followed by identification to the species level by automated bacterial identification and automated antimicrobial susceptibility testing providing MICs (Phoenix, Becton & Dickinson, MD). *Enterococcus* species were identified to the genus level by selective growth on bile esculin agar (BEA) and salt tolerance agar (STA). Enterococcal antimicrobial susceptibility testing was performed with disk diffusion. CLSI breakpoints for MICs and disk diffusion were used for interpretation. When negative, the Uricult™ was not subcultured.

In Leuven, Belgium, the 24 hour incubation period was performed at home by the primary care takers (parents or nurses), using a feeding bottle warmer (Philips®) at 37 °C. If rated positive, the Uricult™ was sent to the laboratory of clinical microbiology for the incubation and identification process. When rated negative at home, the Uricult™ was sent to the trained research nurse for professional review. When she rated the Uricult™ positive, it was yet sent to the laboratory for incubation.

Significant bacteriuria (SBU) was defined as more than 10,000 colony forming units of a single specimen per milliliter in the catheterized urine sample. Urinary tract infection (UTI) was defined as an SBU combined with a positive reading of leukocyturia on the dip stick and clinical symptoms, such as increasing incontinence, foul smell or cloudiness of the catheterized urine. Cultures presenting more than one species of bacteria, regardless of clinical symptoms, were considered as a contamination rather than SBU or UTI.

To avoid repeated calculations for bacterial resistance patterns on one period of persistent SBU, we considered multiple consecutive positive cultures (SBU) without clinical signs of UTI, and therefore no antibiotic treatment, as one ongoing colonization.

Primary outcome

The primary outcome in this analysis was bacterial resistance of uropathogens in children with spina bifida on clean intermittent catheterization to commonly used antibiotics.

Statistical methods

Main treatment effect analyses were published previously [12]. In brief, differences in rates of UTI between the two treatment groups were analyzed using Poisson regression and pointed at no clinically relevant difference in risk of SBU/UTI after stopping AP.

The present analysis represents a secondary analysis of bacterial resistance patterns observed in incubated cultures of urine samples of children with spina bifida and SBU or UTI and the influence of AP. Bacterial species, type of AP used and antibiotic susceptibility (both AP and non-AP antibiotic) were described according to the randomization group (intention-to-treat) and according to the actual use of antibiotics (per protocol).

Prevalence of AP and non-AP resistance in positive urine cultures was calculated as the number of cultures with resistant pathogens divided by the total number of positive cultures. In this calculation we assumed independence of multiple cultures within patients, which was deemed appropriate given the fact that we only included incident episodes of SBU/UTI. Results were stratified for actual AP use (yes/no) and type of AP used.

Differences in prevalence of pathogenic resistance between cultures with and without AP were statistically tested using the Generalized Linear Mixed Model (GLMM) module of SPSS which takes into account the repeated assessments in patients. We applied the binary logistic link function and a random effect for the individual intercept. As primary predictor of interest we included AP use (yes/no) at the time of SBU/UTI to explore the effect of AP use on the risk of resistance against non-AP antibiotics. In addition we explored the effect of country (the Netherlands vs. Belgium), SBU or UTI and gender as potential confounders by adding these variables to the model with AP. Results from this analysis were expressed as odds ratio (OR) with 95% confidence intervals (95% CI).

All analyses were performed using SPSS, version 19.0 and statistical significance was accepted at a two-sided p-value of 0.05.

Results

Of the 176 participants, 88 were randomized to continue AP and 88 to stop using AP. In the latter group, 38 restarted AP during the 18 month study period, due to recurrent UTIs or specific parental request.

Not all patients complied with the fortnightly cultures in the entire study period of eighteen months. From a possible 6864 cultures if all 176 patients had complied with the protocol during the entire study period, 4917 urine samples were sent to and evaluated by the laboratories. Seven hundred and thirteen (14.5%) of these were positive single-strain cultures, of which 315 (44.2%) were considered a UTI due to clinical symptoms and leukocyturia on the dip stick. The remaining 398 (55.8%) were considered SBU, lacking clinical symptoms or leukocyturia (Table 1). No significant differences were seen between boys and girls.

The most common pathogen seen in about half of both SBU and UTI was *Escherichia coli (E.coli)* (54.3%). The other 45.7% consisted of other well-known uropathogens, like *Klebsiella* species (8.8%), *Enterococcus* species (7.9%), *Pseudomonas aeruginosa* (6.6%), *Proteus mirabilis* (4.8%) and 17.6% of less common pathogens (Table 1). Of the 713 single strain cultures only 82 (11.5%) were Gram-positive bacteria, mostly *Enterococcus* species and *Staphylococcus aureus*. Again, there were no differences between boys and girls in pathogens in either group.

Almost half of the cultures were performed in patients randomized to continue AP ($n = 343$, 48.1%), the remaining 370 cultures (51.9%) were from patients randomized to stopping AP. However, 79 (21%) cultures in the stop group were performed after AP was restarted due to recurrent UTIs or specific parental request. Thus, the majority of SBU and UTI occurred while using AP ($N = 422$, 59.2%), mostly trimethoprim and/or nitrofurantoin (Table 2).

Microbial resistance

Microbial resistance against any antibiotic was present in 65.2% of SBU/UTIs, and significantly more prevalent in urine cultures taken in children with spina bifida on AP (72.2%) than in children without AP (53.3%).

In Table 3, determination of resistance patterns to commonly used antibiotics performed on positive urinary cultures with Gram negative bacterial species, tested more than ten times in our patient group, is shown. There were too few Gram positive urinary cultures results to significantly differentiate resistance percentages between the groups on and off AP. The main result shown in this table is that use of AP increases the risk of resistance compared to stopping AP: the percentages of resistance to a specific antibiotic in any bacteria found in the urine cultures were higher when using AP.

Table 1 Frequency of positive cultures and percentages of uropathogens in 176 children with spina bifida on clean intermittent catheterization on and off antibiotic prophylaxis

	Total		Stop group		Continuing group		
	Number	%	Number	%	Number	%	p-value for stop versus continue
Patients with only negative urine tests	23	13.1	11	12.5	12	13.6	
Patients with one or more positive cultures	153	86.9	77	87.5	76	86.4	Pearson chi-square 0.635
SBU	137	77.8	70	79.5	67	76.1	1,000
UTI	107	60.8	55	62.5	52	59.1	0.643
Number of positive cultures	713	14.5	370		343		
SBU	398	55.8	199	53.8	199	58.0	
UTI	315	44.2	171	46.2	144	42.0	
		CI		CI		CI	
Mean number of positive cultures per patient (95% CI)	4.66	(4.1-5.2)	4.81	(4.1-5.5)	4.51	(3.8-5.2)	negative binominal analysis 0.573
SBU	2.60	(2.3-2.9)	2.58	(2.2-3.0)	2.62	(2.1-3.1)	0.915
UTI	2.06	(1.7-2.4)	2.22	(1.7-2.7)	1.89	(1.4-2.4)	0.364
Uropathogens in positive cultures (% of positive cultures)		%		%		%	
E.coli	387	54.3	200	54.1	187	54.5	Pearson chi-square 0.429
Non E.coli	326	45.7	170	45.9	156	45.5	
Gram negative	631	88.5	326	88.1	305	88.9	0.901
Enterobacteriaceae							
AmpC negative							
E.coli	387	54.3	200	54.1	187	54.5	
Klebsiella pneumoniae	42	5.9	21	5.7	21	6.1	
Proteus mirabilis	34	4.8	15	4.1	19	5.5	
Klebsiella oxytoca	21	2.9	16	4.3	5	1.5	
AmpC positive							
Enterobacter cloacae	18	2.5	10	2.7	8	2.3	
Citrobacter freundii	17	2.4	11	3.0	6	1.7	
Non fermenting bacilli							
Pseudomonas auroginosa	47	6.6	29	7.8	18	5.2	
Other	65	9.1	24	6.5	41	12.0	
Gram positive	82	11.5	44	11.9	38	11.1	0.762
Enterococcal species	56	7.9	30	8.1	26	7.6	
Staphylococcus aureus	18	2.5	10	2.7	8	2.3	
Other gram positive	8	1.1	4	1.1	4	1.2	

CI = 95% confidence interval

SBU = significant bacteriuria

UTI = urinary tract infection

GLMM analysis estimated the risk of resistance against one or more antibiotics (including the AP) to be 2.3 (95% CI 1.6-3.1) fold higher while using AP relative to not using AP. Adding country, gender or type of culture (SBU or UTI) in the GLMM analysis did not change this estimate. Excluding resistance to the administered AP changed the estimate slightly to OR 1.7 (95% CI 1.2-2.3) for AP use relative to no AP use.

Table 2 depicts the association between type of AP on resistance patterns in 624 Gram negative cultures. Due to statistical insignificance, we left out the few Gram-negative cultures on other AP than trimethoprim,

Table 2 Percentages of resistance of gram-negative uropathogens against commonly used antibiotics per administered antibiotic prophylaxis

	No prophylaxis	Nitrofurantoin prophylaxis	Trimetoprim prophylaxis	Nitrofurantoin and trimetoprim prophylaxis	Ciprofloxacin prophylaxis
Number of gram-negative cultures	228	166	131	84	15
Antibiotic tested	% resistant				
Amoxicillin	57.0	57.3	71.3*	79.0**	55.6
Amoxicillin/clavulanic acid	23.2	21.5	26.7	40.9**	46.2
Piperacillin	56.6	38.6*	62.5	70.4	41.7
Piperacillin/tazobactam	5.6	4.9	3.4	23.3***	8.3
Cefazolin	17.3	14.0	14.9	29.0	66.7**
Cefuroxim	9.0	21.5**	5.2	14.3	70.0***
Ceftazidim	3.4	12.9*	1.7	5.5	9.1
Ceftriaxon	1.4	7.9*	0.0	3.1	10.0
Meropenem	0.0	2.4	1.6	1.2	8.3
Amikacin	0.6	9.5**	0.8	2.5	0.0
Gentamicin	3.2	4.4	2.6	6.3	0.0
Tobramycin	3.1	6.0	1.6	8.6*	0.0
Ciprofloxacin	3.8	7.2	12.0	2.5	58.3***
Norfloxacin	5.1	8.9	11.6	3.8	63.6***
Levofloxacin	5.9	10.2	11.8	2.5	53.8***
Trimetoprim	38.5	38.7	90.5***	83.3***	55.6
Co-trimoxazol	32.1	30.9	79.1***	71.8***	38.5
Nitrofurantoin	13.2	56.1***	11.6	14.3	77.8***

Legend: GLMM used to compare risk of resistance relative to no prophylaxis used, * $p < 0.05$, ** $p < 0.01$, *** $p < 0.001$

nitrofurantoin, ciprofloxacin or a combination of trimethoprim and nitrofurantoin.

Antibiogram of uropathogens and the influence of antibiotic prophylaxis on resistance
Penicillins
In our study cohort, resistance against amoxicillin and piperacillin was common with a overall prevalence of 66.7% and 68.2% in *E.coli* UTIs (Table 3). Stopping AP decreased the percentage of resistance in *E.*coli UTIs against amoxicillin and piperacillin from respectively 73.8 and 73.5% to 56.3% and 59.5%. Resistance against amoxicillin/clavulanic acid (29.7%) and piperacillin/tazobactam (7.8%) was less common in *E. coli* UTIs, as well as in other Gram negative UTIs. When discontinuing AP, the prevalence of resistance against amoxicillin/clavulanic acid and piperacillin / tazobactam decreased to respectively 22.7 and 5.5% (Table 2).

Cephalosporins
Gram negative bacteria such as *E.coli* showed moderate resistance for first and second generation cephalosporins (17.9% and 11.4% respectively) in our cohort of spina bifida patients, whereas for third generation cephalosporins *E.coli* had significantly lower resistance of 1.7-1.9%

(Table 3). In UTIs with the uropathogen *Klebsiella pneumoniae* however, one in five is resistant to a third generation cephalosporin. Compared to not using AP, trimethoprim (0% and 5%) and nitrofurantoin alternating with trimethoprim (3% and 15%) as AP did not significantly influence resistance to second and third generation cephalosporins. However, the resistance for second generation cephalosporins increased significantly when using nitrofurantoin (21%) or ciprofloxacin (70%) as AP (Table 2).

Fluoroquinolones
In our cohort there was an overall low resistance of around 5% for fluoroquinolones in Gram negative bacteria while not using AP (Table 2). This was negatively influenced by prophylaxis: nitrofurantoin and trimethoprim prophylaxis doubled the resistance percentage (7.1 and 13.0% for ciprofloxacin respectively) (Table 2). When trimethoprim and nitrofurantoin were taken alternately, the resistance rate remained as low as without AP. The use of ciprofloxacin as AP was associated with a sharp increase in fluoroquinolones resistance (58.3-63.6%) (Table 2).

Trimethoprim/sulfamethoxazole
Even without AP, in our cohort *E.coli* bacteria had high resistance for both trimethoprim (42.9%) and trimethoprim/

Table 3 Percentages of resistance against commonly used antibiotics in positive gram-negative urine cultures on and off antibiotic prophylaxis

		Gram negative uropathogens				AmpC positive		Non-fermenting	
		AmpC negative							
		E.coli	Klebsiella pneumoniae	Proteus mirabilis	Klebsiella oxytoca	Enterobacter cloacae	Citrobacter freundii	Pseudomonas aeroginosa	p-value AP+ vs AP-
	Number of cultures	387	42	34	21	18	17	47	
Antibiogram									
Penicillines									
Amoxicillin	total	66.7	NC	24.2	NC	NC	NC	NC	0.031
	AP+	73.8	NC	11.5	NC	NC	NC	NC	
	AP-	56.3	NC	#	NC	NC	NC	NC	
Amoxicillin/clavulanic acid	total	29.7	9.5	6.1	9.5	NC	NC	NC	0.172
	AP+	32.8	9.1	7.7	#	NC	NC	NC	
	AP-	25.3	#	#	14.3	NC	NC	NC	
Piperacillin	total	68.2	NC	9.1	NC	NC	NC	2.6	0.950
	AP+	73.5	NC	9.5	NC	NC	NC	3.1	
	AP-	59.5	NC	#	NC	NC	NC	#	
Piperacillin/tazobactam	total	7.8	17.1	3.0	5.3	#	#	2.2	0.176
	AP+	10.3	15.6	3.8	#	#	#	2.7	
	AP-	4.0	#	#	7.7	#	#	#	
Cephalosporines									
Cefazolin (1)	total	17.9	43.8	4.5	56.3	NC	NC	NC	0.346
	AP+	20.6	54.5	0.0	#	NC	NC	NC	
	AP-	13.5	#	#	50.0	NC	NC	NC	
Cefuroxim (2)	total	11.4	45.2	3.0	14.3	NC	NC	NC	0.016
	AP+	13.5	51.5	0.0	#	NC	NC	NC	
	AP-	8.2	#	#	9.1	NC	NC	NC	
Ceftazidim (3)	total	1.7	21.7	4.3	5.9	NC	NC	4.3	0.161
	AP+	2.6	29.4	4.5	#	NC	NC	2.6	
	AP-	0.0	#	#	4.5	NC	NC	#	
Ceftriaxon (3)	total	1.9	19.4	0.0	5.9	#	NC	#	0.148
	AP+	2.5	25.0	0.0	#	#	NC	#	
	AP-	0.8	#	#	9.1	#	NC	#	
Other bactolactam									
Meropenem	total	0.0	0.0	0.0	0.0	0.0	0.0	7.5	0.461
	AP+	0.0	0.0	0.0	#	#	#	9.1	
	AP-	0.0	#	#	0.0	#	?	#	
Aminoglycosides									
Amikacin	total	1.9	19.0	4.2	0.0	0.0	0.0	2.5	0.054
	AP+	2.6	26.7	4.3	#	#	#	3.0	
	AP-	0.9	#	#	0.0	#	?	#	
Gentamicin	total	4.7	2.4	0.0	0.0	0.0	0.0	0.0	0.500
	AP+	4.4	3.0	0.0	#	#	#	0.0	
	AP-	4.8	#	#	0.0	#	0.0	#	

Table 3 Percentages of resistance against commonly used antibiotics in positive gram-negative urine cultures on and off antibiotic prophylaxis *(Continued)*

Tobramicin	total	4.9	4.8	3.0	0.0	0.0	0.0	2.1	0.194
	AP+	4.8	6.1	3.8	#	#	#	2.6	
	AP-	4.4	#	#	0.0	#	0.0	#	
Fluorquinolones									
Ciprofloxacin	total	7.8	52.9	0.0	0.0	0.0	0.0	5.0	0.021
	AP+	10.2	63.6	0.0	#	#	#	6.1	
	AP-	3.6	#	#	0.0	#	0.0	#	
Norfloxacin	total	7.7	52.9	0.0	0.0	0.0	0.0	9.4	0.047
	AP+	9.7	63.6	0.0	#	#	#	11.1	
	AP-	4.5	#	#	0.0	#	0.0	#	
Levofloxacin	total	9.4	29.3	0.0	0.0	0.0	0.0	9.4	0.057
	AP+	10.6	33.3	0.0	#	#	#	11.1	
	AP-	7.7	#	#	0.0	#	0.0	#	
Other antibiotics									
Trimetoprim	total	66.6	88.2	34.8	23.5	16.7	66.7	NC	<0.001
	AP+	80.7	63.6	36.4	#	#	#	NC	
	AP-	42.9	#	#	18.2	#	90.9	NC	
Cotrimoxazol	total	55.7	52.4	33.3	19.0	11.8	47.1	NC	<0.001
	AP+	69.7	51.5	30.8	#	#	#	NC	
	AP-	35.4	#	#	14.3	#	10.1	NC	
Nitrofurantoin	total	16.4	90.5	NC	28.6	64.7	0.0	NC	<0.001
	AP+	22.4	93.9	NC	#	#	#	NC	
	AP-	7.7	#	NC	21.4	#	0.0	NC	

Legend: # = not calculated as less than ten samples tested, NC = Not considered due to intrinsic resistance or uncommon clinical drug/bug combination

sulfamethoxazole (35.4%) (Table 3). Resistance obviously increased when using AP involved trimethoprim (90.1% and 77.7% respectively) (Table 2). Nitrofurantoin as AP however was not associated with increased resistance for trimethoprim (38.1%) or trimethoprim/sulfamethoxazole (30.7%) in Gram negative bacteria, whereas ciprofloxacin as AP only mildly increased resistance to trimethoprim (45.5%) and trimethoprim/sulfamethoxazole (33.3%) (Table 2).

Aminoglycosides

There was a low resistance rate for intravenous aminoglycosides in our cohort (3%), not influenced by AP nitrofurantoin (4%) or trimethoprim (3%). When using ciprofloxacin as AP, the Gram negative bacteria also remained sensitive to gentamicin, amikacin or tobramycin (Table 3).

Nitrofurantoin

Without AP, 13.2% of UTIs were resistant for nitrofurantoin treatment (Table 2). This resistance for nitrofurantoin treatment remained stable when using trimethoprim as AP (11.6%), while resistance significantly increased when using ciprofloxacin (77.8%) or nitrofurantoin itself (56.1%) as AP (Table 2).

The presence of resistance was not associated with age or gender. Microbial resistance against the prophylactic AP was not 100%: bacterial pathogens were still sensitive for treatment with the used AP in 43.9% of nitrofurantoin, 41.7% of ciprofloxacin and 9.5% of trimethoprim prescribed patients (Table 2).

Discussion

Bacterial resistance is an emerging and hazardous phenomenon occurring with ever-increasing use of antibiotics. Antibiotic prophylaxis (AP) administered to prevent recurrent urinary tract infections (UTIs) contributes to this resistance [13], although it has been proven that AP does not decrease the risk of renal scarring [1].

We compared bacterial susceptibility patterns in positive urine cultures in children with spina bifida and CIC continuing or stopping AP. Overall, our study showed a decrease in resistance to commonly used antibiotics when AP is stopped, confirming our hypothesis. Even when the administered AP is excluded from these calculations, the number of antibiotics to which the cultured pathogen is resistant remains higher in the continuing group. These findings in spina bifida patients on CIC is in accordance with previous studies for resistance patterns comparing AP to no AP in patients with community-acquired UTIs [14–18]. The fact that a particular class of antibiotics is associated with resistance towards other classes of antibiotics might be explained by the observation that bacterial resistance traits can be linked [19, 20].

E.coli accounts for 75-90% of community-acquired UTIs [21, 22], whereas *E.coli* is responsible for only 54.3% of the SBUs and UTIs in our specific population of children with spina bifida, with higher percentages of other uropathogens causing SBU/UTI. This difference is a common feature in non community-acquired UTIs, as described in previous studies in non-spina bifida patients, from Landhani et al (40% *E.coli* in children with underlying pathology), Lutter et al (58% *E.coli* in non-spina bifida children on AP) and Wagenlehner et al (35-60% *E.coli* in adult hospital-acquired UTIs due to catheterization with introduction of alternative pathogens) [15, 16, 23].

Choice of antibiotic prophylaxis in children with spina bifida
Our SPIN UTI study has shown that, whenever safe according to urological care, AP to prevent UTIs should be stopped in children with spina bifida. In a previous article we have shown that every child has to take two years of daily AP to prevent one extra non-febrile, non-scarring UTI [12], and this current study reveals a significant improvement in susceptibility to any necessary antibiotic treatment for a UTI when stopping AP. This article therefore emphasizes the necessity to stop the use of AP in children whenever possible to prevent bacterial resistance, especially since AP has proven not to prevent renal scarring [1].

When however, for reasons of recurrent UTIs, a persistent overactive bladder or high grade vesico-ureteral reflux, AP is a necessity, the choice of prophylaxis has impact on the bacterial resistance to commonly used therapeutic antibiotics. Trimethoprim as AP has the least negative influence on bacterial resistance: in our study cohort, the susceptibility of most therapeutic antibiotics remains relatively stable, except for fluoroquinolones, trimethoprim itself and trimethoprim/sulfamethoxazole. In our study, the use of nitrofurantoin as AP is associated with an increased resistance to cephalosporines, aminoglycosides and fluoroquinolones, with an increased risk of treatment failure, compared to non-AP patients. Particularly AP with fluoroquinolones is associated with a high percentage of resistance, especially to therapeutic oral antibiotic possibilities when necessary, and should therefore be discouraged.

Choice of therapeutic antibiotics in children with spina bifida
First consideration in choosing an appropriate antibiotic when a UTI is suspected or confirmed is the manner of administration: when clinically not ill, oral antibiotic treatment is adequate, whilst in sick children with spina bifida due to a UTI intravenous administration of antibiotics is often necessary. This determines the choice of antibiotic treatment, along with previous culture results and resistance patterns, presence or absence of fever and recently prescribed AP. In our study cohort, nitrofurantoin is first choice medication for a UTI without fever or recent AP. Without fever but with prophylaxis, in children with trimethoprim as AP nitrofurantoin is still first choice. In other AP and in children with fever on or off AP, oral treatment for UTI depends on local susceptibility, with ciprofloxacin and cefuroxim as antibiotics with high a priori chance of treatment success in our study cohort. When intravenous treatment is warranted, a third generation cephalosporin, fluoroquinolon or carbapenem is possible. However, we emphasize that the choice of therapeutic antibiotics depends on local susceptibility and individual resistance patterns in previous urinary cultures.

The strength of this study is the large number of adequate catheterized urinary cultures in a cohort of susceptible children with spina bifida. Remarkable is the relatively high percentage of susceptibility of bacteria for the already administered AP.

Conclusion
Discontinuation of antibiotic prophylaxis decreases bacterial resistance for commonly used antibiotics in children with spina bifida on clean intermittent catheterization should be pursued to prevent bacterial resistance, long term side effects of prophylactic antibiotics and the need for hospital admissions for broad spectrum intravenous antibiotics.

Abbreviations
AP: Antibiotic prophylaxis; CI: Confidence interval; CIC: Clean intermittent catheterization; GLMM: Generalized Linear Mixed Model; OR: Odds ratio; SBU: Significant bacteriuria; UTI: Urinary tract infection

Funding
Full funding was provided by the Wilhelmina Children's Hospital's Scientific Foundation at the University Medical Center Utrecht, the Netherlands.

Authors' contribution
SZ, JK and CJ had a substantial contribution to conception, design, acquisition of data, analysis and interpretation of data. SZ, JD and TB were involved in drafting and revising the manuscript. JK and CJ provided the final approval of the manuscript. All authors read and approved the final manuscript.

Competing interests
All authors state no conflict of interest due to financial, consultant, institutional or other relationships.

Author details
[1]Máxima Medical Center, Post box 77775500 MB Veldhoven, The Netherlands. [2]University Medical Center, Utrecht, The Netherlands. [3]Wilhelmina Children's Hospital, University Medical Center, Utrecht, The Netherlands.

References
1. RIVUR Trial Investigators, Hoberman A, Greenfield SP, Mattoo TK, Keren R, Mathews R, Pohl HG, Kropp BP, Skoog SJ, Nelson CP, Moxey-Mims M, Chesney RW, Carpenter MA. Antimicrobial prophylaxis for children with vesicoureteral reflux. N Engl J Med. 2014;370(25):2367–76.
2. Dayan N, Dabbah H, Weissman I, Aga I, Even L, Glikman D. Urinary tract infections caused by community-acquired extended-spectrum beta-lactamase-producing and nonproducing bacteria: a comparative study. J Pediatr. 2013;163(5):1417–21.
3. Ilic K, Jakovljevic E, Skodric-Trifunovic V. Social-economic factors and irrational antibiotic use as reasons for antibiotic resistance of bacteria causing common childhood infections in primary healthcare. Eur J Pediatr. 2012;171(5):767–77.
4. Shepherd AK, Pottinger PS. Management of urinary tract infections in the era of increasing antimicrobial resistance. Med Clin North Am. 2013;97(4):737–57. xii.
5. Beetz R, Westenfelder M. Antimicrobial therapy of urinary tract infections in children. Int J Antimicrob Agents. 2011;38(Suppl):42–50.
6. Pruitt LJ. Living with spina bifida: a historical perspective. Pediatrics. 2012;130(2):181–3.
7. Lapides J. Urinary diversion. Surgery. 1971;69(0039-6060; 0039-6060; 1):142–54.
8. Schlager TA, Dilks S, Trudell J, Whittam TS, Hendley JO. Bacteriuria in children with neurogenic bladder treated with intermittent catheterization: natural history. J Pediatr. 1995;126(0022-3476; 3):490–6.
9. Schlager TA, Anderson S, Trudell J, Hendley JO. Nitrofurantoin prophylaxis for bacteriuria and urinary tract infection in children with neurogenic bladder on intermittent catheterization. J Pediatr. 1998;132(0022-3476; 4):704–8.
10. Dik P, Klijn AJ, van Gool JD, de Jong-de Vos van Steenwijk CC, De Jong TP. Early start to therapy preserves kidney function in spina bifida patients. Eur Urol. 2006;49(0302-2838; 5):908–13.
11. Zegers BS, Winkler-Seinstra PL, Uiterwaal CS, de Jong TV, Kimpen JL, van de Jong-de Vos van Steenwijk CC. Urinary tract infections in children with spina bifida: an inventory of 41 European centers. Pediatr Nephrol. 2009;24(0931-041; 4):783–8.
12. Zegers B, Uiterwaal C, Kimpen J, van Gool J, de Jong T, Winkler-Seinstra P, Houterman S, Verpoorten C, de Jong-de Vos van Steenwijk C. Antibiotic prophylaxis for urinary tract infections in children with spina bifida on intermittent catheterization. J Urol. 2011;186(6):2365–70.
13. Bitsori M, Maraki S, Galanakis E. Long-term resistance trends of uropathogens and association with antimicrobial prophylaxis. Pediatr Nephrol. 2014;29(6):1053–8.
14. Conway PH, Cnaan A, Zaoutis T, Henry BV, Grundmeier RW, Keren R. Recurrent urinary tract infections in children: risk factors and association with prophylactic antimicrobials. JAMA. 2007;298(1538-3598; 2):179–86.
15. Lutter SA, Currie ML, Mitz LB, Greenbaum LA. Antibiotic resistance patterns in children hospitalized for urinary tract infections. Arch Pediatr Adolesc Med. 2005;159(10):924–8.
16. Ladhani S, Gransden W. Increasing antibiotic resistance among urinary tract isolates. Arch Dis Child. 2003;88(1468-2044; 5):444–5.
17. Narchi H, Al-Hamdani M. Uropathogen resistance to antibiotic prophylaxis in urinary tract infections. Microb Drug Resist. 2010;16(1931-8448; 1076-6294; 2):151–4.
18. Nelson CP, Hoberman A, Shaikh N, Keren R, Mathews R, Greenfield SP, Mattoo TK, Gotman N, Ivanova A, Moxey-Mims M, Carpenter MA, Chesney RW: Antimicrobial Resistance and Urinary Tract Infection Recurrence. Pediatrics 2016, 137(4):10.1542/peds.2015-2490. Epub 2016 Mar 11.
19. Stokes HW, Gillings MR. Gene flow, mobile genetic elements and the recruitment of antibiotic resistance genes into Gram-negative pathogens. FEMS Microbiol Rev. 2011;35(5):790–819.
20. Alekshun MN, Levy SB. Molecular mechanisms of antibacterial multidrug resistance. Cell. 2007;128(6):1037–50.
21. Friedman S, Reif S, Assia A, Mishaal R, Levy I. Clinical and laboratory characteristics of non-E. coli urinary tract infections. Arch Dis Child. 2006; 91(10):845–6.
22. Edlin RS, Shapiro DJ, Hersh AL, Copp HL. Antibiotic resistance patterns of outpatient pediatric urinary tract infections. J Urol. 2013;190(1):222–7.
23. Wagenlehner FM, Cek M, Naber KG, Kiyota H, Bjerklund-Johansen TE. Epidemiology, treatment and prevention of healthcare-associated urinary tract infections. World J Urol. 2012;30(1):59–67.

Characteristics of gram-negative urinary tract infections caused by extended spectrum beta lactamases: pivmecillinam as a treatment option within South Dublin, Ireland

Fardod O'Kelly[2†], Siobhan Kavanagh[1†], Rustom Manecksha[2], John Thornhill[2] and Jérôme P. Fennell[1*]

Abstract

Background: The prevalence of urinary tract infections (UTIs) caused by extended-spectrum β-lactamase (ESBL)-producing Enterobacteriaceae is increasing and the therapeutic options are limited, especially in primary care. Recent indications have suggested pivmecillinam to be a suitable option. This pilot study aimed to assess the viability of pivmecillinam as a therapeutic option in a Dublin cohort of mixed community and healthcare origin.

Methods: A prospective measurement of mean and fractional inhibitory concentrations of antibiotic use in 95 patients diagnosed with UTI caused by ESBL-producing Enterobacteriaceae was carried out. 36 % patients were from general practice, 40 % were admitted to hospital within south Dublin, and 25 % samples arose from nursing homes. EUCAST breakpoints were used to determine if an isolate was sensitive or resistant to antibiotic agents.

Results: Sixty-nine percent of patients ($N = 66$) with urinary ESBL isolates were female. The mean age of females was 66 years compared with a mean age of 74 years for males. Thirty-six percent of isolates originated from primary care, hospital inpatients (26 %), and nursing homes (24 %). The vast majority of ESBL isolates were *E. coli* (80 %). The E tests for mecillinam and co-amoxiclav had concentration ranges from 0.16 mg/L up to 256 mg/L. The mean inhibitory concentration (MIC) of mecillinam ranged from 0.25 to 256 mg/L, while co-amoxiclav MICs ranged from 6 to 256 mg/L. The percentage of isolates resistant to mecillinam and co-amoxiclav was found to be 5.26 and 94.74 % respectively.

Conclusions: This is the first study exploring the use of pivmecillinam in an Irish cohort and has demonstrated that its use in conjunction with or without co-amoxiclav is an appropriate and useful treatment for urinary tract infections caused by ESBL-producing organisms.

Keywords: Extended-spectrum beta lactamase, Pivmecillinam, Antibiotic resistance, Urinary tract infection, Mean inhibitory concentration, *Escherichia coli*

* Correspondence: jfennell@tcd.ie; jerome.fennell@amnch.ie
†Equal contributors
[1]Department of Clinical Microbiology, AMNCH, Tallaght Hospital, Dublin 24, Ireland
Full list of author information is available at the end of the article

Background

Microorganisms constantly evolve resistance to antimicrobials, rendering current agents ineffective. This is compounded by the reality that there are few new antimicrobials in development. Extended-spectrum beta lactamase (ESBL) producing organisms are one of the resistance types of most concern. ESBLs were first recognized in the 1980s due to point mutations of Temoneira (TEM) and Sulphydryl Variable (SHV) broad-spectrum enzymes genes. A common causes of hospital-acquired infections especially in the intensive care unit, ESBLs also commonly carry resistance to other antimicrobials such as quinolones, cotrimoxazole and the aminoglycosides. This further limits treatment options. Laboratory diagnosis of ESBLs is complex and normally performed by screening and phenotypic tests [1].

Traditionally ESBL producing bacteria were associated with nosocomial infection, but they are now widespread in the community. In the UK, community ESBLs were mostly isolated during urinary infections the elderly, who had recent hospitalisation [2]. In contrast, an Irish study found that 42 % of community isolates that were ESBL producing, were from individuals not in long term care or hospitalised in the previous year [3]. Risk factors for acquiring community associated ESBL infections include recurrent UTI, previous antibiotic usage, diabetes and prior instrumentation to urinary tract [1, 4].

ESBLs were first detected in Western Europe, where β-lactam antibiotics were first used, with prevalence varying between countries. In 2001, the Netherlands had a low percentage of ESBL producing Enterobacteriaceae with only 1 % of E. coli and K. pneumoniae being ESBL positive. In contrast 40 % of France's K. pneumoniae were ceftazidime resistant. ESBL producers are normally multiple drug resistant and have become an important mechanism of β-lactam resistance in community uropathogens [5]. Production of β-lactamase is the most common resistance mechanism of bacteria to β-lactam antibiotics [6]. E. coli resistance is mostly due to production of β-lactamases, which hydrolyze the beta-lactam ring of beta-lactam antibiotics such as penicillin. Resistance to ampicillin and amoxicillin is normally due to plasmid-coded β-lactamases the majority of which is the TEM type [7]. ESBLs have resistance to β-lactams, ampicillin, amoxicillin and third generation cephalosporins. The ESBL carrying plasmid often carries other resistance genes as well, e.g. resistance genes to quinolones and aminoglycosides. When this occurs usage of any of the classes of antimicrobials that the plasmid encodes resistance to will select for this multiple resistant isolate. The first ESBLs in E. coli were variants of the TEM or SHV β-lactamases, which could hydrolyze cefotaxime, ceftriaxone and ceftazidime, however the CTX-M-type bla gene has now become the commonest type. The CTX-M enzymes also appear to have a greater ability to spread and cause outbreaks [2, 8, 9]. CLSI recommendations state to only check for ESBLs in E. coli, Klebsiella pneumoniae, K. oxytoca and Proteus mirabilis, but all Gram-negative bacteria can be ESBL positive. In 2006, two E. coli ESBL isolates were associated with UTIs from two residents in an Irish nursing home. On review, five more patients in that nursing home were found to be ESBL positive [10]. This is a typical example of the transmission of antibiotic resistant bacteria in a vulnerable group of patients where long-term isolation is not viable and there is a need to control the spread of these organisms. A more recent study surveyed an Irish nursing home and found over 55 % of residents were colonized by ESBL producers [11]. In Ireland in 2015, 10.6 % of invasive E. coli and 13.3 % of invasive K. pneumoniae isolates were found to be ESBL Positive, the highest annual percentage to date [12].

There is a lack of effective therapeutic options to combat ESBLs. Carbapenems, often regarded the antibiotic of choice, should be used when there are no other options available but their use inevitably leads to the emergence of carbapenem-resistant enterobacteriaciae (CRE). Fluoroquinolones, can be effective against ESBLs, but are not recommended for routine use due to resistance rates. Aminoglycosides, also effective, should not be used for monotherapy in serious infections, as they are bacteriostatic. Colistin should be used with caution, as it is a broad-spectrum agent. The potential nephrotoxicity of these agents is another concern in this setting and is another reason to limit their use. Tigecycline demonstrates good in vitro activity against ESBLs but the FDA has warned against its use due to the increased mortality in Tigecycline-treated patients, as well as its relative inefficacy in pneumonia and bacteraemia, as well as limited GU tract concentrations [13, 14]. Fosfomycin, an old broad-spectrum antibiotic, has been re-evaluated for the treatment of UTIs due to multidrug resistant organisms. It is only licensed for lower uncomplicated UTIs and may develop resistance [15].

Pivmecillinam, a β-lactam antibiotic, the prodrug of mecillinam, is hydrolyzed to the active agent mecillinam [16]. Mecillinam must be administered parentally but oral pivmecillinam is available. Its mode of action is to bind to penicillin-binding protein 2 in Enterobacteriaceae and inhibit bacterial cell wall synthesis [17]. It has high activity against many Gram-negative bacteria such as E. coli, Klebsiella sp., Salmonella sp. and Enterobacter sp. and has limited activity against some Gram positives. The use of pivmecillinam for more than 20 years in Nordic countries confirms its efficiency and safety in treating UTIs. Its oral bioavailability makes it an attractive option without requiring hospital admission for intravenous treatment [16, 18].

Antibiotic resistance is a concerning public health problem that increases morbidity and mortality. Novel drug development is time-consuming, but re-evaluating antibiotics already licensed is more time-effective [17]. Combination therapy is of interest as multi drug resistant microorganisms may require more than one antibiotic to treat successfully [19]. Unfortunately, there are limited oral antibiotics available for complicated UTIs caused by ESBL and AmpC producing bacteria [15].

This clinical study examines the antimicrobial susceptibility of 95 ESBL producing isolates to pivmecillinam and co-amoxiclav in a tertiary referral center, to determine if our catchment population could benefit with combination treatment of ESBL urinary tract infection.

Methods

This study received approval from the hospital ethics committee and the research carried out was also in compliance with the Helsinki Declaration. Clinico-demographic data was collated on 95 patients that had tested positive for ESBL urinary infection at the department of Microbiology, Tallaght hospital (2012–2013). Isolates had previously been confirmed as ESBLs by MASTDISCS ID AmpC and ESBL inhibitors and MASTDISCS cefepime ESBL ID for the Vitek 2. E-tests were performed on ESBLs that were initially stored on beads in an –18 °C freezer, and then plated on MacConkey agar and incubated at 37 °C for 24 h. All isolates were then subcultured onto nutrient agar slopes. One mecillinam and one co-amoxiclav E test were then each applied with forceps onto the plate. The elliptical zones of inhibition were read to determine the MIC of *E. coli* according to the manufacturer instructions. The MIC was read as the point where the ellipse intersected the E test strip. If the intersect was different on both sides the greater value was taken as the MIC.

A checkerboard method was also used to assess the mean inhibitory concentrations (MIC) of each positive ESBL sample by measuring the spectrophotometric absorbance of each well 16 to 24 h following inoculation using an ELX800 universal micro plate reader at a wavelength of 630 nm. The percentage of growth was calculated on the basis of colour absorbance using (OD630 of wells that contained the drug/OD630 of the drug-free well). The MICs of the drugs alone and of in combination were determined as the lowest drug concentrations showing <10 % of the growth of an untreated control [20, 21].

For each combination of antibiotics the fractional inhibitory concentration was calculated which is a predictor of synergy [22]. The fractional inhibitory concentration (FIC) was used to evaluate the effectiveness of the combinations. The formulas used were FIC of drug A (mecillinam) = MIC drug A in combination/ MIC drug A alone; FIC of drug B (co-amoxiclav) = MIC drug B in combination/ MIC drug B alone and FIC index = FIC drug A + FIC drug B. Synergy was defined as FIC index of ≤0.5, indifference of FIC as >0.5 but of ≤4. Antagonism was defined as FIC index of >4. All experiments were performed in triplicate.

EUCAST (European Committee on Antimicrobial Susceptibility Testing) breakpoints for Enterobacteriaceae for both mecillinam and co-amoxiclav were given as ≤8 mg/L as sensitive and ≥8 mg/L as resistant. However the British Society of Antimicrobial Chemotherapy states that an MIC of ≥32 mg/L for co-amoxiclav is suitable for UTIs but not systemic infections, due to the activity of clavulanate alone. Mecillinam concentrations in urine after 400 mg taken orally has been reported to be above 100 mg/L after 6-h. Co-amoxiclav has also been found to have levels above the MIC in human serum during the first 6 h [23]. Therefore the EUCAST breakpoints were used to determine if the isolate was sensitive or resistant to both antibiotic agents. The red line in Figs. 1 and 2 illustrate the EUCAST breakpoint of 8 mg/L.

Results

Sixty-nine percent of patients (*N* = 66) with urinary ESBL isolates were female. The mean age of females was 66 years compared with a mean age of 74 years for males. Thirty-six percent of isolates originated from primary care, hospital inpatients (26 %), and nursing homes (24 %). The vast majority of ESBL isolates were *E. coli* (80 %) (Tables 1 and 2).

The E tests for mecillinam and co-amoxiclav had concentration ranges from 0.16 mg/L up to 256 mg/L. The mean inhibitory concentration (MIC) of mecillinam ranged from 0.25 to 256 mg/L, while co-amoxiclav MICs ranged from 6 to 256 mg/L. The MICs of mecillinam and co-amoxiclav were recorded and the total counts of the MIC were calculated. Distribution charts were constructed from this data (Figs. 1 and 2).

The percentage of isolates resistant to mecillinam and co-amoxiclav was found to be 5.26 % and 94.74 % respectively [24]. Four of five isolates were *E. coli* and were resistant to co-amoxiclav. Isolate number 513 was a *Klebsiella* species. These isolates were tested using the checkerboard technique for synergy between co-amoxiclav and mecillinam. The MIC was reduced significantly in isolates 842 and 513 in comparison to the E tests where only one drug was used. In the checkerboard method isolate 842 was inhibited with 24ug/ml of co-amoxiclav in combination with 12ug/ml of mecillinam. In the E test isolate 842 was inhibited by 12ug/ml alone but was not inhibited by co-amoxiclav until a concentration of 48 mg/L was used. Isolate 513 was inhibited at 24ug/ml of co-amoxiclav in combination with 64ug/ml mecillinam in the 96 well plate. In the E test isolate 513 was not inhibited by co-amoxiclav

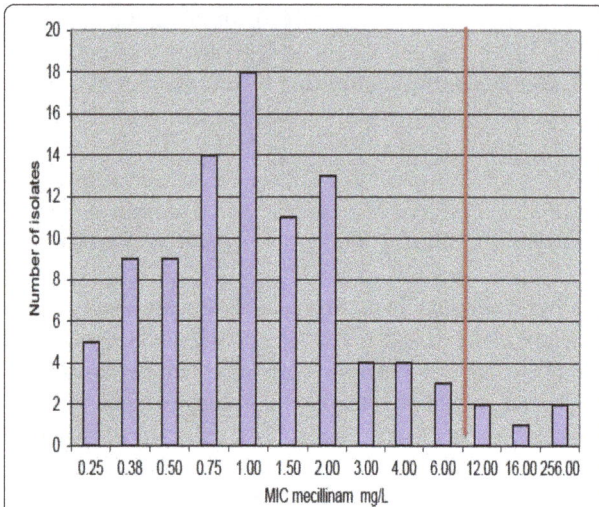

Fig. 1 Distribution of the mean inhibitory concentration (MIC) of 95 Extended spectrum beta-lactamase (ESBL) producing isolates. EUCAST break-point of 8 mg/L demonstrated by *red vertical line*

Table 1 Clinico-demographic profile of patients isolated with extended-spectrum beta lactamase producing urinary infections

Average age of patients (yrs)	%	N =
Female	66.25	n.a.
Male	74.65	n.a.
Source of Isolation of UTI		
Emergency Department	14	13
General Practice	36	34
Inpatient Wards	26	25
Nursing Home	24	23
Species Isolated		
Klebsiella pneumoniae	20	19
Escherichia coli	80	76

even at 256 mg/L. Isolates 779 and 031 did not achieve levels of 10 % of the growth of the control. Therefore the MIC for either or both drugs in combination was higher than 256ug/ml. In contrast the E test results showed isolate 779 was inhibited by co-amoxiclav at 128 mg/L but the results agreed with the checkerboard for mecillinam (>256 mg/L). The E test showed that 031 was inhibited by 12 mg/L of mecillinam but was not inhibited by co-amoxiclav even at 256 mg/L. The FIC is correct in that no positive difference occurred when the two antibiotics were used in combination. Isolate 349 was inhibited by 128 mg/L of mecillinam alone and also in combination with co-amoxiclav (between 6-256 ug/ml) in the 96 well

plate. The E test results showed mecillinam did not inhibit the isolate at even 256 mg/L but co-amoxiclav inhibited 349 at 128 mg/L alone.

Discussion
The increasing prevalence of clinically significant antibiotic resistant bacteria, especially for those resistant to multiple classes of antibiotics, makes appropriate antimicrobial treatment challenging [25, 26]. Many pathogens resistant to first line agents, then require broader spectrum, more expensive agents with less favorable safety profiles, which in turn accelerates the generation of multi drug resistant (MDR) pathogens, where no agents may be available to treat infections caused by these microorganisms. As the ESBL resistance mechanism is commonly expressed by plasmid encoded B lactamases, resistance can be easily transferred between other bacterial species by horizontal gene transfer. These plasmids frequently carry genes encoding for resistance to other antibiotic classes. Unlike methicillin resistant *Staphylococcus aureus*, the resistant Gram-negative bacteria commonly colonise the bowel and there is no available decolonization procedure. Long-term colonization by these bacteria ensures these patients remain a potential source of transmission for many years, with potentially indefinite requirement for isolation and contact precautions [27, 28].

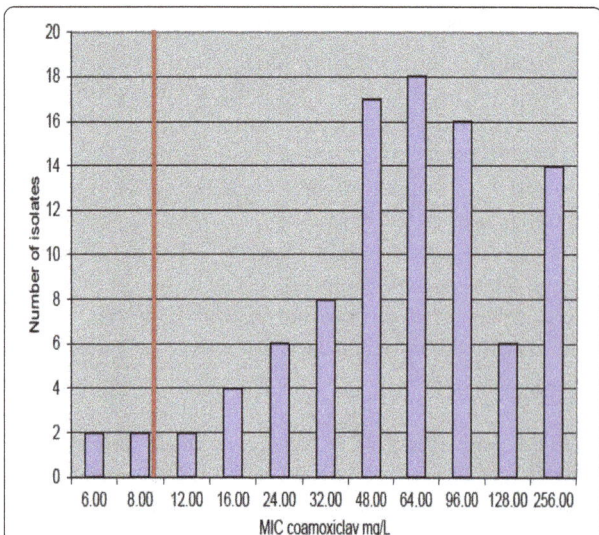

Fig. 2 Distribution of the mean inhibitory concentration (MIC) of 95 Extended spectrum beta-lactamase (ESBL) producing isolates. EUCAST break-point of 8 mg/L demonstrated by *red vertical line*

Table 2 Fractional inhibitory concentration (FIC) of the five extended-spectrum beta lactamase producing isolates which were resistant to mecillinam monotherapy

Isolate	FIC
842	Synergy
513	Synergy
779	Indifference
349	Indifference
031	Indifference

There is an urgent need for more research into new agents that are effective against ESBLs and other resistant bacteria. With the increase in multidrug and carbapenem-resistant microorganisms, there is a need to minimize carbapenem use and they should not be first-line choice for treating ESBLs [29]. Europe-wide antimicrobial drug resistance rates remain high. A Greek study carried out in 2007 demonstrated CRE in 70 % of hospitals. Pan-drug resistant *K. pneumoniae* have also been reported in the same population. The use of mecillinam for UTIs is promising as pivmecillinam achieves high levels in urine, has a low resistance profile and inhibited 94.74 % of the ESBLs in this study. However, a broader clinical evaluation in an Irish patient population is required before clinical use can be advocated. Mecillinam like other penicillins, has low toxicity like other penicillins and is also safe to use for the treatment of UTIs in pregnancy [30]. Mecillinam is poorly absorbed from the gastrointestinal tract but pivmecillinam is well absorbed. Pivmecillinam reaches serum concentrations of 3ug/ml 1.5 h after 200 mg taken orally [31].

Inappropriate use of broad-spectrum antibiotics such as carbapenems adds to the problem of antimicrobial resistance as well as being responsible for a rise in *C. difficile* infections and healthcare costs. This study showed that mecillinam alone has good in vitro activity against clinical isolates of ESBL producing *E. coli* and *Klebsiella*.

Carbapenems are often used to treat UTIs caused by ESBLs; however this has been shown to lead to further resistance and will exacerbate the CRE problem. Invasive CRE infections have limited therapeutic options with mortality rates in excess of 40 % [32]. Pivmecillinam, widely used in Scandinavian countries for treating uncomplicated UTIs has a good safety profile [33]. Side effects of mecillinam include rash, nausea and vomiting. Surveillance in countries that strictly limit pivmecillinam for acute uncomplicated UTIs has shown low resistance in the community despite widespread use for more than 20 years [16]. There are reports of mecillinam resistance in *E. coli*; one mechanism is increased levels of ppGpp, a nucleotide effector [34]. Other studies have shown a low probability of future clonal spread of mecillinam resistance due to little association of resistance due to specific clonal groups. Other authors found that mecillinam resistance is not associated with ESBL production [35, 36].

In this study only 5.36 % of ESBLs that were E tested were resistant to mecillinam according to the EUCAST breakpoints with only two isolates having an MIC of >256 mg/L. This may be due the fact that mecillinam is only slightly affected by TEM and SHV1, which are the most frequent beta lactamases found in *E. coli*. In a French study, clinical efficiency was high with pivmecillinam and independent of MIC, which suggests susceptibility testing for UTIs caused by *E. coli* is not required with pivmecillinam, and could possibly be given empirically [17]. The results of the E tests with coamoxiclav show that only 2.11 % of isolates were susceptible to the drug according to the CLSI breakpoints, however according to the BSAC breakpoints, 25 % would be effective treatment of UTIs. Resistance to coamoxiclav is common and in a Spanish study 30.6 % of its ESBLs population were non-susceptible. The principle risk factor in that study was previous use of coamoxiclav, confirming that increased consumption leads to increased resistance. Resistance mechanisms of *E. coli* to coamoxiclav include B-lactamase overproduction, AmpC cephalosporinase hyperproduction and inhibitor-resistant penicillinases [37]. Resistance is acquired by clonal and non-clonal spread, dissemination of mobile elements with different *bla* genes and eventual mutations in individuals organisms [38].

Coamoxiclav alone was ineffective against 97.89 % of the isolates tested and should not be used alone for treatment of ESBL positive UTIs, however, the combination of coamoxiclav and mecillinam decreased the MIC significantly compared to mecillinam or coamoxiclav alone in three isolates. However two isolates had higher MICs with the combination of the two antibiotics compared to treatment with one antibiotic. For isolate 779 the coamoxiclav MIC increased from 128 mg/L alone to >256ug/ml when combined with mecillinam. Similarly but more worryingly isolate 031 was inhibited by 12 mg/L of mecillinam alone in the E test but was not inhibited by 256ug/ml in combination with coamoxiclav. The results for the mecillinam and coamoxiclav only in the 96 well plate differed to the results of the drugs alone in the E test. It is conceivable that some of these infections could represent identical bacterial strains, however, patients were disparate in time and place, and therefore it is likely that they represent different strains. This demonstrates that the combination of coamoxiclav and pivmecillinam on different species that produce ESBLs could be beneficial. However, further studies using mecillinam monotherapy or in combination with clavulanic acid, would benefit with a larger sample size to improve statistical power.

Conclusion

Pivmecillinam alone appears to be a suitable treatment for UTIs due to ESBL producing Enterobacteriaceae especially lower UTIs. Resistance to this agent has been low even though it has been used for treating UTIs in Nordic countries for more than 20 years. In the future pivmecillinam in combination with coamoxiclav, would seem to be an appropriate treatment alternative for Irish ESBL infections and will also help reduce carbapenem usage, which in turn should help reduce the generation of CRE producing organisms. However for combination therapy further clinical evaluation would be required before clinical use could be advocated.

Abbreviations

CRE: Carbapenem Resistant Enterobacteriaceae; ESBL: Extended spectrum beta lactamase; EUCAST: European Committee on Antimicrobial Susceptibility Testing; FIC: Fractional inhibitory concentration; MIC: Mean inhibitory concentration; PBP: Penicillin binding protein; SHV: Sulfhydryl variable beta-lactamases; TEM: Temoneira beta-lactamases; UTI: Urinary tract infection

Acknowledgements

We would like to acknowledge the tremendous work of the laboratory microbiologists who identified all the organisms and conducted the original susceptibility testing for all the organisms used in this study.

Funding

No funding was received at any stage for this study.

Authors' contributions

All authors have read and approved the manuscript. FOK, SK and JF made substantial contributions to conception and design, or acquisition of data, or analysis and interpretation of data. RPM and JAT were involved in drafting the manuscript or revising it critically for important intellectual content. JAT and JF gave final approval of the version to be published.

Competing interests

The authors declare that they have no competing interests.

Consent for publication

Not applicable.

Author details

[1]Department of Clinical Microbiology, AMNCH, Tallaght Hospital, Dublin 24, Ireland. [2]Department of Urological Surgery, AMNCH, Tallaght Hospital, Dublin 24, Ireland.

References

1. Dhillon RH-P, Clark J. ESBLs: a clear and present danger? Crit Care Res Pract. 2012;2012:625170.
2. Livermore DM, Hawkey PM. CTX-M: changing the face of ESBLs in the UK. J Antimicrob Chemother. 2005;56:451–4.
3. Fennell J, et al. Increasing prevalence of ESBL production among Irish clinical Enterobacteriaceae from 2004 to 2008: an observational study. BMC Infect Dis. 2012;12:116.
4. Linhares I, Raposo T, Rodrigues A, Almeida A. Frequency and antimicrobial resistance patterns of bacteria implicated in community urinary tract infections: a ten-year surveillance study (2000–2009). BMC Infect Dis. 2013;13:19.
5. Thomson KS. Extended-spectrum-beta-lactamase, AmpC, and Carbapenemase issues. J Clin Microbiol. 2010;48:1019–25.
6. Kanj SS, Kanafani ZA. Current concepts in antimicrobial therapy against resistant gram-negative organisms: extended-spectrum beta-lactamase-producing Enterobacteriaceae, carbapenem-resistant Enterobacteriaceae, and multidrug-resistant Pseudomonas aeruginosa. Mayo Clin Proc. 2011;86:250–9.
7. Pobiega M, et al. Molecular characterization and drug resistance of Escherichia coli strains isolated from urine from long-term care facility residents in Cracow, Poland. Med Sci Monit. 2013;19:317–26.
8. Martinez P, Garzón D, Mattar S. CTX-M-producing Escherichia coli and Klebsiella pneumoniae isolated from community-acquired urinary tract infections in Valledupar, Colombia. Braz J Infect Dis. 2012;16:420–5.
9. Azap OK, et al. Risk factors for extended-spectrum beta-lactamase positivity in uropathogenic Escherichia coli isolated from community-acquired urinary tract infections. Clin Microbiol Infect. 2010;16:147–51.
10. Pelly H, et al. Outbreak of extended spectrum beta-lactamase producing E. coli in a nursing home in Ireland, May 2006. Euro Surveill. 2006;11:E060831.1.
11. Ludden C, et al. Colonisation with ESBL-producing and carbapenemase-producing Enterobacteriaceae, vancomycin-resistant enterococci, and meticillin-resistant Staphylococcus aureus in a long-term care facility over one year. BMC Infect Dis. 2015;15:168.
12. EARS-Net Report, Quarter 1-4 2015. Health Protection Surveillance Centre 2016. http://www.hpsc.ie/A-Z/MicrobiologyAntimicrobialResistance/European AntimicrobialResistanceSurveillanceSystemEARSS/EARSSSurveillanceReports/ 2015Reports/File,15214,en. Accessed June 2016.
13. Al-Assil B, Mahfoud M, Hamzeh AR. Resistance trends and risk factors of extended spectrum β-lactamases in Escherichia coli infections in Aleppo, Syria. Am J Infect Control. 2013;41:597–600.
14. Hoşbul T, et al. In vitro activity of fosfomycin trometamol in the treatment of Escherichia coli related uncomplicated urinary tract infections. Mikrobiyol Bul. 2009;43:645–9.
15. Pallett A, Hand K. Complicated urinary tract infections: practical solutions for the treatment of multiresistant Gram-negative bacteria. J Antimicrob Chemother. 2010;65(Suppl 3):iii25–33.
16. Auer S, Wojna A, Hell M. Oral treatment options for ambulatory patients with urinary tract infections caused by extended-spectrum-beta-lactamase-producing Escherichia coli. Antimicrob Agents Chemother. 2010;54:4006–8.
17. Thomas K, Weinbren MJ, Warner M, Woodford N, Livermore D. Activity of mecillinam against ESBL producers in vitro. J Antimicrob Chemother. 2006; 57:367–8.
18. Graninger W. Pivmecillinam–therapy of choice for lower urinary tract infection. Int J Antimicrob Agents. 2003;22(Suppl 2):73–8.
19. Papp-Wallace KM, Endimiani A, Taracila MA, Bonomo RA. Carbapenems: past, present, and future. Antimicrob Agents Chemother. 2011;55:4943–60.
20. Meletiadis J, Pournaras S, Roilides E, Walsh TJ. Defining fractional inhibitory concentration index cutoffs for additive interactions based on self-drug additive combinations, Monte Carlo simulation analysis, and in vitro-in vivo correlation data for antifungal drug combinations against Aspergillus fumi. Antimicrob Agents Chemother. 2010;54:602–9.
21. Hall MJ, Middleton RF, Westmacott D. The fractional inhibitory concentration (FIC) index as a measure of synergy. J Antimicrob Chemother. 1983;11:427–33.
22. White RL, Burgess DS, Manduru M, Bosso JA. Comparison of three different in vitro methods of detecting synergy: time-kill, checkerboard, and E test. Antimicrob Agents Chemother. 1996;40:1914–8.
23. Prieto J, et al. In vitro activities of co-amoxiclav at concentrations achieved in human serum against the resistant subpopulation of heteroresistant Staphylococcus aureus: a controlled study with vancomycin. Antimicrob Agents Chemother. 1998;42:1574–7.
24. Neuzillet Y, Naber KG, Schito G, Gualco L, Botto H. French results of the ARESC study: clinical aspects and epidemiology of antimicrobial resistance in female patients with cystitis. Implications for empiric therapy. Med Mal Infect. 2012;42:66–75.
25. Cullen IM, et al. The changing pattern of antimicrobial resistance within 42,033 Escherichia coli isolates from nosocomial, community and urology patient-specific urinary tract infections, Dublin, 1999–2009. BJU Int. 2012;109: 1198–206.
26. Frakking FNJ, et al. Appropriateness of empirical treatment and outcome in bacteremia caused by extended-spectrum-β-lactamase-producing bacteria. Antimicrob Agents Chemother. 2013;57:3092–9.
27. Fan N-C, et al. Rise of community-onset urinary tract infection caused by extended-spectrum β-lactamase-producing Escherichia coli in children. J Microbiol Immunol Infect. 2013. doi:10.1016/j.jmii.2013.05.006.
28. Yamamoto A. Extended-spectrum β-lactamase (ESBL)-producing Escherichia coli is frequently detected as a pathogen of urinary tract infection in nursing home residents. Nihon Ronen Igakkai Zasshi. 2011;48:530–8.
29. Dewar S, Reed LC, Koerner RJ. Emerging clinical role of pivmecillinam in the treatment of urinary tract infection in the context of multidrug-resistant bacteria. J Antimicrob Chemother. 2014;69:303–8.

30. Heikkilä A, Pyykkö K, Erkkola R, Iisalo E. The pharmacokinetics of mecillinam and pivmecillinam in pregnant and non-pregnant women. Br J Clin Pharmacol. 1992;33:629–33.
31. Andrews J, Kendall MJ, Mitchard M. Factors influencing the absorption and disposition of mecillinam and pivmecillinam in man. Br J Clin Pharmacol. 1976;3:627–32.
32. Kumarasamy KK, et al. Emergence of a new antibiotic resistance mechanism in India, Pakistan, and the UK: a molecular, biological, and epidemiological study. Lancet Infect Dis. 2010;10:597–602.
33. Lampri N, et al. Mecillinam/clavulanate combination: a possible option for the treatment of community-acquired uncomplicated urinary tract infections caused by extended-spectrum β-lactamase-producing Escherichia coli. J Antimicrob Chemother. 2012;67:2424–8.
34. Poulsen HO, Johansson A, Granholm S, Kahlmeter G, Sundqvist M. High genetic diversity of nitrofurantoin- or mecillinam-resistant Escherichia coli indicates low propensity for clonal spread. J Antimicrob Chemother. 2013;68:1974–7.
35. Sougakoff W, Jarlier V. Comparative potency of mecillinam and other beta-lactam antibiotics against Escherichia coli strains producing different beta-lactamases. J Antimicrob Chemother. 2000;46(Suppl 1):9–14. discussion 63–5.
36. Kariuki S, et al. Escherichia coli from community-acquired urinary tract infections resistant to fluoroquinolones and extended-spectrum beta-lactams. J Infect Dev Ctries. 2007;1:257–62.
37. Rodríguez-Baño J, et al. Epidemiological and clinical complexity of amoxicillin-clavulanate-resistant Escherichia coli. J Clin Microbiol. 2013;51:2414–7.
38. Miyakis S, Pefanis A, Tsakris A. The challenges of antimicrobial drug resistance in Greece. Clin Infect Dis. 2011;53:177–84.

Antimicrobial susceptibilities of aerobic and facultative gram-negative bacilli isolated from Chinese patients with urinary tract infections between 2010 and 2014

Qiwen Yang[1†], Hui Zhang[1†], Yao Wang[1], Zhipeng Xu[1], Ge Zhang[1], Xinxin Chen[1], Yingchun Xu[1*], Bin Cao[2], Haishen Kong[3], Yuxing Ni[4], Yunsong Yu[5], Ziyong Sun[6], Bijie Hu[7], Wenxiang Huang[8], Yong Wang[9], Anhua Wu[10], Xianju Feng[11], Kang Liao[12], Yanping Luo[13], Zhidong Hu[14], Yunzhuo Chu[15], Juan Lu[16], Jianrong Su[17], Bingdong Gui[18], Qiong Duan[19], Shufang Zhang[20], Haifeng Shao[21] and Robert E. Badal[22]

Abstract

Background: The objective of this study was to investigate the distribution and susceptibility of aerobic and facultative Gram-negative bacilli isolated from Chinese patients with UTIs collected within 48 h (community acquired, CA) or after 48 h (hospital acquired, HA) of hospital admission.

Methods: From 2010 to 2014, the minimum inhibitory concentrations (MICs) of 12 antibiotics for 4,332 aerobic and facultative Gram-negative bacilli, sampled in 21 hospitals in 16 cities, were determined by the broth microdilution method.

Results: *Enterobacteriaceae* composed 88.5% of the total isolates, with *Escherichia coli* (*E. coli*) (63.2%) the most commonly isolated species, followed by *Klebsiella pneumoniae* (*K. pneumoniae*) (12.2%). Non-*Enterobacteriaceae* accounted for only 11.5% of all isolates and included mainly *Pseudomonas aeruginosa* (*P. aeruginosa*) (6.9%) and *Acinetobacter baumannii* (*A. baumannii*) (3.3%). Among the antimicrobial agents tested, the susceptibility rates of *E. coli* to the two carbapenems, ertapenem and imipenem as well as amikacin and piperacillin-tazobactam ranged from 92.5 to 98.7%. Against *K. pneumonia*, the most potent antibiotics were imipenem (92.6% susceptibility), amikacin (89.2% susceptibility) and ertapenem (87.9% susceptibility).

Although non-*Enterobacteriaceae* did not show high susceptibilities to the 12 common antibiotics, amikacin exhibited the highest in vitro activity against *P. aeruginosa* over the 5-year study period, followed by piperacillin-tazobactam, imipenem, ceftazidime, cefepime, ciprofloxacin, and levofloxacin. The Extended Spectrum Beta-Lactamase (ESBL) rates decreased slowly during the 5 years in *E. coli* from 68.6% in 2010 to 59.1% in 2014, in *K. pneumoniae* from 59.7 to 49.2%, and in *Proteus mirabilis* (*P. mirabilis*) from 40.0 to 26.1%. However, the ESBL rates were different in 5 regions of China (Northeast, North, East, South and Middle-China).

(Continued on next page)

* Correspondence: xuyingchunbm@163.com
†Equal contributors
[1]Department of Clinical Laboratory, Peking Union Medical College Hospital, Peking Union Medical College, Chinese Academy of Medical Sciences, Beijing 100730, China
Full list of author information is available at the end of the article

(Continued from previous page)

Conclusion: *E. coli* and *K. pneumonia* were the major pathogens causing UTIs and carbapenems and amikacin retained the highest susceptibility rates over the 5-year study period, indicating that they are good drug choices for empirical therapies, particularly of CA UTIs in China.

Keywords: Urinary tract infections, Extended spectrum beta-lactamases (ESBLs), Carbapenems, Antimicrobial resistance

Background

Several national and international surveillance programs have been initiated for monitoring susceptibilities of clinically important pathogens in urinary tract infections (UTIs) [1–3]. The Study for Monitoring Antimicrobial Resistance Trends (SMART) is a surveillance program designed to monitor globally susceptibilities of aerobic and facultative Gram-negative bacilli collected from intra-abdominal infections and UTIs (initiated in 2002) [4]. UTIs are frequently encountered in clinical practice and include uncomplicated and complicated pyelonephritis, ureteritis, cystitis and urethritis [5]. The etiologies of these infections arise from Gram-negative bacilli, especially *Enterobacteriaceae,* and some Gram-positive bacteria [6]. During the last decade, multidrug-resistant Gram-negative Enterobacteriaceae have become a challenge for physicians [7] and particularly *E. coli* and *K. pneumonia* strains isolated from UTIs have been reported to increasingly produce ESBLs in the recent years [8–10]. The choice of an empiric UTI antimicrobial therapy should be based on knowledge of the pathogen distribution and the resistance extent of common microorganisms, in addition to hospital-specific resistance patterns particularly for HA infections. This study, as part of the global SMART project, focused on ESBL-producing rates of UTI isolates from 21 centers in 16 Chinese cities between 2010 and 2014 and on UTI derived sample resistance rates against carbapenems, a combination of drugs containing penicillins with β-lactamase inhibitors, a cephamycin, an aminoglycoside, 3rd and 4th generation cephalosporins as well as 2nd generation fluoroquinolones, in order to provide guidance for antimicrobial therapies of IAIs.

Methods

Clinical isolates

During our study period (2010–2014), a total of 4,332 aerobic and facultative Gram-negative bacilli were consecutively isolated from patients with UTIs in 21 hospitals sited in 16 Chinese cities (Beijing, Shanghai, Hangzhou, Nanjing, Shenyang, Tianjin, Wuhan, Changsha, Jinan, Zhengzhou, Guangzhou, Nanchang, Haikou, Harbin, Changchun and Chongqing).

All isolates were cultured from specimens collected from patients who met both clinical and laboratory criteria of urinary tract infections (3,994 from clean catch midstream urine, 154 from urinary bladder, 136 from ureter, 29 from kidney, 13 from urethra, 6 from prostate). Duplicate isolates (same species and genus from one patient) were excluded.

Standard methods were used by the participating clinical microbiology laboratories for initial bacteria identification, and re-identification was carried out by a central laboratory (Peking Union Medical College Hospital) using Vitek 2 Compact (2010–2011) (Biomerieux, France) and MALDI-TOF MS (2012–2014) (Vitek MS, Biomerieux, France).

Isolates were considered to be community-associated (CA) if they were recovered from a specimen taken less than 48 h after the patient was admitted to a hospital, and hospital-associated (HA) if the specimen was taken 48 or more hours after hospital admission, as previously described [11].

Antimicrobial susceptibility test method

Minimum inhibitory concentration (MIC) determinations were performed in a central lab using dehydrated MicroScan broth microdilution panels (Siemens Medical Solutions Diagnostics (West Sacramento, CA) according to Clinical and Laboratory Standards Institute (CLSI) guidelines [12] and susceptibility interpretations were based on clinical CLSI breakpoints [13]. Twelve commonly used antimicrobial agents for UTI treatments were analyzed namely, imipenem (IPM), ertapenem (EPM), ceftriaxone (CRO), cefotaxime (CTX), ceftazidime (CAZ), cefoxitin (FOX), cefepime (FEP), piperacillin-tazobactam (TZP), ampicillin-sulbactam (SAM), amikacin (AMK), ciprofloxacin (CIP) and levofloxacin (LVX). For each batch of MIC testing, the reference strains *E. coli* ATCC 25922, *P. aeruginosa* ATCC 27853 and *K. pneumonia* ATCC 700603 were used as quality controls. Results were only included in the analysis when corresponding quality control isolate test results were in accordance with CLSI guidelines and therefore within an acceptable range.

Extended-spectrum β-lactamases (ESBLs) detection

Phenotypic identification of ESBL production in *E.coli, K. pneumonia, Klebsiella oxytoca* (*K. oxytoca*), and *P. mirabilis* was carried out according to CLSI recommended methods [13]. If cefotaxime or ceftazidime MICs were ≥ 2 μg/mL, the MICs of cefotaxime + clavulanic acid (4 μg/mL) or ceftazidime + clavulanic acid (4 µg/mL) were comparatively determined. ESBL production was defined as a ≥ 8-fold decrease in MICs for cefotaxime or ceftazidime tested in combination with clavulanic acid, compared to their MICs without clavulanic acid.

Statistical analysis

The susceptibility of all gram-negative isolates combined was calculated using breakpoints appropriate for each species and assuming 0% susceptible for species with no breakpoints for any given drug. Ninety-five percent confidence intervals were calculated using the adjusted Wald method; linear trends of ESBL rates in different years were assessed for statistical significance using the Cochran-Armitage test and comparison of ESBL rates in 6 different geographic areas were assessed using Chi-square test. P values < 0.05 were considered statistically significant.

Results

Distribution of organisms from urinary tract infection

A total of 4,332 isolates were collected from UTIs between 2010 and 2014. The highest distribution of bacteria was *E. coli*, which accounted for 63.2% (2,737 strains), followed by *K. pneumonia* (12.2%, 529 strains) and *P. aeruginosa* (6.9%, 297 strains) (Table 1). We also investigated the distribution of strains from HA ($n = 2765$, 72.16%) and CA ($n = 1039$, 27.11%) ($P < 0.0001$) infections, but most of the isolates were sampled from HA infections (62.59–80.42%) (Table 1). *Enterobacteriaceae* were present in the majority of isolates and accounted for 88.5%, including mainly *E.coli* (63.2%), followed by *K. pneumonia* (12.2%), *P. mirabilis* (3.4%) and *Enterobacter cloacae* (*E. cloacae*) (3.3%), while others were present at a rate < 1.3%. Non-*Enterobacteriaceae* accounted for only 11.5% of all isolates and

included mainly *P. aeruginosa* (6.9%) and *Acinetobacter baumannii* (*A. baumannii*) (3.3%).

In vitro susceptibility of Enterobacteriaceae and non-Enterobacteriaceae during 2010–2014

Among the 12 analyzed antimicrobial agents, the susceptibility rates of ertapenem and imipenem against *E. coli* over 5 years were 96.4% (2,639/2,737) and 98.7% (2,702/2,737), with MIC_{90} values of 0.25 µg/mL for both drugs. Most *E.coli* isolates remained susceptible to amikacin (92.8%) and piperacillin-tazobactam (92.51%). However, the susceptibilities to third- and fourth-generation cephalosporins were relatively low, with rates of 58.5, 38.2, 34.6 and 34.4% for ceftazidime (CAZ), cefepime (FEP), cefotaxime (CTX) and ceftriaxone (CRO), respectively. The susceptibility rates of *E. coli* to fluoroquinolones and ampicillin-sulbactam were also less than 30 and 20%, respectively (Fig. 1, Table 2).

Against *K. pneumonia*, the most potent antibiotics were imipenem (92.6% susceptibility), amikacin (89.2% susceptibility) and ertapenem (87.9% susceptibility), with MIC_{90} values of 1 µg/mL, > 32 µg/mL and 1 µg/mL, respectively. Piperacillin-tazobactam was the fourth most active agent, with a susceptibility of 75.8%. The susceptibility rates of other antibiotics ranged from 30.6% (ampicillin-sulbactam) to 67.5% (cefoxitin) (Fig. 1, Table 2,).

Against *P. mirabilis*, antimicrobial agents with > 90% susceptibility rates included ertapenem (99.3%), piperacillin-tazobactam (99.3%) and amikacin (91.2%), but in HA infections, a > 90% susceptibility rate was found for ceftazidime (90.2%). Cephalosporin susceptibility rates were 55.8–88.4% whereas fluoroquinolones exhibited 41.5–55.1% activity. Imipenem had poor

Table 1 Distribution of the UTI pathogens in China between 2010 and 2014

	Total	CA (n/% of total)	HA (n/% of total)	Not identified (n/% of total)	P-value
Enterobacteriaceae	3,832	1,039 (27.11)	2,765 (72.16)	28 (0.73)	<0.0001
Escherichia coli	2,737	739 (27.00)	1,976 (72.20)	22 (0.80)	<0.0001
Klebsiella pneumoniae	529	129 (24.39)	398 (75.24)	2 (0.38)	<0.0001
Proteus mirabilis	147	54 (36.73)	92 (62.59)	1 (0.68)	0.011
Enterobacter cloacae	141	39 (27.66)	101 (71.63)	1 (0.71)	<0.0001
Citrobacter freundii	54	11 (20.37)	43 (79.63)	0 (0.00)	0.0003
Klebsiella oxytoca	51	18 (35.29)	33 (64.71)	0 (0.00)	0.1205
other	173	49 (28.32)	122 (70.52)	2 (1.16)	<0.0001
Non-Enterobacteriaceae	500	105 (21.00)	391 (78.2)	4 (0.8)	<0.0001
Pseudomonas aeruginosa	297	65 (21.89)	231 (77.78)	1 (0.34)	<0.0001
Acinetobacter baumannii	143	26 (18.18)	115 (80.42)	2 (1.40)	<0.0001
other	60	14 (23.33)	45 (75.00)	1 (1.67)	<0.0001
All	4,332	1,144 (26.41)	3,156 (72.85)	32 (0.74)	<0.0001

Not identified: A total of 32 isolates lacked partial demographic information and could not be identified as CA or HA isolates. They were not included in further analyses

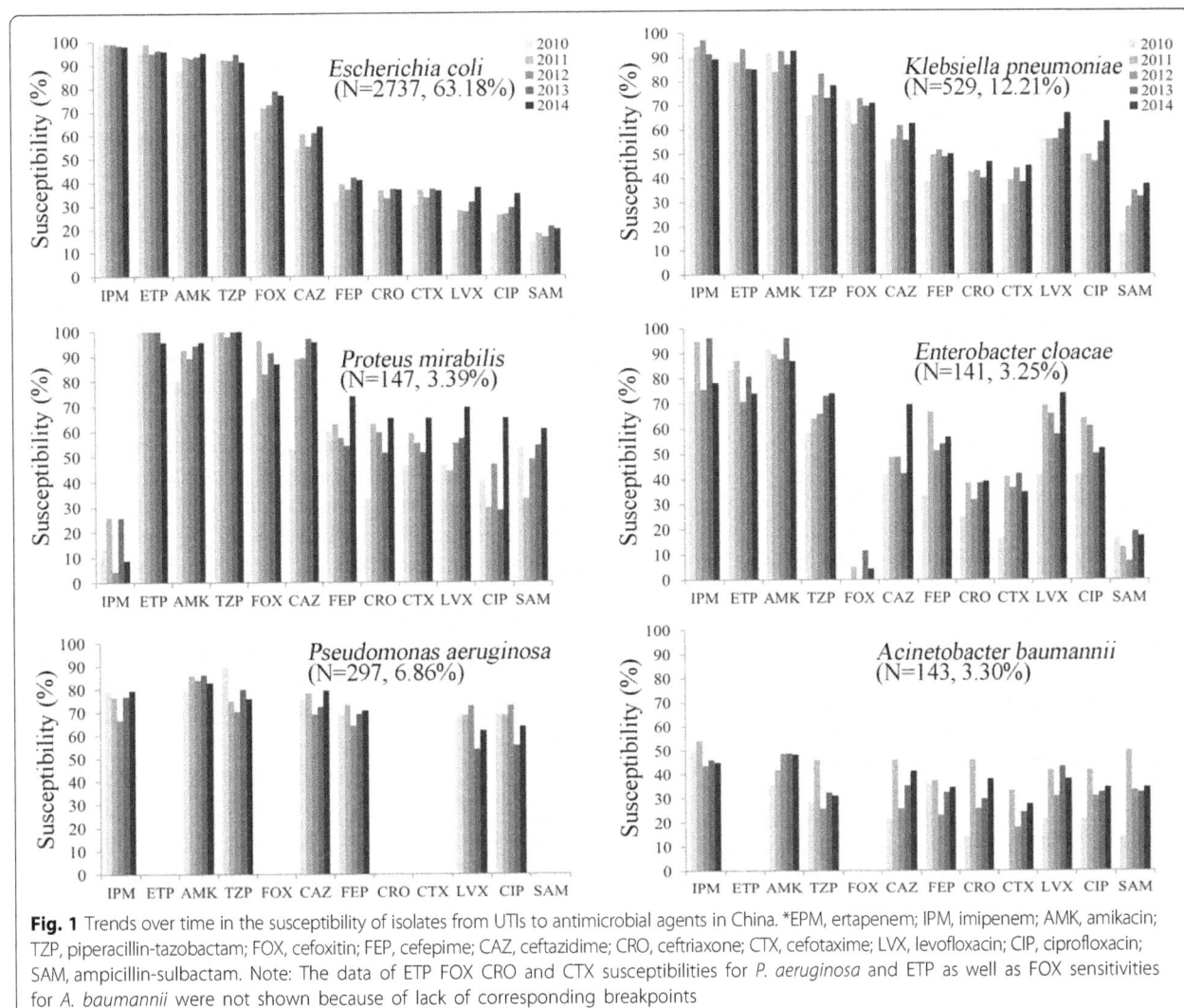

Fig. 1 Trends over time in the susceptibility of isolates from UTIs to antimicrobial agents in China. *EPM, ertapenem; IPM, imipenem; AMK, amikacin; TZP, piperacillin-tazobactam; FOX, cefoxitin; FEP, cefepime; CAZ, ceftazidime; CRO, ceftriaxone; CTX, cefotaxime; LVX, levofloxacin; CIP, ciprofloxacin; SAM, ampicillin-sulbactam. Note: The data of ETP FOX CRO and CTX susceptibilities for *P. aeruginosa* and ETP as well as FOX sensitivities for *A. baumannii* were not shown because of lack of corresponding breakpoints

activity against *P. mirabilis* isolates, with a mean susceptibility rate of only 15.0% in both CA and HA derived isolates (Figs. 1 and 2, Table 2).

Antimicrobial resistance in *Enterobacter cloacae* was more pronounced than in *E. coli* and *K. pneumonia*. The antimicrobial agents with susceptibility rates of > 80% were amikacin (90.1%) and imipenem (85.1%) over the 5-year study period. Particularly in 2014, ertapenem and piperacillin-tazobactam susceptibility rates in HA infections dropped to 53.9%, whereas CA UTIs were still 100% susceptible to both antibiotics (Fig. 2). However, ertapenem was the third most active agent with susceptibilities of 78.7% in all isolates, followed by piperacillin-tazobactam (67.4%), levofloxacin (64.5%), ciprofloxacin (56.7%) and cefepime (55.3%) (Fig. 1, Table 2).

Although non-*Enterobacteriaceae* did not show high susceptibilities to the 12 common antibiotics, amikacin exhibited the highest in vitro activity against *P. aeruginosa*, with a susceptibility rate of 84.2% over the 5-year study period,

followed by piperacillin-tazobactam, imipenem, ceftazidime, cefepime, ciprofloxacin, and levofloxacin. (Figure 1, Table 2).

A. baumannii was the second most frequently isolated non-fermentative Gram-negative bacillus, comprising 3.3% (143/4,332) of all UTIs. The most active agents against *A. baumannii* were imipenem and amikacin, with susceptibility rates of 46.9 and 46.2%, respectively over the entire study period. The other analyzed agents were less effective, with susceptibility rates of < 40% (Fig. 1, Table 2).

The trend of extended spectrum beta-lactamases (ESBL) – producing bacteria occurrence in UTIs from 2010 to 2014

Figure 2a-c shows the frequency of ESBL-producing *E.coli*, *K. pneumonia*, *K. oxytoca* and *P. mirabilis* strains over the study period. The percentage of ESBL positive *E. coli* isolates decreased from 68.6% in 2010 to 59.1% in 2014, while the ESBL rate in *K. pneumonia* decreased from 59.7 to 49.2% and in *P. mirabilis* from 40.0 to 26.1% during the 5-year study period. The susceptibility

Table 2 Susceptibilities of UTI pathogens isolated between 2010 and 2014

	Antibiotics	S%	MIC50 (μg/ml)	MIC90 (μg/ml)
Escherichia coli	IPM	98.72	0.12	0.25
	ETP	96.42	≤0.03	0.25
	AMK	92.88	≤4	16
	TZP	92.51	≤2	16
Klebsiella pneumoniae	IPM	92.63	0.25	1
	AMK	89.22	≤4	>32
	ETP	87.9	≤0.03	1
	TZP	75.8	≤2	>64
Proteus mirabilis	ETP	99.32	≤0.03	0.06
	TZP	99.32	≤2	4
	AMK	91.16	8	16
	CAZ	88.44	≤0.5	8
Enterobacter cloacae	AMK	90.07	≤4	16
	IPM	85.11	0.5	2
	ETP	78.72	0.12	4
	TZP	67.38	4	>64
Pseudomonas aeruginosa	AMK	84.18	8	>32
	TZP	76.43	4	>64
	IPM	74.75	1	>8
	CAZ	74.41	4	64
Acinetobacter baumannii	IPM	46.85	8	>8
	AMK	46.15	>32	>32
	LVX	36.36	>4	>4
	CAZ	34.27	64	>128

differences to ertapenem and imipenem between ESBL and non-ESBL producing strains were generally small, but were greater for other agents, particularly for the third- and fourth-generation cephalosporins, including ceftriaxone (1.1% against ESBL-producing isolates vs 91.0% against ESBL-non-producing isolates), ceftazidime (38.4% vs 93.5%) and cefepime (4.5% vs 96.7%) (data not shown).

Figure 2d-e shows the ESBL rates in *E. coli, K. pneumonia, and P. mirabilis* from UTIs in different regions in China. We categorized the 21 participating sites into 5 different regions in China (Northeast (Haerbin, Changchun and Shenyang), North (Beijing and Tianjing), East (Hangzhou, Nanjing, Jinan, Nanchang and Shanghai), South (Chongqing, Guangzhou and Haikou) and Central China (Changsha, Zhengzhou and Wuhan)). The two sites in the Central China region exhibited higher ESBL rates in *E. coli* (81.5%) and *K. pneumonia* (64.9%), while other regions showed relatively lower ESBL rates in these two species (54.5–65.1% for *E. coli*, and 48.1–56.3% for *K. pneumoniae*). For *P. mirabilis*, the

ESBL rates ranged from 31.4% (South China region) to 47.5% (North China region).

Discussion

Nitrofurantoin, trimethoprim-sulfamethoxazole, fosfomycin, fluoroquinolones and beta-lactams are commonly recommended antimicrobial agents for urinary tract infections [14]. However, fosfomycin and nitrofurantoin are not often used in China [2]. The usage of trimethoprim-sulfamethoxazole for the treatment of UTIs in China is also limited because of a high resistance rate to this agent among *E.coli* isolates [15]. In view of this finding, we focused on the activity of beta-lactams, fluoroquinolones and aminoglycoside against uropathogens in the present study. Since *Enterobacteriaceae* accounted for the majority of aerobic and facultative anaerobic pathogens causing UTIs (88.5% of all isolates) in our study, with *E.coli, K. pneumonia, P. mirabilis* and *Enterobacter cloacae* the most frequently isolated species, knowledge of their resistance pattern is beneficial.

Cephalosporins are commonly recommended as empirical choices for UTIs, but their efficacy is greatly reduced when the pathogens produce ESBL. Over the entire study period, susceptibility rates of *Enterobacteriaceae* to third-generation and fourth-generation cephalosporins were 51.4–66.0% for ceftazidime, 29.4–46.9% for cefotaxime, 29.9–41.2% for ceftriaxone and 35.1–47.1% for cefepime, indicating that these agents might not be the optimum medications for empirical UTI therapies. In the present study, the percentage of ESBL positive *E. coli* isolates decreased from 66.9% in 2010 to 59.1% in 2014, while for *K. pneumonia* it decreased from 59.7 to 48.8% and from 40.0 to 26.1% among *P. mirabilis*. The data were well matched with the non-susceptibility rates to cephalosporins against each species, which indicated that ESBL production might be a reason for cephalosporin resistance [16]. The decrease of ESBL rates in *E. coli, K. pneumonia* and *P. mirabilis* may have been a result of China's antimicrobial stewardship policy on antimicrobial use, which has been promoted for a number of years [17–19]. Our study also highlighted the variation in ESBL rates in different regions of China, with the Central-China region having a higher ESBL prevalence in *E. coli* and *K. pneumonia*. Researchers previously reported that the ESBL genotypes in China were mainly CTX-M types [20–22], especially CTX-M-14, –15, and –55 for *E. coli* and *K. pneumonia*, and CTX-M-65 and –14 for *P. mirabilis* [22]. Plasmids encoding these CTX-M enzymes reached human opportunists, where they have proliferated in community *E. coli* and hospital *K.* species. CTX-M families are dominate in different regions: CTX-M-15 is predominant in most of Europe, North America, the Middle East, and India, but

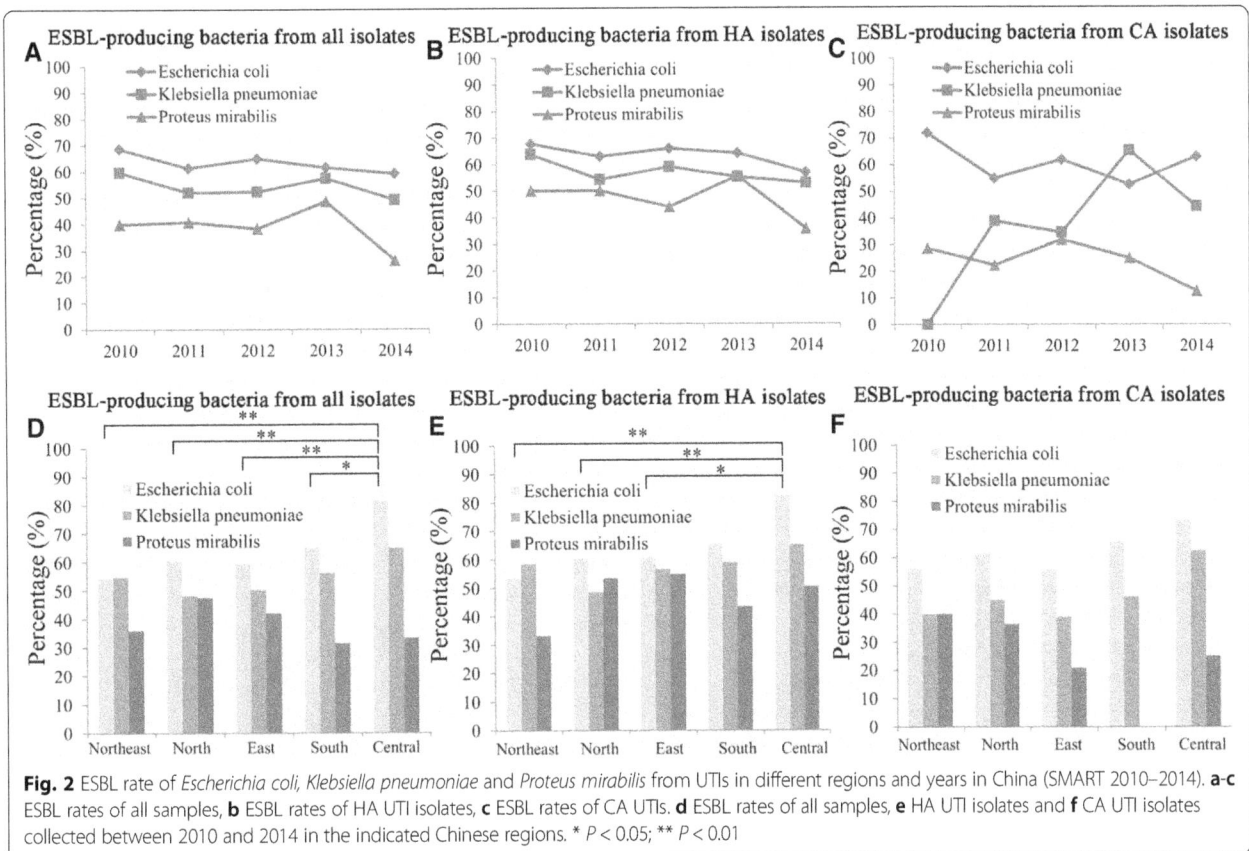

Fig. 2 ESBL rate of *Escherichia coli, Klebsiella pneumoniae* and *Proteus mirabilis* from UTIs in different regions and years in China (SMART 2010–2014). **a-c** ESBL rates of all samples, **b** ESBL rates of HA UTI isolates, **c** ESBL rates of CA UTIs. **d** ESBL rates of all samples, **e** HA UTI isolates and **f** CA UTI isolates collected between 2010 and 2014 in the indicated Chinese regions. * $P < 0.05$; ** $P < 0.01$

CTX-M-14 is most common in China, Southeast Asia and Spain, while CTX-M-2 is predominant in Argentina, Israel, and Japan [23, 24]. Increased numbers of enzyme types and prevalence made determination of resistance profiles more complicated.

Fluoroquinolones, especially ciprofloxacin and levofloxacin, were considered to be effective antimicrobial agents against uropathogens because of high drug concentrations are reached in the urine. However, fluoroquinolone-resistant *E. coli* is also problematic in China. The susceptibility of *E. coli* to fluoroquinolones (ciprofloxacin and levofloxacin) was 26.9–28.9%, with rates of 30.2–32.1% against CA isolates and 25.7–27.8% against HA isolates. Wang et al. also previously reported about ciprofloxacin-resistant *E. coli* strains with multiple gyrA and parC gene substitutions [25]. Regarding the low effectiveness of fluoroquinolones against *Enterobacteriaceae*, ciprofloxacin and levofloxacin should not be considered as first line agents for empirical therapies of complicated UTIs. Our data also showed that susceptibilities of ESBL-producing *E. coli* and *K. pneumonia* strains to fluoroquinolones were significantly lower than that of ESBL-non-producing strains, which is in agreement with previous findings [26].

Carbapenems can still be considered to be suitable for severe infections and as alternative empiric treatment for UTIs caused by bacterial strains highly suspicious of being ESBL-producing or AmpC-derepressed *Enterobacteriaceae* [27–29]. Although carbapenems were not the first line choices for uncomplicated cystitis and pyelonephritis in women according to the IDSA guideline, they were good alternatives against multidrug resistant Gram-negative bacilli that caused UTIs. Our study showed that ertapenem and imipenem were the most effective agents against *Enterobacteriaceae* causing UTIs, with susceptibility rates of 92.5–96.5% and 89.9–95.2%, respectively (2010–2014). On the other hand, carbapenem-resistant *Enterobacteriaceae* have emerged, which has also been noted in other reports [30–33], especially KPC-producing *K. pneumonia* in the northeastern area of the United States of America [31], KPC/VIM-producing *Enterobacteriaceae* in Greece [32, 33] and KPC-producing isolates in eastern China. In our study, very few *E. coli* isolates (<4%) were non-susceptible to carbapenems, while there was a certain proportion of carbapenem-non-susceptible *K. pneumonia* isolates (13.8% to ertapenem), *P. mirabilis* (85% to imipenem) and *E. cloacae* (21.3% to ertapenem and 14.9% to imipenem), which should be noted by

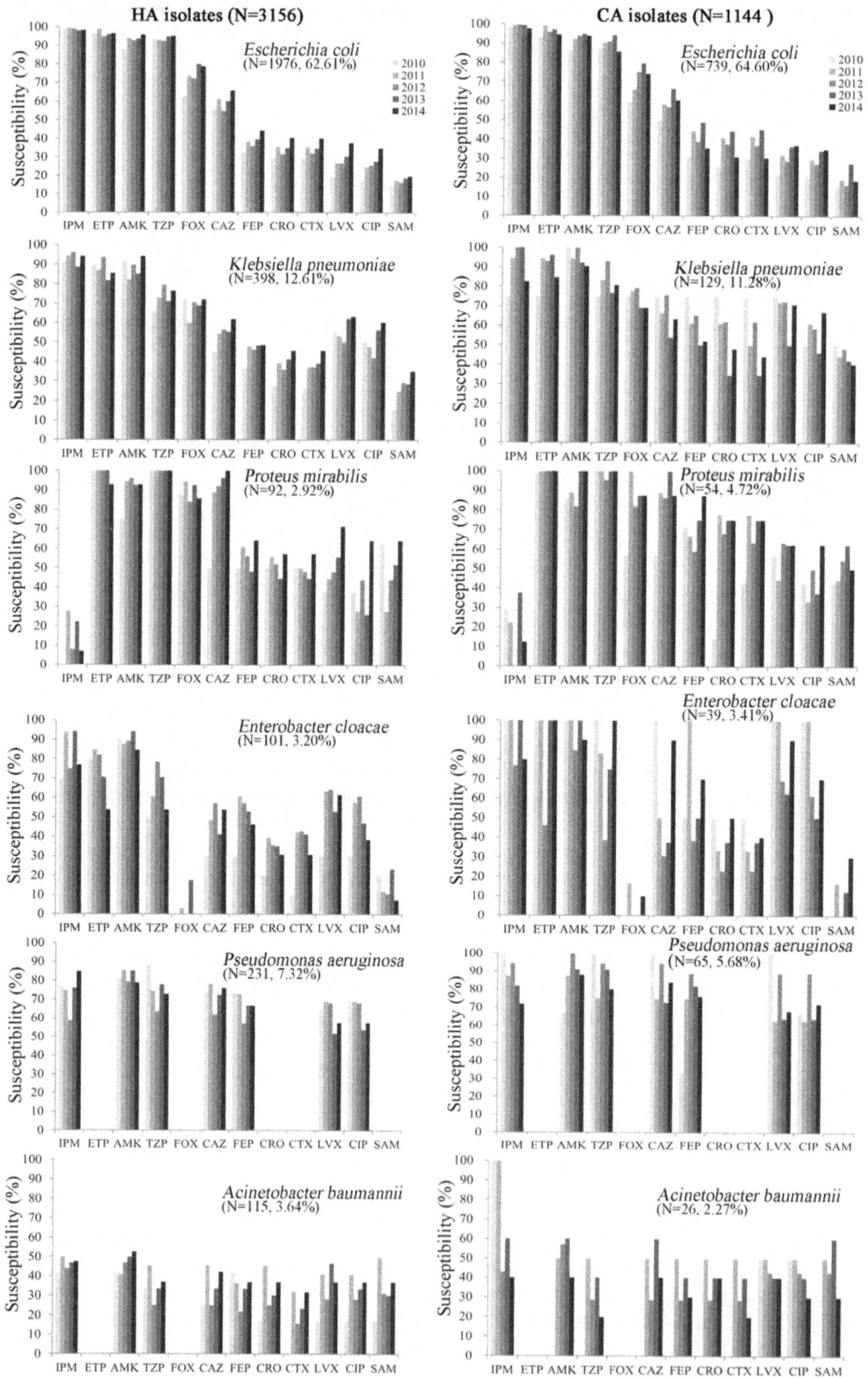

Fig. 3 (See legend on next page.)

(See figure on previous page.)
Fig. 3 Trends over time in the susceptibility of isolates from UTIs to antimicrobial agents in China (CA and HA). *EPM, ertapenem; IPM, imipenem; AMK, amikacin; TZP, piperacillin-tazobactam; FOX, cefoxitin; FEP, cefepime; CAZ, ceftazidime; CRO, ceftriaxone; CTX, cefotaxime; LVX, levofloxacin; CIP, ciprofloxacin; SAM, ampicillin-sulbactam. Note: The data of ETP FOX CRO and CTX susceptibilities for *P. aeruginosa* and ETP as well as FOX sensitivities for *A. baumannii* were not shown because of lack of corresponding breakpoints

clinicians. Especially for *E. cloacae* the susceptibility of HA samples to ertapenem has dropped to 53.9%, while for CA UTIs its susceptibility rate is 100%. Hospital infections caused by *E. cloacae*, which is a typical commensal under normal conditions, have been suggested to be mainly caused by endogenous translocation from the digestive tract in debilitated patients and that under antibiotic therapy, *E. cloacae* strains may selectively reproduce excessively in the gastrointestinal tract [34]. This might be the reason for the high ertapenem resistance in UTIs mainly caused by HA *E. cloacae*. The main resistance mechanism to carbapenem in *Enterobacteriaceae* was reported to be carbapenemase production and porin loss in China [35]. However, the resistance of *P. mirabilis* to imipenem was caused by a mechanism other than carbapenemase [13].

Among the tested antimicrobial agents, amikacin exhibited good activity against most of the uropathogens (80.0–96.2% susceptibility rate against *Enterobacteriaceae* and 83.6% against *P. aeruginosa*). Although the use of this aminoglycoside is limited because of its toxicity, it has also been recommended as an alternative to carbapenems against ESBL-producing isolates that cause UTIs [36].

Conclusion

Carbapenems remain the most effective antimicrobial agents against UTI Gram-negative pathogens, followed by amikacin and piperacillin-tazobactam in China between 2010 and 2014. Due to the reduced susceptibility of *Enterobacteriaceae* to cephalosporins and fluoroquinolones, we recommend that these antibiotics should not be used for empirical UTI therapies in China.

Abbreviations
AMK: Amikacin; CA: Community acquired; CAZ: Ceftazidime; CIP: Ciprofloxacin; CLSI: Clinical and Laboratory Standards Institute; CRO: Ceftriaxone; CTX: Cefotaxime; EPM: Ertapenem; ESBLs: Extended spectrum beta-lactamases; FEP: Cefepime; FOX: Cefoxitin; HA: Hospital acquired; IPM: Imipenem; LVX: Levofloxacin; MICs: Minimum inhibitory concentrations; SAM: Ampicillin-sulbactam; SMART: Study for monitoring antimicrobial resistance trends; TZP: Piperacillin-tazobactam; UTIs: Urinary tract infections

Acknowledgements
We thank all investigators involved in this study. We also thank Shanghai BIOMED Science Technology (Shanghai, China) which was funded by MSD China for providing medical editorial assistance.

Funding
This study was funded by Merck Sharp & Dohme (MSD; Whitehouse Station, NJ, USA) and this study was also funded by CAMS Initiative for Innovative Medicine (2016-I2M-3-014).

Authors' contributions
QWY, HZ and YCX were responsible for the conception and design of the study, drafted the manuscript and revised and commented the draft; QWY, HZ, YW, ZPX, GZ, XXC, YCX, BC, HSK, YXN, YSY, ZYS, BJH, WXH, YW, AHW, XJF, KL, YPL, ZDH, YZC, JL, JRS, BDG, QD, SFZ, HFS and REB performed the data analysis. All authors read and approved the final version of the manuscript and confirm that the content has not been published elsewhere and does not overlap with or duplicate their published work.

Competing interests
The authors declare that they have no competing interests.

Consent for publication
Not applicable.

Author details
[1]Department of Clinical Laboratory, Peking Union Medical College Hospital, Peking Union Medical College, Chinese Academy of Medical Sciences, Beijing 100730, China. [2]Department of Respiratory and Critical Care Medicine, Clinical Microbiology and Infectious Disease Lab., China-Japan Friendship Hospital, Beijing 100029, China. [3]Department of Microbiology, The First Affiliated Hospital of Zhejiang University, Hangzhou 310003, China. [4]Division of Microbiology, Ruijin Hospital, School of Medicine, Shanghai Jiaotong University, Shanghai 200025, China. [5]Department of Infectious Diseases, SirRunRun Shaw Hospital, School of Medicine, Zhejiang University, Hangzhou 310016, China. [6]Department of Laboratory Medicine, Tongji Hospital, Tongji Medical College, Huazhong University of Science and Technology, Wuhan 430030, China. [7]Division of Microbiology, Zhongshan Hospital of Fudan University, Shanghai 200032, China. [8]Division of Microbiology, The First Affiliated Hospital of Chongqing Medical University, Chongqing 400016, China. [9]Department of Laboratory Medicine, Shandong Provincial Hospital Affiliated to Shandong University, Jinan 250021, China. [10]Infection control center, Xiangya Hospital, Central South University, Changsha 410008, China. [11]Division of Microbiology, The First Affiliated Hospital of Zhengzhou University, Zhenzhou 450052, China. [12]Division of Microbiology, The First Affiliated Hospital, Sun Yat-Sen University, Guangzhou 510080, China. [13]Department of Microbiology, The Chinese PLA General Hospital, Beijing 100853, China. [14]Division of Microbiology, Tianjin Medical University General Hospital, Tianjing 300052, China. [15]Division of Microbiology, The First Affiliated Hospital of Chinese Medical University, Shenyang 110001, China. [16]Department of Clinical Laboratory, The First Affiliated Hospital of Harbin Medical University, Harbin 150001, China. [17]Department of Clinical Laboratory, Beijing Friendship Hospital of Capital Medical University, Beijing 100020, China. [18]Clinical Laboratory, The Second Affiliated Hospital of Nanchang University, Nanchang 330006, China. [19]Microbiology Lab, Jilin Province People's Hospital, Changchun 130021, China. [20]Division of Microbiology, Haikou People's Hospital, Haikou 570208, China. [21]Division of Microbiology, General Hospital of Nanjing Military Command, Nanjing 210002, China. [22]Division of Microbiology, International Health Management Associates, Schaumburg, IL 60173-3817, USA.

References
1. Bi XC, Zhang B, Ye YK, He HC, Han ZD, Dai QS, et al. Pathogen incidence and antibiotic resistance patterns of catheter-associated urinary tract infection in children. J Chemother. 2009;21:661–5.
2. Qiao LD, Chen S, Yang Y, Zhang K, Zheng B, Guo HF, et al. Characteristics of urinary tract infection pathogens and their in vitro susceptibility to antimicrobial agents in China: data from a multicenter study. BMJ Open. 2013;3:e004152.

3. Hertz FB, Schonning K, Rasmussen SC, Littauer P, Knudsen JD, Lobner-Olesen A, et al. Epidemiological factors associated with ESBL- and non ESBL-producing E. coli causing urinary tract infection in general practice. Infect Dis (Lond). 2016;48:241–5.

4. Guembe M, Cercenado E, Alcala L, Marin M, Insa R, Bouza E. Evolution of antimicrobial susceptibility patterns of aerobic and facultative gram-negative bacilli causing intra-abdominal infections: results from the SMART studies 2003–2007. Rev Esp Quimioter. 2008;21:166–73.

5. Stapleton AE. Urinary tract infection pathogenesis: host factors. Infect Dis Clin North Am. 2014;28:149–59.

6. Foxman B. Urinary tract infection syndromes: occurrence, recurrence, bacteriology, risk factors, and disease burden. Infect Dis Clin North Am. 2014;28:1–13.

7. Wellington EM, Boxall AB, Cross P, Feil EJ, Gaze WH, Hawkey PM, et al. The role of the natural environment in the emergence of antibiotic resistance in gram-negative bacteria. Lancet Infect Dis. 2013;13:155–65.

8. Caccamo M, Perilli M, Celenza G, Bonfiglio G, Tempera G, Amicosante G. Occurrence of extended spectrum beta-lactamases among isolates of Enterobacteriaceae from urinary tract infections in southern Italy. Microb Drug Resist. 2006;12:257–64.

9. Al Yousef SA, Younis S, Farrag E, Moussa H, Bayoumi FS, Ali AM. Clinical and laboratory profile of urinary tract infections associated with extended Spectrum beta-Lactamase producing Escherichia coli and Klebsiella pneumoniae. Ann Clin Lab Sci. 2016;46:393–400.

10. Bonkat G, Muller G, Braissant O, Frei R, Tschudin-Suter S, Rieken M, et al. Increasing prevalence of ciprofloxacin resistance in extended-spectrum-beta-lactamase-producing Escherichia coli urinary isolates. World J Urol. 2013;31:1427–32.

11. Hawser SP, Bouchillon SK, Hoban DJ, Badal RE. In vitro susceptibilities of aerobic and facultative anaerobic Gram-negative bacilli from patients with intra-abdominal infections worldwide from 2005–2007: results from the SMART study. Int J Antimicrob Agents. 2009;34:585–8.

12. Institute CaLS. Method for dilution antimicrobial susceptibility tests for bacteria that grow aerobically; approved standard. 9th ed. Wayne: PA:CLSI document M7-A9; 2012.

13. Institute CaLS. Performance standards for antimicrobial susceptibility testing. Twenty-fifth informational supplement. Wayne: PA:Document M100-S25; 2015.

14. Gupta K, Hooton TM, Naber KG, Wullt B, Colgan R, Miller LG, et al. International clinical practice guidelines for the treatment of acute uncomplicated cystitis and pyelonephritis in women: a 2010 update by the infectious diseases Society of America and the European society for microbiology and infectious diseases. Clin Infect Dis. 2011;52:e103–20.

15. Zhao L, Chen X, Zhu X, Yang W, Dong L, Xu X, et al. Prevalence of virulence factors and antimicrobial resistance of uropathogenic Escherichia coli in Jiangsu province (China). Urology. 2009;74:702–7.

16. Hope R, Potz NA, Warner M, Fagan EJ, Arnold E, Livermore DM. Efficacy of practised screening methods for detection of cephalosporin-resistant Enterobacteriaceae. J Antimicrob Chemother. 2007;59:110–3.

17. Guo W, He Q, Wang Z, Wei M, Yang Z, Du Y, et al. Influence of antimicrobial consumption on gram-negative bacteria in inpatients receiving antimicrobial resistance therapy from 2008–2013 at a tertiary hospital in Shanghai, China. Am J Infect Control. 2015;43:358–64.

18. Ding H, Yang Y, Wei J, Fan S, Yu S, Yao K, et al. Influencing the use of antibiotics in a Chinese pediatric intensive care unit. Pharm World Sci. 2008; 30:787–93.

19. Zou YM, Ma Y, Liu JH, Shi J, Fan T, Shan YY, et al. Trends and correlation of antibacterial usage and bacterial resistance: time series analysis for antibacterial stewardship in a Chinese teaching hospital (2009–2013). Eur J Clin Microbiol Infect Dis. 2015;34:795–803.

20. Chanawong A, M'Zali FH, Heritage J, Xiong JH, Hawkey PM. Three cefotaximases, CTX-M-9, CTX-M-13, and CTX-M-14, among Enterobacteriaceae in the People's Republic of China. Antimicrob Agents Chemother. 2002;46:630–7.

21. Wang H, Kelkar S, Wu W, Chen M, Quinn JP. Clinical isolates of Enterobacteriaceae producing extended-spectrum beta-lactamases: prevalence of CTX-M-3 at a hospital in China. Antimicrob Agents Chemother. 2003;47:790–3.

22. Yang Q, Zhang H, Cheng J, Xu Z, Xu Y, Cao B, et al. In vitro activity of flomoxef and comparators against Escherichia coli, Klebsiella pneumoniae and Proteus mirabilis producing extended-spectrum beta-lactamases in China. Int J Antimicrob Agents. 2015;45:485–90.

23. Hawkey PM. Prevalence and clonality of extended-spectrum beta-lactamases in Asia. Clin Microbiol Infect. 2008;14 Suppl 1:159–65.

24. Bush K. Extended-spectrum beta-lactamases in North America, 1987–2006. Clin Microbiol Infect. 2008;14 Suppl 1:134–43.

25. Wang H, Dzink-Fox JL, Chen M, Levy SB. Genetic characterization of highly fluoroquinolone-resistant clinical Escherichia coli strains from China: role of acrR mutations. Antimicrob Agents Chemother. 2001;45:1515–21.

26. Ben-Ami R, Rodriguez-Bano J, Arslan H, Pitout JD, Quentin C, Calbo ES, et al. A multinational survey of risk factors for infection with extended-spectrum beta-lactamase-producing enterobacteriaceae in nonhospitalized patients. Clin Infect Dis. 2009;49:682–90.

27. Livermore DM, Oakton KJ, Carter MW, Warner M. Activity of ertapenem (MK-0826) versus Enterobacteriaceae with potent beta-lactamases. Antimicrob Agents Chemother. 2001;45:2831–7.

28. Essack SY. Treatment options for extended-spectrum beta-lactamase-producers. FEMS Microbiol Lett. 2000;190:181–4.

29. Paterson DL. Recommendation for treatment of severe infections caused by Enterobacteriaceae producing extended-spectrum beta-lactamases (ESBLs). Clin Microbiol Infect. 2000;6:460–3.

30. Kaczmarek FM, Dib-Hajj F, Shang W, Gootz TD. High-level carbapenem resistance in a Klebsiella pneumoniae clinical isolate is due to the combination of bla(ACT-1) beta-lactamase production, porin OmpK35/36 insertional inactivation, and down-regulation of the phosphate transport porin phoe. Antimicrob Agents Chemother. 2006;50:3396–406.

31. Bratu S, Landman D, Haag R, Recco R, Eramo A, Alam M, et al. Rapid spread of carbapenem-resistant Klebsiella pneumoniae in New York City: a new threat to our antibiotic armamentarium. Arch Intern Med. 2005;165:1430–5.

32. Vatopoulos A. High rates of metallo-beta-lactamase-producing Klebsiella pneumoniae in Greece–a review of the current evidence. Euro Surveill. 2008;13.

33. Maltezou HC, Giakkoupi P, Maragos A, Bolikas M, Raftopoulos V, Papahatzaki H, et al. Outbreak of infections due to KPC-2-producing Klebsiella pneumoniae in a hospital in Crete (Greece). J Infect. 2009;58:213–9.

34. Keller R, Pedroso MZ, Ritchmann R, Silva RM. Occurrence of virulence-associated properties in Enterobacter cloacae. Infect Immun. 1998;66:645–9.

35. Yang Q, Wang H, Sun H, Chen H, Xu Y, Chen M. Phenotypic and genotypic characterization of Enterobacteriaceae with decreased susceptibility to carbapenems: results from large hospital-based surveillance studies in China. Antimicrob Agents Chemother. 2010;54:573–7.

36. Han SB, Lee SC, Lee SY, Jeong DC, Kang JH. Aminoglycoside therapy for childhood urinary tract infection due to extended-spectrum beta-lactamase-producing Escherichia coli or Klebsiella pneumoniae. BMC Infect Dis. 2015; 15:414.

Oral fosfomycin for treatment of urinary tract infection

Philippa C. Matthews[1,2]*, Lucinda K. Barrett[1], Stephanie Warren[1], Nicole Stoesser[1,2], Mel Snelling[3], Matthew Scarborough[1] and Nicola Jones[1]

Abstract

Background: Fosfomycin is increasingly called upon for the treatment of multi drug-resistant (MDR) organisms causing urinary tract infection (UTI). We reviewed oral fosfomycin use for UTI treatment in a large UK hospital. The primary goal was to audit our clinical practice against current national guidelines. Secondary aims were to identify factors associated with treatment failure, and to investigate the potential for using fosfomycin in patients with co-morbidities.

Methods: We retrospectively studied 75 adult patients with UTI who received 151 episodes of treatment with fosfomycin from March 2013 to June 2015. We collected clinical data from our electronic patient record, and microbiology data pre- and post- fosfomycin treatment. We recorded additional data for patients receiving prolonged courses in order to make a preliminary assessment of safety and efficacy. We also reviewed >18,000 urinary tract isolates of *Escherichia coli* and *Klebsiella spp.* processed by our laboratory over the final year of our study period to determine the prevalence of fosfomycin resistance.

Results: There was a significant increase in fosfomycin treatment episodes over the course of the study period. Co-morbidities were present in 71 % of patients. The majority had *E. coli* infection (69 %), of which 59 % were extended spectrum beta-lactamase (ESBL)-producers. *Klebsiella* infections were more likely than *E. coli* to fail treatment, and more likely to be reported as fosfomycin resistant in cases of relapse following treatment. There were no adverse events in five patients treated with prolonged fosfomycin. Among all urinary isolates collected over a year, fosfomycin resistance was documented in 1 % of *E. coli* vs. 19 % of *Klebsiella* spp. ($p < 0.0001$).

Conclusions: We report an important role for oral fosfomycin for MDR UTI treatment in a UK hospital population, and based on the findings from this study, we present our own local guidelines for its use. We present preliminary data suggesting that fosfomycin is safe and effective for use in patients with complex comorbidities and over prolonged time periods, but may be less effective against *Klebsiella* than *E. coli*.

Keywords: Gram-negative, UTI, *Escherichia coli*, Uropathogens, Urosepsis, Fosfomycin, Antibacterials, Antibacterial resistance

Background

Urinary tract infections (UTI) are common and account for a significant burden of hospital admissions and associated healthcare expenditure [1]. Treatment has become more challenging due to an ageing population, high rates of comorbid disease and polypharmacy, allergy or intolerance to antimicrobial drugs, a growing number of patients with underlying immunological or anatomical defects, and the increasing prevalence of multi-drug resistant pathogens [1, 2]. Re-evaluation of 'neglected' antibacterial drugs is one approach to tackling this complicated burden of disease [3, 4]. One such agent, fosfomycin, is being called back into play in the UK for treating UTI [5, 6].

Characteristics that make fosfomycin appealing for the treatment of UTI include rapid absorption after oral administration, concentration for excretion in urine, biofilm activity [7, 8], and its efficacy against many

* Correspondence: p.matthews@doctors.org.uk
[1]Department of Infectious Diseases and Microbiology, Oxford University Hospitals NHS Foundation Trust, John Radcliffe Hospital, Headley Way, Headington, Oxford OX3 9DU, UK
[2]Nuffield Department of Medicine, University of Oxford, Peter Medawar Building for Pathogen Research, South Parks Road, Oxford OX1 3SY, UK
Full list of author information is available at the end of the article

multi-drug resistant organisms, including extended spectrum beta-lactamase (ESBL) and AmpC-producing Enterobacteriaceae [9]. Oral fosfomycin is well tolerated and largely free of serious adverse effects [10, 11], with only 5 % of patients reporting side-effects, most commonly diarrhoea [12].

Until recently, the only preparation of fosfomycin available in the UK was unlicensed Monuril (fosfomycin trometamol) imported from Germany. However, a licensed product has now become available (Mercury Pharmaceuticals). National guidelines have been published by two UK agencies, NICE (National Institute for Health and Care Excellence) and PHE (Public Health England); fosfomycin is recommended for uncomplicated UTI (defined as no fever/flank pain) caused by ESBL-producing *E. coli* in adults, if the prescription is endorsed by a microbiologist [13–15].

Approaches to dosing vary: NICE guidelines suggest a single dose of 3 g in women and two 3 g doses (at an interval of 3 days) in men [14], but the UK product licence is for a single dose only and European guidelines produced by the European Association of Urology do not recommend fosfomycin for use in men at all [16]. Although the UK recommendation is restricted to uncomplicated lower UTI [3, 14, 17, 18], and the focus of existing guidance is for out-patient treatment, fosfomycin has also been used with some success in patients with risk factors for persistent or recurrent UTI [11, 12, 19].

Nitrofurantoin is a potential alternative treatment for UTI caused by MDR *E. coli* [13], but is not recommended in the third trimester of pregnancy, and should be used with caution in patients with significant renal impairment. Guidance on the estimated glomerular filtration rate (eGFR) threshold for use has varied, generally being set at 45 ml/min, but also sanctioned for use in certain circumstances down to 30 ml/min [20]. Pivmecillinam is another potential choice of oral agent, but susceptibility testing has only recently been introduced in our institution, and was not in routine use until after the time period described by this study.

We retrospectively studied the use of fosfomycin in our large teaching hospital by auditing local prescribing against existing guidelines [14, 16], with the primary aim of developing a clear picture of the context in which this agent is currently used, and identifying ways in which prescribing can be optimized. Secondly, having identified a small group of patients receiving prolonged or recurrent treatment, we scrutinized these cases to gain insights into special situations that are not covered by current guidance, but in which fosfomycin may have a useful role. Finally, within the constraints of a retrospective study, we sought to identify preliminary evidence for factors predictive of treatment failure, in order to inform ongoing research efforts and to guide treatment decisions.

Methods
Study design
We undertook a retrospective observational study of oral fosfomycin use for UTI. We included all episodes of oral fosfomycin use for the treatment of UTI in adults age ≥16 years, from March 2013 (when this agent was first added to our local formulary) through to the end of June 2015, irrespective of urine culture results.

Characteristics of patient cohort
The study centre is a large tertiary referral teaching hospital in Oxfordshire, UK, with >1400 in-patient beds serving a population of 805,000 (http://www.ouh.nhs.uk). Our population of individuals with complex, recurrent, resistant or persistent UTI is inflated by a tertiary referral service for urology, a large renal dialysis unit, and a regional renal transplant unit.

This cohort represents a group of patients who were all deemed well enough to receive treatment with an oral antibacterial agent. Routine clinical practice would be to admit any patient unwell with signs of systemic sepsis or clinical suspicion of pyelonephritis for monitoring, imaging, and treatment with intravenous antimicrobial therapy (this is a clinical assessment based on the whole picture, but would hinge on features such as fever >38 °C, tachycardia, hypotension, loin or back pain, and raised inflammatory markers).

We identified fosfomycin treatment episodes retrospectively using electronic records held by pharmacy. Based on the complex and changing product licence of fosfomycin, as well as recommendations made by NICE guidelines [14], local policy is that all fosfomycin prescriptions should be authorized by the infectious diseases/microbiology team. During the period of this study, general practitioners were not able to access fosfomycin, so all prescriptions were generated by hospital clinicians. Our practice is to give oral fosfomycin as monotherapy for UTI treatment.

Data collection methods
We collected data on patient demographics, co-morbid diagnoses and laboratory parameters from the hospital electronic patient record (EPR, Powerchart), and culture results from electronic microbiology records (Sunquest). We were unable to gain access to sufficient paper records to review in detail the clinical symptoms at the time of every treatment episode. However, in the five patients who each received >10 fosfomycin doses, we did obtain paper-based clinical notes as an additional source of information.

Analysis of fosfomycin resistance

In order to develop an overview of fosfomycin resistance in our region, we also reviewed antibacterial susceptibility data from *E. coli* and *Klebsiella* spp. isolated from all urine cultures processed by our laboratory during the final twelve-month period of our study. These represent unselected samples submitted from both primary and secondary care settings. We focused our analysis on these two organisms as they collectively account for >80 % of UTIs treated with fosfomycin (see 'Microbiology of UTI treated with fosfomycin' in results).

Standards for evaluation of prescribing

We used guidance published by Public Health England (PHE) [15] and NICE [14] as standards against which to evaluate our own prescribing.

Laboratory methods

Antimicrobial susceptibilities for uropathogens were determined using the BD Phoenix Automated Microbiology System (Becton Dickinson, Franklin Lakes, New Jersey; NMIC-75 panel. For fosfomycin, this contains Glucose-6-Phosphate). BD Phoenix utilises an optimised colorimetric redox indicator to detect active growth of an organism in the presence of the antimicrobial. The organism to be tested is grown on a non-selective medium in appropriate conditions (37 °C in O_2 for *E. coli* / *Klebsiella* spp.) for 16–18 h, before a 0.5 MacFarland suspension is prepared (BD AutoPrep). This suspension is inoculated into the appropriate antimicrobial susceptibility testing panel (gram negative NMIC-75) that contains microwells pre-lined with increasing concentrations of antimicrobial. The panel is incubated at 35 °C on the instrument for up to 16 h, and automatically read every 20 min for growth. The MIC (minimum inhibitory concentration) for each antimicrobial is then determined by the concentration at which the organism fails to grow. The breakpoint for fosfomycin susceptibility was ≤32 mg/L for oral treatment of uncomplicated UTI based on breakpoint data published both by the European Committee for Antimicrobial Susceptibility Testing (EUCAST), available on-line at www.eucast.org, and the British Society for Antimicrobial Chemotherapy (BSAC) Standing Committee on Susceptibility Testing, available on line at http://bsac.org.uk.

ESBL-production was detected by BD Phoenix. For *E. coli* and *Klebsiella pneumoniae*, ESBL-positivity is reported based on an ESBL test (a differential response between the inhibitory effect of 2nd/3rd generation cephalosporins used alone or in combination with clavulanic acid) and/or an ESBL phenotypic pattern (resistance to piperacillin in combination with resistance to any of the ESBL screening drugs, cefotaxime, ceftriaxone, ceftazidime, cefpodoxime or aztreonam in organisms that are carbapenem-susceptible).

Other oral antibacterial agents for which susceptibility was routinely tested include amoxicillin, co-amoxiclav (amoxicillin/clavulanate), cephalexin, trimethoprim, nitrofurantoin and ciprofloxacin. During the study period, our laboratory did not routinely test susceptibility to pivmecillinam.

Definitions for treatment outcome

Due to the retrospective, observational approach, this study was not designed to provide robust assessment of clinical cure. However we set out to interrogate the microbiology dataset for any preliminary evidence of outcome following fosfomycin treatment.

We divided the potential laboratory outcomes into the following five endpoint categories:

(i) No follow-up sample available;
(ii) Sterile urine;
(iii) Isolation of an indistinguishable organism compared to pre-treatment cultures (may represent relapse);
(iv) Isolation of a different organism compared to pre-treatment cultures (may represent re-infection);
(v) Mixed growth (may represent either a contaminated sample, or relapse/re-infection).

We used these five endpoints to group patients into the following two broad outcome categories:

(a) 'Microbiological cure' was our stringent cure definition, classifying only individuals for whom there was a sterile urine sample following their treatment episode as being cured (endpoint (ii) from the list above).
(b) 'Functional cure' was a more relaxed definition. Those classified as 'cured' in this case included those with microbiological cure as defined above (endpoint (ii)), but was also expanded to include patients for whom there was no follow-up sample (endpoint (i), suggesting likely clinical cure).

We excluded analysis of those for whom repeat cultures showed either pure growth of a different organism from baseline (endpoint (iv)) or mixed growth (endpoint (v)). This approach was based on the rationale that in patients with a different organism at follow-up, re-infection is the most likely explanation. This scenario is not suggestive of failure of index treatment with fosfomycin (and is rather a marker of the nature of this cohort in which patients have complex underlying reasons for recurrence of UTI, that is not related to failure of the antibacterial agent). Mixed cultures are of uncertain significance, potentially representing contamination of the urine sample, or recurrent infection with more than one organism; neither of these outcomes can be regarded as robust evidence of fosfomycin failure.

Data analysis

We recorded and analysed our data in a Microsoft Excel spreadsheet (Microsoft 2011; v14.5.7). Additional analysis was undertaken using Prism v6.0f, and on-line at http://graphpad.com. We used open access regression analysis tools in Google sheets to produce Fig. 1.

For univariate analysis of factors associated with cure, we used the Mann–Whitney U-test to assess the statistical significance of differences between groups for continuous variables, and Chi-square/Fisher's Exact Test for categorical variables (depending on sample size).

For multivariate analysis, we selected variables to enter based on those reaching statistical significance at univariate level (*Klebsiella* infections) and variables that we predicted *a priori* to predict fosfomycin treatment failure, namely in vitro fosfomycin resistance, creatinine clearance and comorbidity. Analysis was undertaken using a logistic regression approach in Google sheets (https://docs.google.com/spreadsheets).

Study approval

This study was registered and approved by the Audit Department at Oxford University Hospitals NHS Foundation Trust. Informed consent was not deemed to be required.

Results

Characteristics of patient cohort

During the study period, 75 patients received oral fosfomycin, undergoing 151 treatment episodes (for raw data, see Additional file 1). There was a significant increase in fosfomycin prescriptions by month over the time period studied (Fig. 1). Females outnumbered males (57 vs. 18). The median age was 73 years (IQR 55–80; range 16–94), with no difference in age according to sex ($p = 0.7$, Mann Whitney U test).

Co-morbidities or risk factors for UTI were present in 52/75 patients (71 %), most commonly underlying renal tract disease (Table 1). eGFR was ≥10 mL / min in all patients. There was documented evidence of input from the microbiology/infectious diseases team in the EPR for 57/75 (76 %) index treatment episodes.

Microbiology of UTI treated with fosfomycin

We analysed microbiology data initially focusing just on the first treatment episode for each patient. The majority had urine cultures positive for *E. coli* (52/75, 69 %; Table 2). ESBL-production was reported in 31/52 of the *E. coli* isolates (59 %) and 6/9 *K. pneumoniae* (67 %); (Table 2). Overall, therefore, only 31/75 (41 %) of all isolates met the microbiological criterion (ESBL *E. coli*) for fosfomycin treatment stipulated by NICE guidance [14]. This result reflects a discrepancy between our own clinical practice and current guidelines.

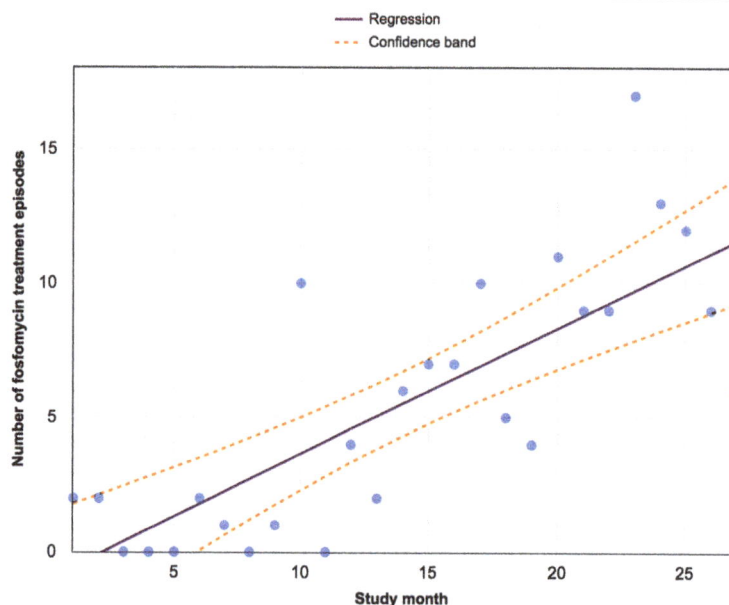

Fig. 1 Number of fosfomycin treatment episodes by month in a cohort of adults treated for UTI in a UK teaching hospital. Each data point represents the number of unique fosfomycin prescriptions (irrespective of total dose) issued each month, from the time fosfomycin was first introduced to our formulary (March 2013) over 27 months to the end of the study period (May 2015). The solid line represents the trend computed by linear regression (slope = 0.46, 95 % CI 0.31-0.62, R^2 = 0.6, $p < 0.0001$); the dashed lines indicate 95 % confidence intervals around the regression line

Table 1 Risk factors for urinary tract infection in a cohort of 75 adults treated with oral fosfomycin

Risk factor	Number of cases (% of all individuals treated)
GU tract pathology (stones, cancer of prostate/bladder/kidneys, urethral disease, self catheterisation)	25 (33.3)
Renal transplant	12 (16.0)
Systemic disease (non-renal tract malignancy, steroids, diabetes, cardiovascular disease, GI tract disease)	12 (16.0)
Pregnant	3 (4.0)
No documented risk factor(s) [a]	23 (30.7)
TOTAL	75

[a] No cases of recent urological intervention or patients with indwelling urethral catheters were identified on the basis of retrospective review of electronic records

Unexpectedly, fosfomycin was prescribed for two patients with a urinary isolate that was reported as fosfomycin resistant in vitro; one of these was *E. coli* and the other *Enterobacter aerogenes*. There were a further two isolates for which an in vitro fosfomycin susceptibility was not reported (both *E. coli*).

Treatment episodes and dose schedules
The majority of individuals ($n = 53/75$; 71 %) had just one fosfomycin treatment episode during the study period; eight patients had two treatment episodes and fourteen patients received ≥3 treatment courses. There was no relationship between age or sex and receipt of >1 treatment episode ($p = 0.9$ and $p = 0.2$, respectively).

NICE guidelines recommend a single dose of fosfomycin for females, and two doses (off-licence) for males [13, 15]. Among females in this study cohort, 45/57 (79 %) first treatment episodes adhered to the single dose recommendation [13, 15] with the remaining 12 being prescribed two or three doses. In contrast, among males, only 8/18 (44 %) received the recommended ≥2 doses. However, across all 151 treatment episodes, men were more likely to be prescribed additional fosfomycin doses (median 1 dose in women, versus median 3 doses in men $p < 0.0001$; data not shown).

Potential for treatment with nitrofurantoin
Among index treatment episodes, 31/75 (41 %) patients had an isolate that was nitrofurantoin susceptible; 30/31 of these were *E. coli* (Table 2). Among the 31 patients with nitrofurantoin-susceptible isolates, 30 had contemporaneous measurement of renal function. Of these 30, four were ineligible for nitrofurantoin due to eGFR <30 mL/min, one was pregnant, and another had previously failed to respond to nitrofurantoin. This leaves a total of 24 individuals for whom there was no documented contra-indication to nitrofurantoin, but who received fosfomycin instead.

Prolonged or recurrent fosfomycin treatment
In five individuals, treatment with standard short-course fosfomycin failed to sterilize the urinary tract, and longer courses were used (Table 3). There were no documented concerns about safety or tolerability, and infection was either cured or suppressed sufficiently to keep the patient out of hospital during the treatment course, although two subsequently relapsed and have been re-treated.

Treatment outcomes
Although this study was not specifically designed to ascertain outcomes, we sought preliminary evidence for

Table 2 Urine culture results obtained at index episode of UTI in 75 adults treated with oral fosfomycin

Urine culture result	Number (% of all patients)[a]	Number with ESBL (% of cases with this organism)[b]	Number nitrofurantoin sensitive (% of cases with this organism)[b]	Number fosfomycin sensitive (% of cases with this organism)[b]
Escherichia coli	52/75 (69.3)	31/52 (58.5)	30/52 (56.6)	49/50 (98.0)
Klebsiella pneumoniae	9/75 (12.0)	6/9 (66.7)	1/9 (11.1)	9/9 (100.0)
Other Enterobacteriaceae in pure growth	6/75 (8.0)	0/6 (0)	0/6 (0)	5/6 (83.3)
Pseudomonas	1/75 (1.3)	n/a	n/a	n/d
Mixed growth	4/75 (5.3)	n/a	n/a	n/a
No significant growth	2/75 (2.7)	n/a	n/a	n/a
No data	1/75 (1.3)	n/a	n/a	n/a
Total	75/75	37/61	31/61	63/65

n/a not applicable, *n/d* no data

[a]The denominator in this column is the total number of patients with a urinary isolate ($n = 75$)

[b]The denominator in these columns is adjusted according to data availability / relevance. Note that fosfomycin susceptibility data were missing for two *E. coli* isolates

Table 3 Summary of five patients treated with more than ten 3 g doses of oral fosfomycin for UTI

Study number	Age group at first dose (years)	Gender	Clinical background, including possible risk factors for UTI	Urine culture result	Total number of 3 g fosfomycin doses	eGFR at baseline	Any reported side-effects	Notes on outcome
FOS015	80–89	M	Vasculopath; bilateral below knee amputations. Recurrent *E. coli* bacteraemia with unclear source despite extensive investigation. Relapsed after a treatment course of iv ertapenem	ESBL *E. coli*	36	79	None reported	Well when reviewed following end of treatment course; discharged from clinic
FOS038	60–69	M	History of recurrent UTI for > 10 years. Dilatation for urethral stricture, followed by TURP. Prostate cancer confirmed; treated post-op with radiotherapy	ESBL *E. coli*	81	>90	None reported	Interval free of infection, followed by recurrence of UTI (different organisms)
FOS060	60–69	M	Relapsing urosepsis following TRUS biopsy (negative for prostate cancer). Presumed prostatitis as focus of infection.	ESBL *E. coli*	33	79	Reported shortness of breath during treatment, but thought unlikely to be related to fosfomycin	Well when reviewed following end of treatment course; discharged from clinic
FOS098	70–79	M	Transitional cell carcinoma treated with nephroureterectomy. Regular surveillance cystoscopy complicated by recurrent UTI; recurred after completing treatment with meropenem.	ESBL *E. coli*	49	41	None reported	Interval free of infection, followed by recurrence and re-treatment with fosfomycin
FOS140	40–49	F	Recurrent UTI following sling procedure and botox treatment for stress/urge incontinence. Intermittent self-catheterisation. Good symptomatic relief with fosfomycin.	*E. coli*	15	>90	None reported	Ongoing prophylaxis while awaiting urogynaecology surgery

eGFR estimated glomerular filtration rate, *TURP* trans-urethral resection of the prostate, *TRUS* trans-rectal ultrasound guided prostate biopsy

the success of treatment, using two different definitions, 'functional' cure and 'microbiological' cure (see Methods). Follow-up culture results were obtained at a median of 13 days following the first fosfomycin dose (range 2–241 days; IQR 7–40 days).

Follow-up outcomes based on urine cultures were divided into five categories as follows: no follow-up sample available (22/75; 29.3 %), sterile urine at follow-up (21/75; 28 %), isolation of the same organism compared to pre-treatment cultures (19/75; 25.3 %), isolation of a different organism compared to pre-treatment cultures (8/75, 10.6 %) and mixed growth (5/75; 6.6 %).

(i) Microbiological cure: Using this stringent definition of cure, only 40/75 cases could be classified (the remaining 35 either had no post-treatment culture data ($n = 22$), had culture data more suggestive of reinfection ($n = 8$), or a mixed/contaminated sample ($n = 5$)). Of the 40 that could be classified (Table 4), 21 (53 %) met the criteria for cure, and no factor was statistically associated with failure.

(ii) Functional cure: Among 75 index treatment episodes, 61 patients could be classified using this more relaxed cure definition (the remaining 14

were equivocal due to post-treatment urine culture being unavailable ($n = 1$), growing a different organism ($n = 8$) or a mixed/contaminated sample ($n = 5$). Of these, 42/61 (69 %) were considered cured. The only factor associated with failure on univariate analysis was infection with *K. pneumoniae* ($p = 0.03$; Table 4). This finding should be interpreted with caution as statistical significance is lost when correction for multiple comparisons is undertaken (e.g. by a Bonferroni approach). However, undertaking a multivariate approach to analysis again demonstrated *Klebsiella* as a significant predictor of treatment failure ($p = 0.04$; Table 5).

Selection of fosfomycin resistance within this cohort

On follow-up urine culture, there were 19 instances in which the identification of the organism was the same as that from pre-treatment culture. In five isolates that had been fosfomycin susceptible at baseline, the follow-up culture was reported fosfomycin resistant (four *Klebsiella pneumoniae* and one *Morganella morganii*). Selection of resistance was significantly more frequent in non-*E. coli* Enterobacteriaceae than in *E. coli* (5/6 vs. 0/13; $p = 0.0005$).

Table 4 Univariate analysis of clinical and laboratory variables as predictors of outcome for fosfomycin treatment of urinary tract infection in adults. Cure and fail are classified according to 'functional' definition (results presented in data columns 1–3) or 'microbiological' definition (results presented in data columns 4–6)

Predictor	'Cure' (functional definition) Total n = 42	'Fail' (functional definition) Total n = 19	p-value (functional definition)	'Cure' (microbiological definition) Total n = 21	'Fail' (microbiological definition) Total n = 19	p-value (microbiological definition)
ESBL-positive	20/37	10/19	1.0[a]	12/21	10/19	1[a]
Nitrofurantoin resistant	17/37	12/19	0.3[a]	8/21	12/19	0.2[a]
Fosfomycin resistant	1/35	1/19	1.0[a]	0/20	1/19	0.49[a]
Male	14/42	4/19	0.4[a]	4/21	4/19	0.72[a]
Klebsiella pneumoniae	2/37	5/19	0.03[a]	2/21	5/19	0.22[a]
Comorbidity (any)	32/42	15/19	1.0[a]	12/21	15/19	0.19[a]
Transplant	8/42	3/19	1.0[a]	4/21	3/19	1[a]
Urethral catheter	4/42	3/19	0.66[a]	2/21	3/19	0.65[a]
Median age, years (IQR)	75 (62–81)	64 (42–79)	0.13[b]	70 (58–78)	64 (42–79)	0.47[b]
Median eGFR, ml/min (IQR)	70 (41–87)	>90 (29– > 90)	0.2[b]	64 (38–89)	>90 (29– > 90)	0.26[b]
Median CRP, mg/L (IQR)	21 (3–93)	25 (6–62)	1.0[b]	16 (2–78)	25 (6–62)	0.84[b]

Total number of patients represented is 61 for functional cure ('cure' group (n = 42) is patients with a sterile urine on follow-up culture, or no follow-up culture; 'fail' group (n = 19) is patients with recurrent growth of an indistinguishable organism). Total number of patients is 40 for microbiological cure ('cure' group (n = 21) is patients with a sterile urine on follow-up culture; 'fail' group (n = 19) is patients with recurrent growth of an indistinguishable organism)
The denominator in some rows is smaller than the overall total due to missing data, including no culture / susceptibility data and ESBL-status unknown or not applicable
eGFR estimated glomerular filtration rate, *CRP* C-reactive protein
[a]Fisher's Exact Test; [b] Mann Whitney *U* test

Fosfomycin resistance patterns in all urine isolates of *E. coli* and *Klebsiella*

Of 18,474 urinary *E. coli* and *Klebsiella spp.* isolates processed by our laboratory in the final twelve months of the study, 511 were fosfomycin resistant (3 %). The majority of these were *Klebsiella* spp. (363/1888 (19 %) fosfomycin resistant, versus 148/16586 (1 %) for *E. coli*;

$p < 0.0001$). There was no relationship between ESBL-production and fosfomycin resistance (data not shown).

Mortality

Our electronic patient record did not record any patient deaths. However, this study was not designed to capture mortality data robustly and we cannot exclude the

Table 5 Multivariate analysis of clinical and laboratory variables as predictors of outcome for fosfomycin treatment of urinary tract infection in adults. Cure and fail are classified according to 'functional' definition (results presented in data columns 1–3) or 'microbiological' definition (results presented in data columns 4–6)

Predictor	'Cure' (functional definition) Total n = 33	'Fail' (functional definition) Total n = 19	p-value (functional definition)	'Cure' (microbiological definition) Total n = 20	'Fail' (microbiological definition) Total n = 19	p-value (microbiological definition)
Fosfomycin resistant in vitro	1/33	1/19	0.21	0/20	1/19	0.99
Klebsiella pneumoniae	2/33	5/19	0.04	2/20	5/19	0.13
Comorbidity (any, including transplant/urethral catheter)	21/33	14/19	0.22	15/20	14/19	0.47
Median eGFR, ml/min (IQR)	64 (41–86)	90 (29–90)	0.19	64 (37–87)	90 (29–90)	0.20

Total number of patients represented is 52 for functional cure ('cure' group (n = 33) is patients with a sterile urine on follow-up culture, or no follow-up culture; 'fail' group (n = 19) is patients with recurrent growth of an indistinguishable organism)
Total number of patients represented is 39 for microbiological cure ('cure' group (n = 20) is patients with a sterile urine on follow-up culture; 'fail' group (n = 19) is patients with recurrent growth of an indistinguishable organism)
eGFR estimated glomerular filtration rate

possibility that patients referred for treatment from outside our region may subsequently have died.

Discussion

As the global prevalence of drug resistance increases, fosfomycin is likely to become increasingly called upon for the oral treatment of UTI [21], as well as for other infections of the urogenital tract including prostatitis [22]. This pattern is reflected in our own centre, in which we show that fosfomycin prescriptions have increased over time. Within the constraints of retrospective analysis, it is difficult to be certain what underpins this change, but we can postulate that the increase in treatment episodes is most likely to reflect increased clinician awareness of fosfomycin as a formulary agent, recognition of NICE guidelines, and potentially an increase in the number of patients presenting with MDR organisms over time.

Current NICE guidelines [14] are based on only four small studies (for summary, see Additional file 2) of which two were undertaken in Turkey, one in Spain and one in North America [10, 11, 19, 23]. This cohort is therefore a significant recent addition to the data, and offers a unique snapshot of a UK population. A median age of 73 is likely to reflect the increasing risk of UTI with age [24], as well as the fact that co-morbid problems increase with age.

In our subgroup analysis, only 21 of 40 cases (53 %) met our most stringent definition of cure. Notably, 22 cases were excluded from this analysis as there was no follow-up data; this may well artificially lower the proportion of cases that we were able to report as cured. Low cure rates may also be a result of the complex population described here (co-morbidity, older age, urethral catheters), but due to small numbers none of these factors was found to be independently predictive of treatment failure (Table 4).

We identified several notable patterns in fosfomycin prescribing and outcomes. Firstly, males were significantly less likely to receive the recommended fosfomycin treatment dose than females based on NICE guidance [13]. Secondly, our data suggest a lower chance of cure in UTI caused by *Klebsiella* spp., consistent with higher local in vitro resistance rates, also observed elsewhere [25–27]. Interestingly, however, the failure of fosfomycin in this cohort occurred even with *Klebsiella* isolates that were reported as fosfomycin susceptible pre-treatment. In the absence of robust prospective data collection, we can only speculate why fosfomycin might have been used in two patients with an isolate reported as resistant in vitro. The most likely explanations are that the fosfomycin was prescribed prior to the full susceptibility data being released from the laboratory and/or the patient had a previous urinary isolate that was reported as fosfomycin susceptible.

Thirdly, this cohort is of particular interest in being enriched for individuals with significant risk factors for recurrent, resistant and difficult-to-treat UTI due to the tertiary referral specialties in our centre. We did not find any association between co-morbidities and increased risk of treatment failure in this cohort. This is preliminary evidence that fosfomycin can be safe and effective for treating UTI even in this complex group, although larger numbers and prospective studies are needed to assess this with greater confidence.

Finally, in this cohort, nearly one-third of patients were potentially eligible for treatment with nitrofurantoin, which is licensed, easier to access, and cheaper [14]. However, the retrospective approach to data collection meant it was not possible to identify the proportion of these patients in whom there was a contra-indication to nitrofurantoin. Another alternative agent for the treatment of urinary tract infection caused by ESBL-producing Enterobacteriaceae is pivmecillinam [28], which may increasingly be called into play.

Concerns regarding wider use of fosfomycin include tolerability, cost, and the spread of resistance; we address these issues here in turn.

Regarding tolerability, in our five patients who received multiple fosfomycin doses, the clinical notes suggested the drug was well tolerated. This is consistent with previous reports [19, 22, 23, 29].

In terms of economic implications in the UK, a single sachet of fosfomycin 3 g can currently cost £10-60 depending on the supply route (unlicensed or licensed product) compared to an equivalent three day treatment regimen with nitrofurantoin for which the total is < £3 [14]. Although nitrofurantoin is cheaper, there are potential disadvantages, including uncommon (but potentially serious) side effects, and the need for longer courses (typically four times daily dosing for 3 to 5 days). Alternative oral agents may have been possible in some cases, but 31/75 patients in this cohort had no other oral alternative. In these instances, fosfomycin saves the cost, risks and time taken to provide intravenous therapy.

The issue of selection and spread of resistance is complex [6, 16, 21, 30, 31]. Notably, in this study, the post-treatment isolate in 5/19 cases of microbiological failure was fosfomycin-resistant, all of which were non-*E. coli* Enterobacteriaceae. Fosfomycin resistance can be caused by a number of different mechanisms, including chromosomal mutations in genes encoding membrane transport systems or regulators of these transporters (*uhpA*, *uhpT*, *glpT*, *ptsI*), modification of murA (the drug's target of action), or the presence of catalytic enzymes encoded by *fos* genes, some of which can be transferred on mobile genetic elements [21, 30, 31]. A recent analysis reports a fosfomycin resistance rate of 0.5 % in community-acquired *E. coli* UTI in women in the UK [24]; it is unsurprising that our figure is higher (1 %) as this includes a hospital population at more risk of MDR organisms.

Data from both in vitro and clinical studies suggest that the emergence of resistance during treatment is higher for *Pseudomonas aeruginosa, Proteus, Klebsiella* and *Enterobacter* spp., as opposed to *E. coli*, [21, 27] consistent with what we observed here, and suggesting that fosfomycin should be used with caution in infections caused by these organisms.

In this current study, multivariate analysis is somewhat limited by small patient numbers and by missing data (due to the retrospective approach). Furthermore, the selection of variables entered into a multivariate analysis is characteristically based on those which reach statistical significance at univariate level; in this case only *Klebsiella* infection reached this threshold. Nevertheless, entering factors that could reasonably be hypothesized to be predictive of treatment failure into multivariate analysis, Klebsiella still emerged as significantly associated with failure ($p = 0.04$). A small study from Hong Kong also points to a higher rates of failure in *Klebsiella* compared to *E. coli* UTI [27]. The benefits of more widespread use of fosfomycin therefore have to be balanced against the dual risks of increasing selection pressures for resistance, and these preliminary data suggesting that it may be less efficacious against Klebsiella infection, irrespective of in vitro susceptibility.

There are several caveats and limitations to this study. Although our cohort is larger than previous equivalent studies (Additional file 1: Table S1), our power to derive statistically significant findings is still limited by small numbers of patients in each individual subgroup (highlighted by the breakdown of characteristics presented in Tables 1, 2, 4 and 5). Certain data (e.g. co-morbidities and involvement of the microbiology team) may have been under-reported in the EPR. We did not have access to complete paper records for the full cohort, so we have not been able to provide a detailed description of patient symptoms at the outset of treatment. Thus we have not been able to discriminate between asymptomatic bacteriuria and symptomatic UTI, or to identify features to distinguish between upper and lower UTI.

The retrospective study design also made assessment of clinical and microbiological end-points challenging, and made it impossible to justify why fosfomycin was chosen for treatment in each individual case. A related problem is the tertiary referral nature of our centre, which means that relevant culture data may have been generated elsewhere, and this may have led to missing culture data at the outset of treatment, and a potential over-estimation of cases of functional cure. Further prospective studies are undoubtedly warranted to scrutinize prescribing and outcomes in larger cohorts, to collect more complete and robust clinical data and to provide a more reliable assessment of

final outcome, including seeking information from primary care regarding previous or subsequent courses of antibacterial therapy. Those wishing to apply our conclusions to their own centres should consider carefully the extent to which the cohort and epidemiology described here is comparable to their own patient populations.

Nevertheless, as a consequence of the data presented here, we have reviewed our local approach to fosfomycin prescribing, and have produced new guidelines with a view to making our own use of fosfomycin more rational and consistent. These include the following recommendations:

i. Use of an alternative oral agent, particularly nitrofurantoin, should be considered first; fosfomycin should only be used if other oral options are contraindicated on the grounds of in vitro susceptibility data or clinical factors (drug allergy, pregnancy, renal impairment, previous treatment failure);

ii. Fosfomycin may be used in patients with UTI caused by non-*E. coli* Enterobacteriaceae, but only after careful consideration, particularly considering the potential risk of treatment failure for infection caused by *Klebsiella* spp.;

iii. The number of doses of fosfomycin treatment should be carefully considered: gender-based dosing is suggested by NICE, although this approach is not uniform. Additional doses may be used for patients in whom eradication of infection is difficult.

iv. Underlying medical or surgical risk factors should not be considered a contra-indication to treatment with fosfomycin, and this preliminary evidence suggests that prolonged courses are likely to be safe and well tolerated; however, such patients need to be kept under close expert review.

v. The optimum way to ensure that all of these factors are considered is to reinforce the recommendation that all individuals receiving oral fosfomycin are discussed with the infectious diseases/microbiology team. We have added fosfomycin to the electronic guidelines available to clinicians via the 'Microguide' app (http://microguide.eu/).

vi. We have implemented a protocol for primary care physicians to access fosfomycin for patients in the community, following telephone or email approval from a hospital microbiologist.

Conclusions

Overall, our findings underline the important role of fosfomycin in the antibacterial armamentarium for treatment of UTI. At present, the evidence of benefit is strongest for *E. coli* infections, and careful stewardship is important to reduce the risk of selection of antimicrobial resistance. This study also provides preliminary data to suggest that prolonged courses of this drug are safe and can be effective in suppressing or eradicating multi-resistant organisms even in immunosuppressed patients and in the setting of complex, abnormal renal tract anatomy.

Additional files

Additional file 1: Spreadsheet reporting 75 unique patients treated with fosfomycin for urinary tract infections. This excel file contains anonymised details of 75 unique adult patients treated with fosfomycin for urinary tract infections at Oxford University Hospitals NHS Foundation Trust from March 2013 through June 2015. Our original analysis also included patient sex, but this has been removed from the suppl. data file in order to protect anonymity.

Additional file 2: Tabulated summary of studies that have informed current NICE guidelines for fosfomycin use in UTI. This table contains a brief summary of four studies from Europe/North America that are referenced by current NICE guidelines regarding the use of oral fosfomycin for treatment of UTI, including date of study, cohort location, study design and cure data.

Abbreviations

BSAC: British Society for Antimicrobial Chemotherapy; *E. coli*: *Escherichia coli*; eGFR: Estimated glomerular filtration rate; EPR: Electronic patient record; ESBL: Extended spectrum beta-lactamase; EUCAST: European Committee for Antimicrobial Susceptibility Testing; MIC: Minimum inhibitory concentration; NICE: National Institute for Health and Care Excellence; PHE: Public Health England; UTI: Urinary tract infection

Acknowledgements
We would like to thank the OXMID group and Oxford University Hospitals Antimicrobial Steering Group for helpful feedback on these data, and Mr. Marcus Morgan for his help with laboratory data and protocols.

Funding
No specific funding was obtained for the production of this article. During the period of the study, PCM received a research salary from the NIHR. During the final phases of manuscript production, PCM was funded by a Wellcome Trust Fellowship (grant ref. 110110/Z/15/Z).

Authors' contributions
PM and LB designed the study and collected the data. SW interrogated a year of laboratory records for uropathogens and contributed laboratory methods to the paper. MeS provided pharmacy input for advice on prescribing, helping with interpretation of existing guidelines and production of new recommendations. NS contributed to clinical and laboratory data on multidrug resistance in Enterobacteriaceae. PM, LB and NJ developed new antimicrobial guidelines for local approval. PM analysed the data and wrote the manuscript, with input from LB, NS and MaS. All authors read and approved the final paper.

Competing interests
The authors declare that they have no competing interests.

Consent for publication
Informed consent was not obtained as data were collected and reviewed retrospectively as part of a quality improvement exercise, data were analysed and presented in anonymised form, and there was no intervention. This approach was approved by a local review body (see approval information above).

Author details
[1]Department of Infectious Diseases and Microbiology, Oxford University Hospitals NHS Foundation Trust, John Radcliffe Hospital, Headley Way, Headington, Oxford OX3 9DU, UK. [2]Nuffield Department of Medicine, University of Oxford, Peter Medawar Building for Pathogen Research, South Parks Road, Oxford OX1 3SY, UK. [3]Pharmacy Department, Oxford University Hospitals NHS Foundation Trust, John Radcliffe Hospital, Headley Way, Headington, Oxford OX3 9DU, UK.

References

1. Foxman B. Urinary tract infection syndromes: occurrence, recurrence, bacteriology, risk factors, and disease burden. Infect Dis Clin North Am. 2014;28(1):1–13.
2. Flores-Mireles AL, Walker JN, Caparon M, Hultgren SJ. Urinary tract infections: epidemiology, mechanisms of infection and treatment options. Nat Rev Microbiol. 2015;13(5):269–84.
3. Cassir N, Rolain JM, Brouqui P. A new strategy to fight antimicrobial resistance: the revival of old antibiotics. Front Microbiol. 2014;5:551.
4. Rosso-Fernandez C, Sojo-Dorado J, Barriga A, Lavin-Alconero L, Palacios Z, Lopez-Hernandez I, Merino V, Camean M, Pascual A, Rodriguez-Bano J, et al. Fosfomycin versus meropenem in bacteraemic urinary tract infections caused by extended-spectrum beta-lactamase-producing Escherichia coli (FOREST): study protocol for an investigator-driven randomised controlled trial. BMJ Open. 2015;5(3):e007363.
5. Grigoryan L, Trautner BW, Gupta K. Diagnosis and management of urinary tract infections in the outpatient setting: a review. Jama. 2014;312(16):1677–84.
6. Meier S, Weber R, Zbinden R, Ruef C, Hasse B. Extended-spectrum beta-lactamase-producing Gram-negative pathogens in community-acquired urinary tract infections: an increasing challenge for antimicrobial therapy. Infection. 2011;39(4):333–40.
7. Reffert JL, Smith WJ. Fosfomycin for the treatment of resistant gram-negative bacterial infections. Insights from the Society of Infectious Diseases Pharmacists. Pharmacotherapy. 2014;34(8):845–57.
8. Mikuniya T, Kato Y, Ida T, Maebashi K, Monden K, Kariyama R, Kumon H. Treatment of Pseudomonas aeruginosa biofilms with a combination of fluoroquinolones and fosfomycin in a rat urinary tract infection model. J Infect Chemother. 2007;13(5):285–90.
9. Sultan A, Rizvi M, Khan F, Sami H, Shukla I, Khan HM. Increasing antimicrobial resistance among uropathogens: Is fosfomycin the answer? Urology annals. 2015;7(1):26–30.
10. Pullukcu H, Tasbakan M, Sipahi OR, Yamazhan T, Aydemir S, Ulusoy S. Fosfomycin in the treatment of extended spectrum beta-lactamase-producing Escherichia coli-related lower urinary tract infections. Int J Antimicrob Agents. 2007;29(1):62–5.
11. Senol S, Tasbakan M, Pullukcu H, Sipahi OR, Sipahi H, Yamazhan T, Arda B, Ulusoy S. Carbapenem versus fosfomycin tromethanol in the treatment of extended-spectrum beta-lactamase-producing Escherichia coli-related complicated lower urinary tract infection. J Chemother. 2010;22(5):355–7.
12. Qiao LD, Zheng B, Chen S, Yang Y, Zhang K, Guo HF, Yang B, Niu YJ, Wang Y, Shi BK, et al. Evaluation of three-dose fosfomycin tromethamine in the treatment of patients with urinary tract infections: an uncontrolled, open-label, multicentre study. BMJ Open. 2013;3(12):e004157.
13. National Institute of Health and Care Excellence: Fosfomycin for treating urinary tract infections caused by bacteria that are resistant to more than one antibiotic [https://www.nice.org.uk/guidance/esuom17/resources/fosfomycin-for-treating-urinary-tract-infections-caused-by-bacteria-that-are-resistant-to-more-than-one-antibiotic-17481397957]. Accessed Sept 2015.
14. National Institute of Health and Care Excellence Evidence Summary: Unlicensed or off-label medicine. Multidrug resistant urinary tract infections: fosfomycin trometamol (NICE advice [ESUOM17]) [https://www.nice.org.uk/advice/esuom17/chapter/key-points-from-the-evidence]. Accessed Sept 2015.
15. Public Health England: Management of infection guidance for primary care for consultation and local adaptation [https://www.gov.uk/government/uploads/system/uploads/attachment_data/file/524984/Management_of_infection_guidance_for_primary_care_for_consultation_and_local_adaptation.pdf]. Accessed Sept 2015.
16. European Association of Urology Guidelines on Urological Infections [http://uroweb.org/wp-content/uploads/18_Urological-infections_LR.pdf]. Accessed Sept 2015.

17. Garcia-Tello A, Gimbernat H, Redondo C, Arana DM, Cacho J, Angulo JC. Extended-spectrum beta-lactamases in urinary tract infections caused by Enterobacteria: understanding and guidelines for action. Actas Urol Esp. 2014;38(10):678–84.

18. Falagas ME, Giannopoulou KP, Kokolakis GN, Rafailidis PI. Fosfomycin: use beyond urinary tract and gastrointestinal infections. Clin Infect Dis. 2008;46(7):1069–77.

19. Neuner EA, Sekeres J, Hall GS, van Duin D. Experience with fosfomycin for treatment of urinary tract infections due to multidrug-resistant organisms. Antimicrob Agents Chemother. 2012;56(11):5744–8.

20. British National Formulary [https://www.bnf.org/]. Accessed Sept 2015.

21. Karageorgopoulos DE, Wang R, Yu XH, Falagas ME. Fosfomycin: evaluation of the published evidence on the emergence of antimicrobial resistance in Gram-negative pathogens. J Antimicrob Chemother. 2012;67(2):255–68.

22. Grayson ML, Macesic N, Trevillyan J, Ellis AG, Zeglinski PT, Hewitt NH, Gardiner BJ, Frauman AG. Fosfomycin for Treatment of Prostatitis: New Tricks for Old Dogs. Clin Infect Dis. 2015;61(7):1141–3.

23. Rodriguez-Bano J, Alcala JC, Cisneros JM, Grill F, Oliver A, Horcajada JP, Tortola T, Mirelis B, Navarro G, Cuenca M, et al. Community infections caused by extended-spectrum beta-lactamase-producing Escherichia coli. Arch Intern Med. 2008;168(17):1897–902.

24. Tandogdu Z, Wagenlehner FM. Global epidemiology of urinary tract infections. Curr Opin Infect Dis. 2016;29(1):73–9.

25. Livermore DM, Warner M, Mushtaq S, Doumith M, Zhang J, Woodford N. What remains against carbapenem-resistant Enterobacteriaceae? Evaluation of chloramphenicol, ciprofloxacin, colistin, fosfomycin, minocycline, nitrofurantoin, temocillin and tigecycline. Int J Antimicrob Agents. 2011;37(5):415–9.

26. Cho YH, Jung SI, Chung HS, Yu HS, Hwang EC, Kim SO, Kang TW, Kwon DD, Park K. Antimicrobial susceptibilities of extended-spectrum beta-lactamase-producing Escherichia coli and Klebsiella pneumoniae in health care-associated urinary tract infection: focus on susceptibility to fosfomycin. Int Urol Nephrol. 2015;47(7):1059–66.

27. Tung C, Cheon C. Single-dose Fosfomycin Tromethamine for Treatment of Urinary Tract Infection In Hong Kong Women: a Preliminary Prospective Study. Hong Kong J Gynaecol Obstet Midwifery. 2012;12:37–42.

28. Jansaker F, Frimodt-Moller N, Sjogren I, Dahl Knudsen J. Clinical and bacteriological effects of pivmecillinam for ESBL-producing Escherichia coli or Klebsiella pneumoniae in urinary tract infections. J Antimicrob Chemother. 2014;69(3):769–72.

29. Los-Arcos I, Pigrau C, Rodriguez-Pardo D, Fernandez-Hidalgo N, Andreu A, Larrosa N, Almirante B. Long-Term Fosfomycin-Tromethamine Oral Therapy for Difficult-To-Treat Chronic Bacterial Prostatitis. Antimicrob Agents Chemother. 2015;60(3):1854–8.

30. Oteo J, Bautista V, Lara N, Cuevas O, Arroyo M, Fernandez S, Lazaro E, de Abajo FJ, Campos J, Spanish E-E-NSG. Parallel increase in community use of fosfomycin and resistance to fosfomycin in extended-spectrum beta-lactamase (ESBL)-producing Escherichia coli. J Antimicrob Chemother. 2010;65(11):2459–63.

31. Sorlozano A, Jimenez-Pacheco A, de Dios Luna Del Castillo J, Sampedro A, Martinez-Brocal A, Miranda-Casas C, Navarro-Mari JM, Gutierrez-Fernandez J. Evolution of the resistance to antibiotics of bacteria involved in urinary tract infections: a 7-year surveillance study. Am J Infect Control. 2014;42(10):1033–8.

Randomized controlled trial of piperacillin-tazobactam, cefepime and ertapenem for the treatment of urinary tract infection caused by extended-spectrum beta-lactamase-producing *Escherichia coli*

Yu Bin Seo[1], Jacob Lee[1], Young Keun Kim[2], Seung Soon Lee[3], Jeong-a Lee[3], Hyo Youl Kim[2], Young Uh[4], Han-Sung Kim[5] and Wonkeun Song[6]*

Abstract

Background: Due to limited therapeutic options, the spread of extended-spectrum beta-lactamases (ESBLs) have become a major public health concern. We conducted a prospective, randomized, open-label comparison of the therapeutic efficacy of piperacillin-tazobactam (PTZ), cefepime, and ertapenem in febrile nosocomial urinary tract infection with ESBL-producing *Escherichia coli* (ESBL-EC).

Methods: This study was conducted at three university hospitals between January 2013 and August 2015. Hospitalized adult patients presenting with fever were screened for healthcare-associated urinary tract infection (HA-UTI). When ESBL-EC was solely detected and susceptible to a randomized antibiotic in vitro, the case was included in the final analysis. Participants were treated for 10–14 days with PTZ, cefepime, or ertapenem.

Results: A total of 66 participants were evenly assigned to the PTZ and ertapenem treatment groups. After the recruitment of six participants, assignment to the cefepime treatment group was stopped because of an unexpectedly high treatment failure rate. The baseline characteristics of these participants did not differ from participants in other treatment groups. The clinical and microbiological response to PTZ treatment was estimated to be 94% and was similar to the response to ertapenem treatment. The efficacy of cefepime was 33.3%. In the cefepime group, age, Charlson comorbidity index, genotype, and minimal inhibitory concentration (MIC) did not significantly affect the success of treatment. Similarly, genotype seemed to be irrelevant with respect to clinical outcome in the PTZ group. Expired cases tended to involve septic shock with a high Charlson comorbidity index and high MIC.

Conclusion: Results from this study suggest that PTZ is effective in the treatment of urinary tract infection caused by ESBL-EC when the in vitro test indicates susceptibility. In addition, cefepime should not be used as an alternative treatment for urinary tract infection caused by ESBL-EC.

Keywords: Extended spectrum, Beta-lactamase, Piperacillin-tazobactam, Cefepime, Ertapenem

* Correspondence: swonkeun@hallym.or.kr
[6]Department of Laboratory Medicine, Kangnam Sacred Heart Hospital,
Hallym University College of Medicine, 1 Shingil-ro, Youngdeungpo-gu, Seoul
150-950, Korea
Full list of author information is available at the end of the article

Background

The spread of extended-spectrum beta-lactamase (ESBL)-producing organisms has gradually increased in hospitals and long-term care facilities [1]. ESBLs are enzymes that hydrolyze most beta-lactam antibiotics including penicillins, advanced-generation cephalosporins, and aztreonam. The genes of ESBLs are encoded on transferable plasmids, which can carry multiple co-resistance genes for other non-beta-lactam antibiotics [2, 3]. The spread of ESBLs has become a major public health concern due to limited therapeutic options.

Compared to non-ESBL-producing organism infections, those with ESBL-producing organisms are related to poor clinical outcomes [4]. Carbapenems are generally considered the drug of choice for ESBL-producing organism infections due to their stability against ESBLs [5, 6]. However, their use should be restricted considering the emergence of carbapenem-resistant organisms [7]. Alternative treatments are urgently needed to relieve the selective pressure for carbapenem [8, 9]. Thus, over the past few decades, numerous studies have been conducted to determine possible alternatives.

Currently, the most frequently mentioned alternative treatments are beta-lactam/beta-lactamase inhibitors (BLBLI), cephamycins, cefepime, and aminoglycosides [10–20]. Results have been promising, but several studies have reported suboptimal outcomes of cefepime or piperacillin-tazobactam (PTZ) treatment [21–23]. Because previous studies were conducted with observational methods, these conflicting results could be due to confounding factors, such as mixed sources of infection, variability in dosing, and different patient characteristics. To overcome the limitations of observational studies, we conducted a prospective, randomized, open-label comparison of the therapeutic efficacy of PTZ, cefepime, and ertapenem in patients with febrile nosocomial urinary tract infection (UTI) with ESBL-producing *Escherichia coli* (EBSL-EC).

Methods

Study setting

This study was conducted at three university hospitals between January 2013 and August 2015. Hospitalized adult patients ($\geq$ 19 years of age) presenting with fever were screened for healthcare-associated UTI (HA-UTI), which was defined according to the CDC/NHSN surveillance recommendations [24]. Exclusion criteria were presence of suspicious or confirmatory infectious foci other than HA-UTI, any use of antibiotics within 7 days prior to recruitment for any reason, any complicating urinary factors that could not be effectively treated during the trial (such as obstruction, suspected or confirmed prostatitis, and epididymitis), indwelling urinary catheters expected to remain in place after completion of therapy, and need for renal replacement therapy. After providing written consent, participants were randomly assigned to receive treatment for 10–14 days with PTZ, cefepime, or ertapenem at each institute, in that order. Clinical data on age, gender, comorbidities, Charlson comorbidity index (CCI), and APACHE II score were collected. On day 5–7 of the initial therapy, the investigator at each institute performed a urine culture to determine whether continuation of the study therapy was appropriate. When ESBL-EC was solely detected and was susceptible to a randomized antibiotic regardless of the sensitivities to other antibiotics, the case was included in the final analysis. If a patient receiving a randomized antibiotic dropped out, that antibiotic was given to the next participant. Because randomization was performed at each institute, a laboratory center monitored the balance in sample sizes across the groups over time. This study was performed in accordance with the CONSORT (Consolidated Standards of Reporting Trials) statement.

Antibiotic regimen

All patients received doses adjusted according to renal function. For PTZ, patients with creatinine clearance (Ccr) > 40 mL/min were treated with 4.5 g every 6 h, those with Ccr of 20-40 mL/min received 2.25 g every 6 h, and those with Ccr < 20 mL/min received 8 g every 8 h. For cefepime, patients with Ccr > 60 mL/min were treated with 2 g every 12 h, those with Ccr of 30-60 mL/min received 2 g every 24 h, and those with Ccr < 30 mL/min received 1 g every 24 h. For ertapenem, patients with Ccr > 30 mL/min were treated with 1 g every 24 h, and those with Ccr $\leq$ 30 mL/min received 500 mg daily.

Bacterial isolates

Urine and blood cultures were conducted in the microbiological laboratory at each hospital prior to antibiotic therapy. To evaluate the microbiological response, urine culture was repeated on day 10–14. At each hospital, microbiological identification was carried out using the Vitek 2 system (bioMérieux Vitek, Hazelwood, MO). Vitek GNI cards containing an ESBL test were used. Susceptibility to multiple antibiotics (including amikacin, ampicillin, ampicillin-sulbactam, aztreonam, cefepime, cefotaxime, cefotetan, ceftazidime, cephalothin, ciprofloxacin, ertapenem, gentamicin, imipenem, PTZ, and trimethoprim-sulfamethoxazole) was recorded. When an ESBL-EC was isolated, the sub-cultured specimen was delivered to Kangnam Sacred Heart Hospital for genotyping of ESBLs, AmpC beta-lactamases, and carbapenemases. For ESBLs-positive isolates, a PCR and sequencing strategy was used to characterize enzymes related to the ESBLs (TEM, SHV, CTX-M, and GES), AmpC beta-lactamases (DHA, MOX, and CMY), and carbapenemases (KPC, NDM, IMP, VIM, and OXA-48) using primers previously described [25–29]. CTX-M type sequencing primers used in this study are summarized in Table 1. Using two primer pairs, we amplified genes included in the CTX-M-1 ($bla_{CTX-M-1}$, $bla_{CTX-M-3}$, and $bla_{CTX-M-15}$) and CTX-M-9 groups ($bla_{CTX-M-9}$, $bla_{CTX-M-14}$, and $bla_{CTX-M-27}$). Then we sequenced the PCR products using identical primer pairs to identify each specific bla_{CTX-M} gene. The identified nucleotide sequences were compared with reference bla_{CTX-M} alleles (http://www.lahey.org/studies/). We performed species identification using the Vitek 2 system but did not identify the strain using multilocus sequence typing or pulsed field gel electrophoresis.

Clinical and microbiological efficacy
Clinical and microbiological responses were evaluated by the investigators on day 3–5, 10–14, and 28–30. Clinical success was defined as resolution of fever and symptoms of UTI present at entry with no development of new symptoms. If clinical improvement was not achieved until day 3–5, the case was defined as a clinical failure. Microbiological success was defined as elimination of ESBL-producing E. coli on a urine culture performed on day 10–14. Emergence of E. coli resistance to randomized antibiotic treatment, relapse rate, reinfection rate, and 28-day mortality were evaluated on day 28–30.

Statistical analysis
One-way analysis of variance (ANOVA) with post-hoc Bonferroni analysis was used to compare continuous variables among the three groups. Chi-square and Fisher's exact tests were used for bivariate analyses. To identify risk factors for treatment failure, multivariate analysis is generally used. However, there were too few failure cases to conduct this analysis. Therefore, a descriptive approach was used in the genotype and MIC analyses. All p-values were two sided and accepted when $p < 0.05$. Statistical analysis was performed using SPSS 18.0 software (SPSS Korea, Seoul, Korea).

Results
Study subjects
During the study period, a total of 72 participants were enrolled. Of these, 66 participants were evenly assigned to the PTZ and ertapenem treatment groups. After recruitment of six participants to the cefepime treatment group, allocation to this treatment group was stopped due to an unexpectedly high treatment failure rate.

Table 2 shows the baseline characteristics of the participants. The average age of participants (65 years) did not vary among the three groups. There were more female than male participants assigned to both the PTZ (female 90.9%) and ertapenem (female 78.8%) treatment groups, but significant gender differences were not observed between the two groups ($p = 0.303$). In the cefepime group, there was an equal distribution of female and male participants, and the gender ratio was significantly different from the two other groups ($p = 0.049$). With respect to comorbidities, the Charlson comorbidity index was similar among the three groups. Almost 65% of the participants had at least one or more underlying disease. Septic shock and concomitant bacteremia were presented in 20–30% of participants in the PTZ and ertapenem groups and did not show statistical differences. APACHE II scores were similar among the three groups. Septic shock and bacteremia were not detected in the cefepime group.

Clinical and microbiological outcomes
Clinical and microbiological outcomes are summarized in Table 3. Clinical success rate was 93.9% (31/33) with PTZ and 97.0% (32/33) with ertapenem; the rates were not statistically different ($p = 0.500$). However, the clinical success rate with cefepime was 33.3% (2/6), which was significantly lower than those of the other antibiotic groups ($p < 0.001$). The microbiological success rates of PTZ and ertapenem were the same at 97.0% (32/33), while the cefepime group achieved a 33.3% success rate (2/6). The 28-day mortality was also the same between the PTZ and ertapenem groups with a rate of 6.1% (2/33) in both groups. On the other hand, the rate was 33.3% (2/6) in the cefepime group ($p = 0.108$). There were no cases of emergence of E. coli resistance to randomized antibiotics, relapse, or reinfection. In the case of microbiological failure, the MICs of late cultures at 10–14 days were not different from early cultures. All patients with a positive culture at test of cure had clinical symptoms that were consistent with UTI.

Genotypic analysis in the cefepime and piperacillin-tazobactam groups
There were no ESBL-EC isolates combined with AmpC or carbapenemase enzymes in this study. In the cefepime group, only two participants achieved clinically successful recovery (Table 4). There were four failure cases and

Table 1 Primers used for PCR amplification and sequencing of bla_{CTX-M} genes

Target	Name of primer	Sequence (5' → 3')	Expected size of amplicon (bp)	Reference
CTX-M-1 group	CTX-M-1F CTX-M-1R	GCAGCACCAGTAAAGTGATGGGCTGGGTGAAGTAAGTGACC	591	[28]
CTX-M-9 group	CTX-M-9F CTX-M-9R	GCTGGAGAAAAGCAGCGGAGGTAAGCTGACGCAACGTCTG	474	[29]

Table 2 Demographic characteristics of study subjects

	Piperacillin/tazobactam (N = 33)	Cefepime (N = 6)	Ertapenem (N = 33)	p-value
Age	68.8 ± 14.4	75.3 ± 6.6	65.2 ± 16.9	0.281
Female	30 (90.9)	3 (50.0)	26 (78.8)	0.049
Comorbidity, n (%)				
Ischemic heart disease	0 (0)	0 (0)	1 (3.0)	1.000
Diabetes mellitus	12 (36.4)	1 (16.7)	15 (45.5)	0.474
Cerebrovascular accident	5 (15.2)	1 (16.7)	2 (6.1)	0.420
Dementia	3 (9.1)	0 (0)	2 (6.1)	1.000
Hemiplegia	2 (6.1)	0 (0)	2 (6.1)	1.000
Congestive heart failure	5 (15.2)	1 (16.7)	1 (3.0)	0.230
COPD	1 (3.0)	0 (0)	1 (3.0)	1.000
Chronic kidney disease	2 (6.1)	0 (0)	2 (6.1)	1.000
Liver cirrhosis	2 (6.1)	0 (0)	4 (12.1)	0.809
Solid tumor	6 (18.2)	1 (16.7)	7 (21.2)	1.000
Lymphoma	1 (3.0)	0 (0)	2 (6.1)	1.000
None	12 (36.4)	2 (33.3)	12 (36.4)	1.000
Charlson comorbidity index	4.7 ± 3.0	4.7 ± 1.0	4.5 ± 3.0	0.951
Bacteremia, n (%)	9 (27.3)	0 (0)	7 (21.2)	0.477
Septic shock, n (%)	9 (24.2)	2 (33.3)	11 (33.3)	0.928
APACH II score	12.9 ± 2.9	16.5 ± 6.4	16.6 ± 5.6	0.298

two deaths. While the MIC of cefepime was 1 μg/mL or 2 μg/mL, the successful cases all had an MIC of 2 μg/mL. The genotype was predominantly CTX-M-9, but one case was detected as SHV-2. The genotype did not appear to significantly affect the success of treatment. In addition, age and Charlson comorbidity index did not seem to be directly related to clinical success. All mortality cases occurred under conditions of septic shock.

In the PTZ group, treatment was successful except in two cases (Table 4). In most cases, the MIC was 16 μg/mL and accounted for 72.7% of the total. Although the clinical outcome was satisfactory in most cases of 16 μg/mL MIC, all failure and mortality cases were in the 16 μg/mL MIC group. Ten samples were lost during transport or over the course of the experiment. CTX-M-14, CTX-M-15, and CTX-M-27 were frequently observed. The genotypes of the mortality cases were CTX-M-15 or CTX-M-27. Similar to cefepime, the genotype seemed to be irrelevant with respect to clinical outcome. Deaths tended to

be associated with septic shock with high Charlson comorbidity index and high MIC.

Discussion

This is the first randomized study comparing the efficacy of PTZ, cefepime, and ertapenem. Although the sample size was small, results from the study showed that PTZ was as effective as ertapenem for the treatment of ESBL-EC UTI. Clinical and microbiological response to PTZ treatment was estimated to be 94%. Unexpectedly, the efficacy of cefepime was only 33.3%, suggesting that cefepime is not an appropriate therapeutic alternative for ESBL-EC UTI.

ESBLs might be inhibited by beta-lactamase inhibitors; thus, it is theoretically attractive to use BLBLI combinations to treat ESBL infections. In fact, a large, multicenter, prospective observational study has reported that outcomes using BLBLIs were comparable to those with carbapenem in the treatment of ESBL-EC blood stream

Table 3 Clinical and microbiological outcomes according to the antibiotic groups

	Piperacillin/tazobactam (N = 33)	Cefepime (N = 6)	Ertapenem (N = 33)	p-value
Clinical success, n (%)	31 (93.9)	2 (33.3)	32 (97.0)	<0.001
Microbiological success, n (%)	32 (97.0)	2 (33.3)	32 (97.0)	<0.001
Clinical and microbiological success, n (%)	31 (93.9)	2 (33.3)	32 (97.0)	<0.001
28-days mortality, n (%)	2 (6.1)	2 (33.3)	2 (6.1)	0.108

Table 4 Schematic description of clinical outcomes according to MIC, genotype, age, Charlson comorbidity index (CCI), presence of concomitant bacteremia and septic shock in cefepime, piperacillin/tazobactam and ertapenem groups

Case	MIC (µg/mL)	ESBLs genotype	CCI	Bacteremia	Septic shock	Clinical outcome
A. Cefepime (N = 6)						
Patient 1	2	CTX-M-14	5	No	No	Success
Patient 2	2	CTX-M-14	3	No	No	Success
Patient 3	1	CTX-M-14	4	No	No	Failure
Patient 4	2	CTX-M-14	6	No	No	Failure
Patient 5	1	SHV-12	5	No	Yes	Failure and expired
Patient 6	2	CTX-M-14	5	No	Yes	Failure and expired
B. Piperacillin/tazobactam (N = 33)						
Patient 1	4	CTX-M-14	6	No	No	Success
Patient 2	4	CTX-M-15	5	No	Yes	Success
Patient 3	4	CTX-M-15	0	No	No	Success
Patient 4	4	CTX-M-15	1	No	No	Success
Patient·5	4	CTX-M-27	9	No	No	Success
Patient 6	4	CTX-M-27	9	No	No	Success
Patient 7	4	CTX-M-27	9	No	No	Success
Patient 8	8	CTX-M-14	3	Yes	Yes	Success
Patient 9	8	CTX-M-14	1	No	No	Success
Patient 10	16	CTX-M-1	4	No	No	Success
Patient 11	16	CTX-M-3	2	No	Yes	Success
Patient 12	16	CTX-M-14	3	No	No	Success
Patient 13	16	CTX-M-14	3	Yes	Yes	Success
Patient 14	16	CTX-M-15	1	No	Yes	Success
Patient 15	16	CTX-M-15	4	No	No	Success
Patient 16	16	CTX-M-27	0	No	No	Success
Patient 17	16	CTX-M-15	3	No	No	Success
Patient 18	16	CTX-M-14	5	No	No	Success
Patient 19	16	CTX-M-14	7	No	No	Success
Patient 20	16	CTX-M-14	1	Yes	No	Success
Patient 21	16	CTX-M-14	8	No	No	Success
Patient 22	16	Not tested	5	No	No	Success
Patient 23	16	Not tested	2	No	Yes	Success
Patient 24	16	Not tested	7	No	No	Success
Patient 25	16	Not tested	3	No	No	Success
Patient 26	16	Not tested	7	No	No	Success
Patient 27	16	Not tested	8	No	No	Success
Patient 28	16	Not tested	5	No	No	Success
Patient 29	16	Not tested	5	No	No	Success
Patient 30	16	Not tested	3	Yes	No	Success
Patient 31	16	Not tested	7	Yes	Yes	Success
Patient 32	16	CTX-M-15	9	Yes	Yes	Failure and expired
Patient 33	16	CTX-M-27	10	No	Yes	Failure and expired

Table 4 Schematic description of clinical outcomes according to MIC, genotype, age, Charlson comorbidity index (CCI), presence of concomitant bacteremia and septic shock in cefepime, piperacillin/tazobactam and ertapenem groups *(Continued)*

C. Ertapenem (N = 33)						
Patient 1	0.5	CTX-M-15	0	No	No	Success
Patient 2	0.5	CTX-M-27	0	No	No	Success
Patient 3	0.5	CTX-M-14	1	No	No	Success
Patient 4	0.5	CTX-M-15	1	No	No	Success
Patient 5	0.5	CTX-M-14	1	Yes	No	Success
Patient 6	0.5	CTX-M-15	1	No	Yes	Success
Patient 7	0.5	CTX-M-3	2	No	Yes	Success
Patient 8	0.5	CTX-M-14	2	Yes	Yes	Success
Patient 9	0.5	CTX-M-14	3	No	No	Success
Patient 10	0.5	CTX-M-15	3	No	No	Success
Patient 11	0.5	CTX-M-15	3	No	No	Success
Patient 12	0.5	CTX-M-14	3	Yes	No	Success
Patient 13	0.5	CTX-M-14	3	Yes	Yes	Success
Patient 14	0.5	CTX-M-14	3	Yes	Yes	Success
Patient 15	0.5	CTX-M-1	4	No	No	Success
Patient 16	0.5	CTX-M-15	4	No	No	Success
Patient 17	0.5	CTX-M-14	5	No	No	Success
Patient 18	0.5	CTX-M-14	5	No	No	Success
Patient 19	0.5	CTX-M-15	5	No	No	Success
Patient 20	0.5	CTX-M-14	5	Yes	No	Success
Patient 23	0.5	CTX-M-15	5	No	Yes	Success
Patient 21	0.5	CTX-M-14	6	Yes	No	Success
Patient 22	0.5	CTX-M-14	7	No	No	Success
Patient 24	0.5	CTX-M-14	7	No	No	Success
Patient 25	0.5	CTX-M-14	7	No	No	Success
Patient 26	0.5	CTX-M-14	8	No	No	Success
Patient 27	0.5	CTX-M-14	8	No	No	Success
Patient 28	0.5	CTX-M-27	9	No	No	Success
Patient 29	0.5	CTX-M-27	9	No	No	Success
Patient 30	0.5	CTX-M-27	9	No	No	Success
Patient 31	0.5	CTX-M-27	10	No	No	Success
Patient 32	0.5	CTX-M-14	9	Yes	Yes	Failure and expired
Patient 33	0.5	CTX-M-15	7	Yes	Yes	Failure and expired

Not tested: The isolate was ESBLs-positive by Vitek-2 system but not tested the ESBLs genotyping due to loss of the isolate

infection [10]. In addition, a recent meta-analysis found no statistical differences in mortality between carbapenem treatment and BLBLI treatment in patients with bacteremia caused by ESBL-producing pathogens [30]. However, in another study, BLBLI appeared to be inferior to carbapenem for treatment of bacteremia [31]. These inconclusive results might be due to differences in the proportion of bacteremia sources among the various studies since the infection site can significantly influence the therapeutic efficacy of antibiotics. To overcome issues due to infection heterogeneity, this study focused on the treatment of UTIs.

According to our results, PTZ is a reliable alternative in the treatment of ESBL-EC-proven UTI. An inoculum effect has been proposed as a major limitation of PTZ [32]. PTZ has some merits for use in cases of UTI. Tazobactam is mainly excreted in the urine, and its high concentration in the urine is noted in the presence of piperacillin [33]. In addition, UTIs can have a relatively lower bacterial burden than other infectious diseases, such as pneumonia, complicated intra-abdominal infection, and blood stream infection. Therefore, PTZ might be able to overcome the inoculum effect in UTIs. Interestingly, mortality cases were found in participants with a high MIC who received PTZ treatment. Due to the small sample size, it was difficult to determine whether a higher MIC of PTZ is an important risk factor for treatment failure. However, in this study, multiple cases with a 16 µg/mL MIC of PTZ were successfully treated. As discussed in a previous study, the MIC might not be a significant risk factor in UTIs [16]. Treatment failure seems to be closely related to the patient's baseline conditions, irrespective of the MIC.

Cefepime is frequently used for treatment of healthcare associated infections and shows greater stability in vitro against ESBL-producing pathogens than other cephalosporins [34]. Some clinical studies have reported successful treatment using cefepime in cases of ESBL-producing bacterial infection [19, 35]. However, several other studies have shown disappointing outcomes when using cefepime to treat bacteremic conditions [20, 23]. Cefepime is highly vulnerable to the inoculum effect, and a high MIC is an important risk factor for treatment failure [32]. As seen in our study, cefepime was not effective in the treatment of UTIs even in non-bacteremic conditions. Treatment failure was also observed despite an MIC of 1 µg/mL or 2 µg/mL. Thus, a lower MIC does not predict clinical success in cefepime treatment. Although cefepime is excreted mostly unchanged in urine, it can be easily inactivated by ESBLs in UTIs. Otherwise, the results we observed might be due to the emergence of phenotypic heterogeneous resistance to cefepime during treatment [36]. Another cause of treatment failure could be under-dosing of cefepime. In Korea, cefepime has been approved to be administered at 1 g twice a day for mild or moderate infection, 2 g twice a day for severe infection, and 2 g three times a day for neutropenic patients if renal function is normal. The recommended dose is the same in most other countries. However, some studies recommended higher doses of cefepime than usual for clinical doses. One study reported that doses of at least 2 g every 8 h are required to treat infections considering clinical pharmacodynamics [37]. However, that study enrolled patients with non-urinary tract infections, and the pathogen of focus was *Pseudomonas aeruginosa*. Therefore, it is difficult to infer the same conclusion from this study. Other studies using a series of 5000-subject Monte Carlo simulations mentioned that a cefepime dose of 2 g every 6 h provided favorable probability [38]. Considering results from existing studies, further clinical studies increasing the dose of cefepime seem to be necessary to clarify the failure of cefepime.

This study has several limitations. First, the statistical power was low due to the small number of participants. To estimate the sample size for clinical research studies, the variance or standard deviation is obtained from previous studies. When there are no previous studies, a formal sample size calculation might not be appropriate. We decided to complete the study according to the study period regardless of the sample size, as in the pilot study. During the study period, the number of patients susceptible in vitro to PTZ was unexpectedly small. Furthermore, the exclusion criteria were strict in order to reduce possible confounding factors. Accordingly, the sample size was only 33 participants in each group except the cefepime group; however, this is a common pilot sample study size for a two-arm trial [39]. In order to have more confidence in the outcome, a larger sample size is needed in future studies. Second, it has been suggested that ESBL-*Klebsiella pneumoniae* is associated with higher mortality than ESBL-EC bacteremia [40]. Therefore, the results could not be generalized to pathogens other than *E. coli*. Third, the genotype was not determined in some cases due to loss of the isolate. Fourth, the molecular PCR typing was not done for cefepime resistance gene such as OXA-30. Results could be interpreted differently in situations with other ESBL genotypes. In the Republic of Korea, the predominant types of ESBLs in *E. coli* are CTX-M-14 and CTX-M-15, which is consistent with the results of the tested isolates in our study [41]. In our study, the tested isolates demonstrated similar predominance. Therefore, these results could be applied to the situation of high spread of the CTX-M type.

Conclusion

Alternatives for the treatment of ESBL-producing bacteria are urgently needed to suppress the emergence of carbapenem-resistant pathogens. Results from this study suggest that PTZ is effective in the treatment of UTI caused by ESBL-EC when the in vitro test indicates susceptibility. Empirical PTZ therapy for healthcare-associated UTI seems to be reasonable if the hospital epidemiological antimicrobial pattern of ESBLs (especially the CTX-M type) is dominantly in vitro susceptible to PTZ. In addition, cefepime should not be used as an alternative treatment in urinary tract infections caused by ESBL-EC.

Abbreviations
ESBL-EC: ESBL-producing *Escherichia coli*; ESBLs: Extended-spectrum beta-lactamases; HA-UTI: Healthcare-associated urinary tract infection; MIC: Minimal inhibitory concentration; PTZ: Piperacillin-tazobactam; UTI: Urinary tract infection

Funding
This study was supported by a research grant from the Korean Health Technology R&D Project, Ministry of Health & Welfare, Republic of Korea (HI12C0756).

Authors' contributions

YBS, JL: contribution to the study concept and design, analysis of the data, and writing the manuscript. YKK, SSL, JL, HYK, YU, H-SK: contribution to the collection and analysis of data. WS: contribution to the study concept and design and review of the manuscript. All authors gave final approval of the version to be published.

Competing interests

The authors declare that they have no competing interests.

Consent for publication

Not applicable.

Author details

[1]Division of Infectious Diseases, Department of Internal Medicine, Kangnam Sacred Heart Hospital, Hallym University College of Medicine, Seoul, Republic of Korea. [2]Department of Internal Medicine, Yonsei University Wonju College of Medicine, Wonju, Republic of Korea. [3]Division of Infectious Diseases, Department of Internal Medicine, Hallym University Sacred Heart Hospital, Hallym University College of Medicine, Seoul, Republic of Korea. [4]Department of Laboratory Medicine, Yonsei University Wonju College of Medicine, Wonju, Republic of Korea. [5]Department of Laboratory Medicine, Hallym University Sacred Heart Hospital, Hallym University College of Medicine, Seoul, Republic of Korea. [6]Department of Laboratory Medicine, Kangnam Sacred Heart Hospital, Hallym University College of Medicine, 1 Shingil-ro, Youngdeungpo-gu, Seoul 150-950, Korea.

References

1. Thaden JT, Fowler VG, Sexton DJ, Anderson DJ. Increasing incidence of extended-Spectrum beta-Lactamase-producing *Escherichia coli* in community hospitals throughout the southeastern United States. Infect Control Hosp Epidemiol. 2016;37(1):49–54.
2. Schwaber MJ, Navon-Venezia S, Schwartz D, Carmeli Y. High levels of antimicrobial coresistance among extended-spectrum-beta-lactamase-producing Enterobacteriaceae. Antimicrob Agents Chemother. 2005;49(5):2137–9.
3. Morosini MI, Garcia-Castillo M, Coque TM, Valverde A, Novais A, Loza E, et al. Antibiotic coresistance in extended-spectrum-beta-lactamase-producing Enterobacteriaceae and in vitro activity of tigecycline. Antimicrob Agents Chemother. 2006;50(8):2695–9.
4. Ramphal R, Ambrose PG. Extended-spectrum beta-lactamases and clinical outcomes: current data. Clin Infect Dis. 2006;42(Suppl 4):S164–72.
5. Paterson DL, Bonomo RA. Extended-spectrum beta-lactamases: a clinical update. Clin Microbiol Rev. 2005;18(4):657–86.
6. Rodriguez-Bano J, Pascual A. Clinical significance of extended-spectrum beta-lactamases. Expert Rev Anti-Infect Ther. 2008;6(5):671–83.
7. Nordmann P, Naas T, Poirel L. Global spread of Carbapenemase-producing Enterobacteriaceae. Emerg Infect Dis. 2011;17(10):1791–8.
8. Go ES, Urban C, Burns J, Kreiswirth B, Eisner W, Mariano N, et al. Clinical and molecular epidemiology of acinetobacter infections sensitive only to polymyxin B and sulbactam. Lancet. 1994;344(8933):1329–32.
9. Guh AY, Limbago BM, Kallen AJ. Epidemiology and prevention of carbapenem-resistant Enterobacteriaceae in the United States. Expert Rev Anti-Infect Ther. 2014;12(5):565–80.
10. Rodriguez-Bano J, Navarro MD, Retamar P, Picon E, Pascual A, Extended-Spectrum Beta-Lactamases-Red Espanola de Investigacion en Patologia Infecciosa/Grupo de Estudio de Infeccion Hospitalaria G. Beta-Lactam/beta-lactam inhibitor combinations for the treatment of bacteremia due to extended-spectrum beta-lactamase-producing *Escherichia coli*: a post hoc analysis of prospective cohorts. Clin Infect Dis. 2012;54(2):167–74.
11. Lee CH, Su LH, Tang YF, Liu JW. Treatment of ESBL-producing *Klebsiella pneumoniae* bacteraemia with carbapenems or flomoxef: a retrospective study and laboratory analysis of the isolates. J Antimicrob Chemother. 2006;58(5):1074–7.
12. Han SB, Lee SC, Lee SY, Jeong DC, Kang JH. Aminoglycoside therapy for childhood urinary tract infection due to extended-spectrum beta-lactamase-producing *Escherichia coli* or *Klebsiella pneumoniae*. BMC Infect Dis. 2015;15:414.
13. Matsumura Y, Yamamoto M, Nagao M, Komori T, Fujita N, Hayashi A, et al. Multicenter retrospective study of cefmetazole and flomoxef for treatment of extended-spectrum-beta-lactamase-producing *Escherichia coli* bacteremia. Antimicrob Agents Chemother. 2015;59(9):5107–13.
14. Tasbakan MI, Pullukcu H, Sipahi OR, Yamazhan T, Ulusoy S. Nitrofurantoin in the treatment of extended-spectrum-beta-lactamase-producing *Escherichia coli*-related lower urinary tract infection. Int J Antimicrob Agents. 2012;40(6):554–6.
15. Gavin PJ, Suseno MT, Thomson RB Jr, Gaydos JM, Pierson CL, Halstead DC, et al. Clinical correlation of the CLSI susceptibility breakpoint for piperacillin-tazobactam against extended-spectrum-beta-lactamase-producing *Escherichia coli* and Klebsiella species. Antimicrob Agents Chemother. 2006;50(6):2244–7.
16. Retamar P, Lopez-Cerero L, Muniain MA, Pascual A, Rodriguez-Bano J, Group E-RG. Impact of the MIC of piperacillin-tazobactam on the outcome of patients with bacteremia due to extended-spectrum-beta-lactamase-producing *Escherichia coli*. Antimicrob Agents Chemother. 2013;57(7):3402–4.
17. Doi A, Shimada T, Harada S, Iwata K, Kamiya T. The efficacy of cefmetazole against pyelonephritis caused by extended-spectrum beta-lactamase-producing Enterobacteriaceae. Int J Infect Dis. 2013;17(3):e159–63.
18. Ipekci T, Seyman D, Berk H, Celik O. Clinical and bacteriological efficacy of amikacin in the treatment of lower urinary tract infection caused by extended-spectrum beta-lactamase-producing *Escherichia coli* or *Klebsiella pneumoniae*. J Infect Chemother. 2014;20(12):762–7.
19. Labombardi VJ, Rojtman A, Tran K. Use of cefepime for the treatment of infections caused by extended spectrum beta-lactamase-producing *Klebsiella pneumoniae* and *Escherichia coli*. Diagn Microbiol Infect Dis. 2006;56(3):313–5.
20. Lee NY, Lee CC, Huang WH, Tsui KC, Hsueh PR, Ko WC. Cefepime therapy for monomicrobial bacteremia caused by cefepime-susceptible extended-spectrum beta-lactamase-producing Enterobacteriaceae: MIC matters. Clin Infect Dis. 2013;56(4):488–95.
21. Ofer-Friedman H, Shefler C, Sharma S, Tirosh A, Tal-Jasper R, Kandipalli D, et al. Carbapenems versus Piperacillin-Tazobactam for bloodstream infections of Nonurinary source caused by extended-Spectrum Beta-Lactamase-producing Enterobacteriaceae. Infect Control Hosp Epidemiol. 2015;36(8):981–5.
22. Lee NY, Lee CC, Li CW, Li MC, Chen PL, Chang CM, et al. Cefepime therapy for Monomicrobial *Enterobacter cloacae* Bacteremia: unfavorable outcomes in patients infected by Cefepime-susceptible dose-dependent isolates. Antimicrob Agents Chemother. 2015;59(12):7558–63.
23. Chopra T, Marchaim D, Veltman J, Johnson P, Zhao JJ, Tansek R, et al. Impact of cefepime therapy on mortality among patients with bloodstream infections caused by extended-spectrum-beta-lactamase-producing *Klebsiella pneumoniae* and *Escherichia coli*. Antimicrob Agents Chemother. 2012;56(7):3936–42.
24. Horan TC, Andrus M, Dudeck MA. CDC/NHSN surveillance definition of health care-associated infection and criteria for specific types of infections in the acute care setting. Am J Infect Control. 2008;36(5):309–32.
25. Ryoo NH, Kim EC, Hong SG, Park YJ, Lee K, Bae IK, et al. Dissemination of SHV-12 and CTX-M-type extended-spectrum beta-lactamases among clinical isolates of *Escherichia coli* and *Klebsiella pneumoniae* and emergence of GES-3 in Korea. J Antimicrob Chemother. 2005;56(4):698–702.
26. Perez-Perez FJ, Hanson ND. Detection of plasmid-mediated AmpC beta-lactamase genes in clinical isolates by using multiplex PCR. J Clin Microbiol. 2002;40(6):2153–62.
27. Poirel L, Walsh TR, Cuvillier V, Nordmann P. Multiplex PCR for detection of acquired carbapenemase genes. Diagn Microbiol Infect Dis. 2011;70(1):119–23.
28. Abdalhamid B, Pitout JD, Moland ES, Hanson ND. Community-onset disease caused by Citrobacter freundii producing a novel CTX-M beta-lactamase, CTX-M-30, in Canada. Antimicrob Agents Chemother. 2004;48(11):4435–7.
29. Pitout JD, Hossain A, Hanson ND. Phenotypic and molecular detection of CTX-M-beta-lactamases produced by *Escherichia coli* and Klebsiella spp. J Clin Microbiol. 2004;42(12):5715–21.
30. Vardakas KZ, Tansarli GS, Rafailidis PI, Falagas ME. Carbapenems versus alternative antibiotics for the treatment of bacteraemia due to Enterobacteriaceae producing extended-spectrum beta-lactamases: a systematic review and meta-analysis. J Antimicrob Chemother. 2012;67(12):2793–803.
31. Tamma PD, Han JH, Rock C, Harris AD, Lautenbach E, Hsu AJ, Avdic E, Cosgrove SE, Antibacterial Resistance Leadership G. Carbapenem therapy is

associated with improved survival compared with piperacillin-tazobactam for patients with extended-spectrum beta-lactamase bacteremia. Clin Infect Dis. 2015;60(9):1319-25.

32. Thomson KS, Moland ES. Cefepime, piperacillin-tazobactam, and the inoculum effect in tests with extended-spectrum beta-lactamase-producing Enterobacteriaceae. Antimicrob Agents Chemother. 2001;45(12):3548–54.

33. Komuro M, Maeda T, Kakuo H, Matsushita H, Shimada J. Inhibition of the renal excretion of tazobactam by piperacillin. J Antimicrob Chemother. 1994;34(4):555–64.

34. Sanders CC. In vitro activity of fourth generation cephalosporins against enterobacteriaceae producing extended-spectrum beta-lactamases. J Chemother. 1996;8(Suppl 2):57–62.

35. Goethaert K, Van Looveren M, Lammens C, Jansens H, Baraniak A, Gniadkowski M, et al. High-dose cefepime as an alternative treatment for infections caused by TEM-24 ESBL-producing Enterobacter aerogenes in severely-ill patients. Clin Microbiol Infect. 2006;12(1):56–62.

36. Ma W, Sun J, Yang S, Zhang L. Epidemiological and clinical features for cefepime heteroresistant Escherichia coli infections in Southwest China. Eur J Clin Microbiol Infect Dis. 2016;35(4):571–8.

37. Crandon JL, Bulik CC, Kuti JL, Nicolau DP. Clinical pharmacodynamics of cefepime in patients infected with Pseudomonas Aeruginosa. Antimicrob Agents Chemother. 2010;54(3):1111–6.

38. Zasowski E, Bland CM, Tam VH, Lodise TP. Identification of optimal renal dosage adjustments for high-dose extended-infusion cefepime dosing regimens in hospitalized patients. J Antimicrob Chemother. 2015;70(3):877–81.

39. Billingham SA, Whitehead AL, Julious SA. An audit of sample sizes for pilot and feasibility trials being undertaken in the United Kingdom registered in the United Kingdom clinical research network database. BMC Med Res Methodol. 2013;13:104.

40. Apisarnthanarak A, Kiratisin P, Mundy LM. Predictors of mortality from community-onset bloodstream infections due to extended-spectrum beta-lactamase-producing Escherichia coli and Klebsiella pneumoniae. Infect Control Hosp Epidemiol. 2008;29(7):671–4.

41. Song W, Lee H, Lee K, Jeong SH, Bae IK, Kim JS, et al. CTX-M-14 and CTX-M-15 enzymes are the dominant type of extended-spectrum beta-lactamase in clinical isolates of Escherichia coli from Korea. J Med Microbiol. 2009;58(Pt 2):261–6.

Restriction of in vivo infection by antifouling coating on urinary catheter with controllable and sustained silver release

Kedar Diwakar Mandakhalikar[1]*(iD), Rong Wang[2], Juwita N. Rahmat[3], Edmund Chiong[3], Koon Gee Neoh[4] and Paul A. Tambyah[1]

Abstract

Background: Catheter Associated Urinary Tract Infections are among the most common urological infections world-wide. Bacterial biofilms and encrustation cause significant complications in patients with urinary catheters. The objective of the study is to demonstrate the efficacy and safety of an anti-microbial and anti-encrustation silver nanoparticle (AgNP) coating on silicone urinary catheter in two different animal models.

Methods: Antifouling coating (P3) was prepared with alternate layers of polydopamine and AgNP and an outermost antifouling layer. Sixteen C57BL/6 female mice and two female PWG Micropigs® were used to perform the experiments. In mice, a 5 mm long silicone catheter with or without P3 was transurethrally placed into the urinary bladder. Micropigs were transurethrally implanted – one with P3 silicone catheter and the other with commercially available silver coated silicone catheter. Both models were challenged with *E. coli*. Bacteriuria was evaluated routinely and upon end of study (2 weeks for mice, 3 weeks for micropigs), blood, catheters and bladders were harvested and analysed for bacterial colonization and encrustation as well as for toxicity.

Results: Lower bacterial colonization was seen on P3 catheters as well as in bladders of animals with P3 catheter. Bacteriuria was consistently less in mice with P3 catheter than with uncoated catheters. Encrustation was lower on P3 catheter and in bladder of micropig with P3 catheter. No significant toxicity of P3 was observed in mice or in micropig as compared to controls. The numbers were small in this proof of concept study and technical issues were noted especially with the porcine model.

Conclusions: Antifouling P3 coating reduces bacterial colonization on catheter and in animal bladders without causing any considerable toxicity for 2 to 3 weeks. This novel coating could potentially reduce the complications of indwelling urethral catheters.

Keywords: CAUTI, Silver nanoparticles, Urinary catheter, Mouse model, Porcine model, Catheter associated urinary tract infections

* Correspondence: a0092803@u.nus.edu
[1]Department of Medicine, Yong Loo Lin School of Medicine, National University of Singapore, 1E, Kent Ridge Road, NUHS Tower Block, Level 10, Singapore 119228, Singapore
Full list of author information is available at the end of the article

Background

Urinary catheters are among the most common medical devices in clinical use [1]. However, catheter associated urinary tract infections (CAUTI) are among the most common hospital acquired infections [2–4]. The risk of CAUTI is reported to be between 3 and 7% daily and increases with the duration of catheterization [5].

Uropathogenic *Escherichia coli* (UPEC) are responsible for most CAUTI [6]. Many UPEC strains are now resistant to multiple antibiotics, and thus difficult to treat, emphasizing the importance of preventative strategies [7–9].

Intraluminal and extraluminal biofilms, caused by the attachment of bacteria to the catheter, facilitate the entry and persistence of uropathogens in the bladder and thus promote the development of resistance [6]. In addition, urease producing bacteria, especially *P. mirabilis*, contribute significantly to catheter encrustation through precipitation of mineral salts such as calcium phosphate and magnesium ammonium phosphate [10]. These encrustations and biofilms are major contributors to morbidity and mortality in CAUTI [11–14]. They are responsible for the failure of many medical devices [15]. Novel approaches to preventing CAUTI have focussed on preventing the development of biofilms using various techniques including novel coatings [16].

We have previously developed an anti-fouling catheter with controllable and sustained silver release which is effective in resisting encrustation induced by *Proteus mirabilis* in vitro for up to 45 days [17]. The coating comprises multiple layers of silver using polydopamine (PDA) as the surface anchor which reduces the silver ions into silver nanoparticles (AgNPs) and stabilizes and protects the AgNPs from oxidization and aggregation. Therefore, the amount of silver loaded, and its subsequent release profile is readily controllable by changing the number of silver-containing layers. The outermost layer is made of an antifouling polymer, poly (sulfobetaine methacrylate-*co*-acrylamide) [poly (SBMA-*co*-AAm)], which also allows free diffusion of silver. Thus, this novel coating is different in having a higher intrinsic silver release capability than the current commercially available silver coated urinary catheters.

Here, we used a previously described mouse model [18, 19] to study the safety and potential efficacy of this catheter against biofilm formation and colonization by UPEC in vivo. To further test the coating for human catheters, we chose a porcine model for our in vivo experiments as it provides a urinary tract that resembles the macroscopic human urinary tract fairly well and is a very accessible animal for laboratory testing [20]. To our knowledge, this model has not been used for a long-term catheterization study. It was also important to compare the efficacy of our catheter to a silver coated catheter currently in use in patients. Therefore, we used an uncoated control in the mouse model whereas a commercially available silver coated catheter control was used in the porcine model.

This study was funded by Technology Enterprise Commercialisation Scheme-Proof-Of-Concept grant of SPRING Singapore (TI/TECS/POC/14/10).

Methods

Bacteria and growth conditions

E. coli UTI89, an uropathogenic strain known to be a good biofilm developer, isolated from a patient with uncomplicated cystitis, was kindly provided by Dr. Swaine Chen of Genome Institute of Singapore [21]. *E. coli* was cultured in lysogeny broth (LB) (BD Difco, Singapore) at 37 °C with constant agitation at 180–200 rpm. LB agar was used to grow *E. coli* on solid medium and incubated at 37 °C for 12–18 h.

Catheters for mouse model of CAUTI

Small silicone tubing, SIL037 (3 French, 0.5 mm ID × 0.9 mm OD) was obtained from Braintree Scientific, Inc., USA. Anti-fouling coating (P3) was prepared by coating PDA-AgNP-PDA-AgNP-PDA-poly(SBMA-*co*-AAm) layers on the inside as well as outside surfaces of the silicone tubing as described previously [17]. The method was modified to expedite the coating process as polydopamine was coated with oxygen bubbling at 60 °C for 20 min, instead of in air at room temperature for 24 h in our earlier work. Silver content in the coating was determined to be 33.98 ± 1.62 µg/cm^2 using Inductive Coupled Plasma-Optical Emission Spectrometry (ICP-OES, iCAP 6200 duo, Thermo Scientific, USA) as previously described [17]. The tubing was cut in 5 mm long segments, autoclaved and air-dried in a clean biosafety cabinet (BSC) before use in mice. Twelve mm long segments of SIL037 catheter tubing were fitted on sterile 25 G needles (Becton Dickinson). A 5 mm long, either coated or uncoated, sterile segment of SIL037 tubing was then placed on top of the 12 mm segment for implantation.

Catheters for porcine model of CAUTI

Uncoated silicone catheters of 14 Fr size were purchased from Promed Pte. Ltd., Singapore. P3 coated catheter was prepared by coating PDA-AgNP-PDA-AgNP-PDA-poly(SBMA-*co*-AAm) layers on pristine silicone catheter over the interior and exterior of the whole length as described previously with modification to obtain a similar silver content (30.30 ± 1.33 µg/cm^2) as in the mouse work [17]. For a 14 Fr Foley catheter (40 cm long), total silver amount was estimated to be approximately 3 mg per catheter. A commercially available, Dover™ silver coated 100% silicone Foley catheter was purchased from Covidien Pte. Ltd., Singapore.

Since the balloon inflation port of the silicone catheter was not autoclave-compatible, the coated catheters were disinfected by 70% ethanol followed by UV irradiation for 30 min and sealed before the pig study. The Dover™ catheter was used as received since it was in sterile package.

Murine model of CAUTI

All animal experiments were conducted in accordance with the university ethical regulations and were approved by the National University of Singapore Institutional Animal Care and Use Committee (IACUC). All animals were allowed an acclimatization period of at least five days in the animal testing facility after arrival, prior to experimentation. Laboratory feed and drinking water were provided ad libitum during entire duration, including before and during experimentation. The animal subjects were provided with environmental enrichment in accordance to species-specific standards. The temperature and humidity of the housing space was regulated as per international standards, and animals were provided with a cycle of 12 h of light followed by 12 h of darkness.

The mouse model was adapted from a previously published study with modifications mainly in the implant size and bacteria used [19]. Briefly, 18–20 weeks old C57BL/6 female mice (from InVivos Pvt. Ltd., Singapore) were anesthetized and 5 mm long catheter pieces were delivered in the urinary bladders by catheterizing the mice with a covered 25 G needle via the urethra lumen. The mice were re-catheterized with IV Catheters (24 G) and 50 μL bacterial cultures (2 x 10^6 Colony Forming Units (CFU)/ml) were instilled in the urinary bladder. After 30 min dwelling, the bladder was gently pressed to expel the contents.

Urine cultures were collected daily in metabolic cages overnight. Metabolic cages were used so as to collect larger volumes of urine for measurement of silver release from the coating. However, this way of urine collection may increase the risk of contamination of the urine by faeces and feed which we attempted to mitigate by having multiple comparisons. At the end of 14 days, mice were euthanized with CO_2 overdose (method approved by NUS-IACUC), and catheters were collected (if not passed out in urine). Bacterial biofilm was quantified from the collected catheters with a method using vortexing and sonication as reported recently [22]. In addition, bacterial colonization in the urinary bladder was measured. Each bladder was cut in two halves – one for homogenization and bacterial count, the other for histopathology studies.

Porcine model of CAUTI

Female miniature pigs (PWG Micropig®) from Prestige BioResearch Pte Ltd., Singapore (PBR) were used for this study. The work was carried out at PBR in accordance with approval by PBR-IACUC. During acclimation, animals were group housed. After the Foley catheter implantation, the animals were individually housed in well labelled steel cages. A standard nutrient and micro-ingredient composition of laboratory animal pig diet ration (pellets - 400 g, Altromin 9029, Altromin Spezialfutter GmbH & Co.KG, Germany) was available to each animal daily. Ultraviolet-irradiated municipal tap water was provided ad libitum to the animals. The animal room environment was controlled: a temperature of 16–27 °C, humidity of 50–80% and approximately 12 h of the light/dark cycle with 150–300 lx.

The study was conducted in compliance with the principles specified in national and international regulatory authority test guideline: ISO 10993:2006 "Biological Evaluation of Medical Devices – Part 11: Tests for Systemic Toxicity". This guideline largely deals with standardization of biological and clinical methods for evaluation of medical devices [23].

This proof of concept experiment comprised of two animals – one implanted with P3 coated catheter and the other animal with the commercially available silver coated Dover™ catheter for comparison. Implantation of the catheters was performed aseptically under general anaesthesia induced by isoflurane inhalation. The Foley catheter was inserted into the urinary bladder with long surgical forceps via the transurethral route with the animal in dorsal recumbency. The balloon was inflated with 5–6 ml of sterile distilled water according to the manufacturer's instructions. Subsequently, the inner lumen and outer surface were inoculated with 20 μL each of E. coli (10^5 CFU/ml) in 1X PBS at the outlet. After waiting approximately 10 min for bacteria to attach to the catheter surface, the external part of the catheter was tied to the tail of the pig with suitable adhesives.

Initially a urine reservoir bag was attached to the catheter at all times to maintain a closed system of urine collection as is the case in humans. We were not successful in securing the bag to the animal and observed that the catheter was pulled out or dropped out due to additional pressure from the bag. Therefore, subsequently, this was modified to an open catheter system. The outlet of the Foley catheter was anchored via suturing to skin in a dependent position and the urine bag was used only for urine sample collection.

Animals were euthanized at the endpoint (20 days post inoculation (dpi) for P3 catheter and 21 dpi for Dover™ catheter) by exsanguination of the vena cava and thoracic vein/artery under deep barbiturate anaesthesia (pentobarbitone sodium) as approved by PBR-IACUC. Catheters and organs of urinary tract were collected for evaluation of bacterial colonization and encrustation.

Assays used for analysis

In mice, efficacy of the coating was analysed using bacterial quantification in urine, on catheters and in tissues, scanning electron microscopy (SEM) and by measuring IL-6 levels in urine. Moreover, safety of the coating was assessed by monitoring body weight, kidney function tests and histopathology examination. Additionally, in the porcine model, encrustation was qualitatively examined visually as well as quantified using ICP-OES to measure calcium and magnesium deposition on catheters and in tissues.

Bacteria in urine and from catheter or tissue samples were counted using Miles and Misra method [24]. SEM was performed as published elsewhere [25] with some modifications and visualised using JEOL JSM-6701F Field Emission Scanning Electron Microscope. IL-6 levels were measured by ELISA to assess the degree of inflammation (Mouse IL-6, Cat# 88–7064-88, eBioscience Inc., USA).

Results and discussion
Euthanasia and harvesting
Mice

Out of 8 mice implanted with uncoated catheters, two mice were terminated early in the experiment due to bladder outlet obstruction as there was no urine output. An enlarged bladder was observed during post-mortem examination (Additional file 1: Figure S1). Catheters and bladders were collected and processed to assess bacterial colonization. One mouse was terminated 10dpi due to weight loss more than 25% and catheter and organs were collected and processed. The remaining 5 mice were euthanized at the endpoint (14 dpi). All 8 uncoated catheters were recovered.

Among the 8 mice implanted with P3 coated catheters, all mice survived till the endpoint. However, two catheters were lost, possibly, passed with urine from the bladder, hence only 6 catheters were recovered.

Pigs

Dover™ catheter in the pig was collected after euthanizing the animal 21 dpi. The P3 catheter did drop out once at two dpi, which was replaced with a new catheter and reinoculated with *E. coli* and the catheter was collected at the endpoint for the animal (20 dpi). It should be noted the pig was implanted with the P3 catheter for 23 days in total.

Anti-biofilm activity of P3 coating
Mice

After the mice were sacrificed, bacterial colonization on the catheter as well as in the bladder was quantified (Table 1). It was found that only one out of four P3 coated catheters had *E. coli* biofilm, whereas five out of six uncoated catheters had developed biofilm. On bacterial quantification, while median values showed a reduction of 10^7 CFU, average CFU values demonstrated a 50% reduction in bacterial load on P3 coated catheter. Moreover, both uncoated catheters recovered from mice terminated 3–4 dpi due to bladder obstruction were seen to be colonized by high numbers of bacteria (10^7). The majority of urinary bladders (5 out of 6) implanted with P3 coated catheters did not show any bacterial colonization. In comparison, more than half of the bladders (5 out of 8) implanted with uncoated catheters had bacterial colonization. Moreover, if the two bladders (implanted with uncoated catheters) that were harvested 3–4 dpi were excluded from analysis, the median value of CFU/bladder would be 1.2×10^2 (range: 0 to 6×10^7).

Biofilm formation on mouse catheters was visualized by SEM and the differences in coated and uncoated catheters can be seen in Fig. 1. Comparison between uncoated and P3 coated catheters at low magnification in Fig. 1a and b shows the difference in surface area covered with a layer or a film. At high magnification, a few rod-shaped structures resembling *E. coli* shape (and size)

Table 1 Catheter recovery, bladder harvesting and *E. coli* colonization

	Uncoated Up to 14dpi[a]	P3 coated 14dpi
Number of mice euthanized (total 8 mice per group)	8	8
Catheters collected (catheters lost)	8 (0)	6 (2)
Number of catheters processed for biofilm extraction assay (catheters processed for SEM[b])	6 (2)	4 (2)
Number of catheters with viable biofilm	5	1
Median values of CFU[c]/catheter (range)	6.58×10^7 (0 to 1.52×10^8)	0 (0 to 1.18×10^8)
Number of urinary bladders collected with catheters	8	6
Number of bladders with viable bacteria	5	1
Median values of CFU/bladder (range)	5.0×10^2 (0 to 1.4×10^8)	0 (0 to 1.03×10^5)

[a]Days post inoculation
[b]Scanning electron microscopy
[c]Colony forming units

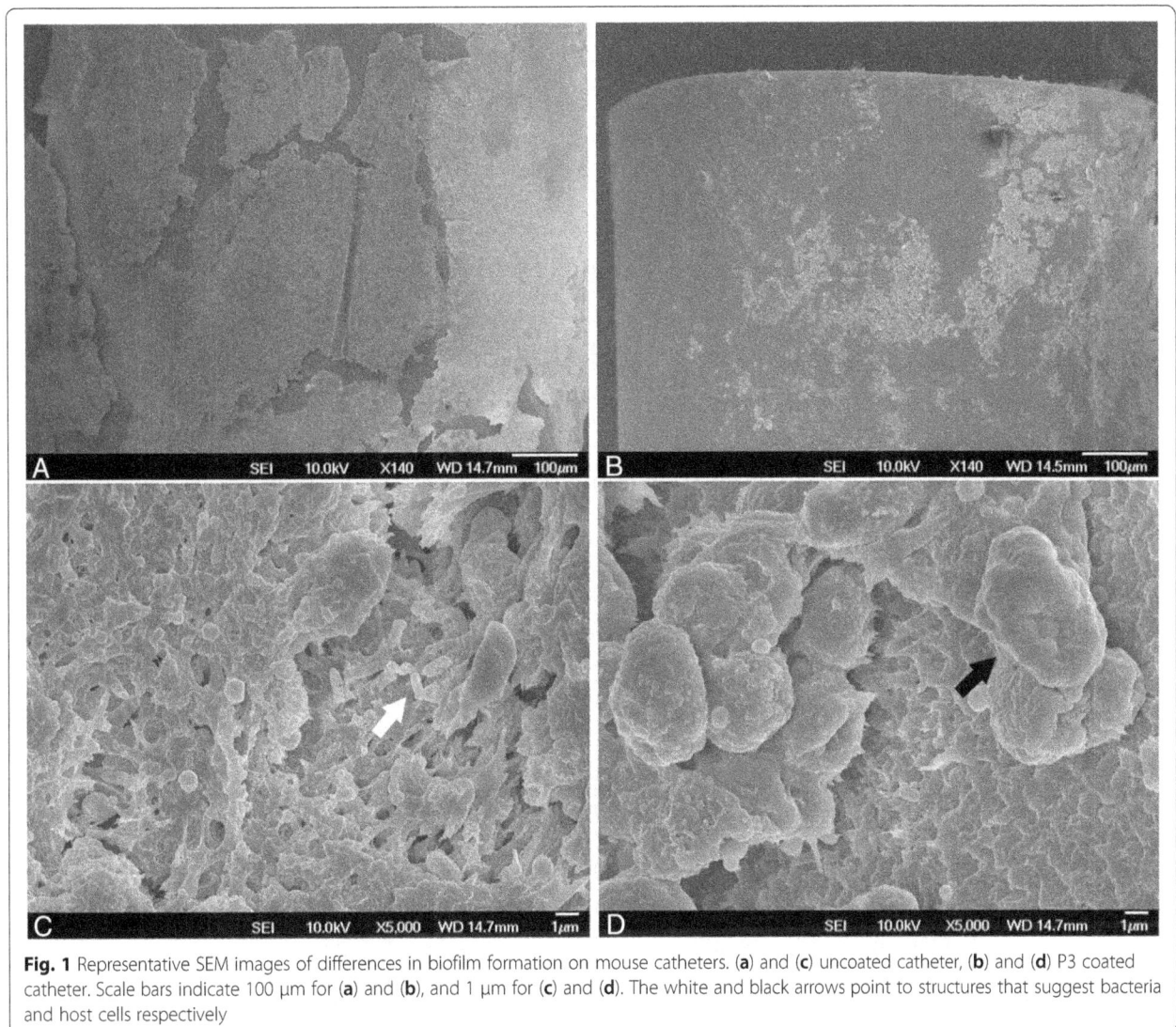

Fig. 1 Representative SEM images of differences in biofilm formation on mouse catheters. (**a**) and (**c**) uncoated catheter, (**b**) and (**d**) P3 coated catheter. Scale bars indicate 100 μm for (**a**) and (**b**), and 1 μm for (**c**) and (**d**). The white and black arrows point to structures that suggest bacteria and host cells respectively

can be seen on the uncoated catheter (Fig. 1c – indicated by white arrow), suggesting that these are bacterial biofilms. On the other hand, the size of the cell-like structures seen on P3 coated catheters (Fig. 1d – indicated by black arrow) suggests that they are host cells.

Pigs
The human catheter in the porcine model also showed promising results as average bacterial counts from the catheter collected from the pig with the P3 catheter (20 dpi) were 2.4 times lower than that on the silver coated Dover™ catheter (21 dpi). Biofilm extracted from three segments near tip of the catheters recovered from both animals yielded mostly *E. coli* colonies whereas two segments near the urethral exit yielded a polymicrobial biofilm.

Comparison between *E. coli* inoculated micropigs in Fig. 2 showed a significant (~ 700 fold) reduction in

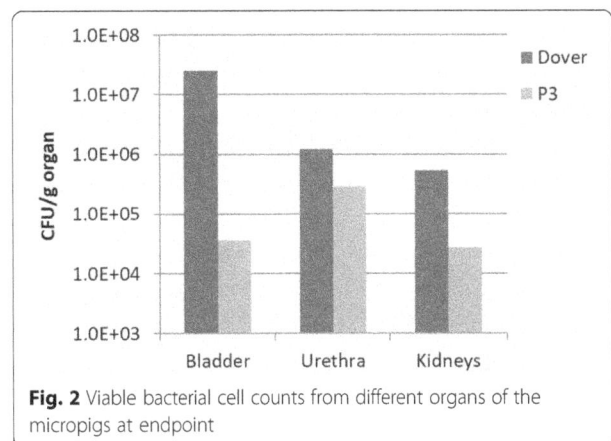

Fig. 2 Viable bacterial cell counts from different organs of the micropigs at endpoint

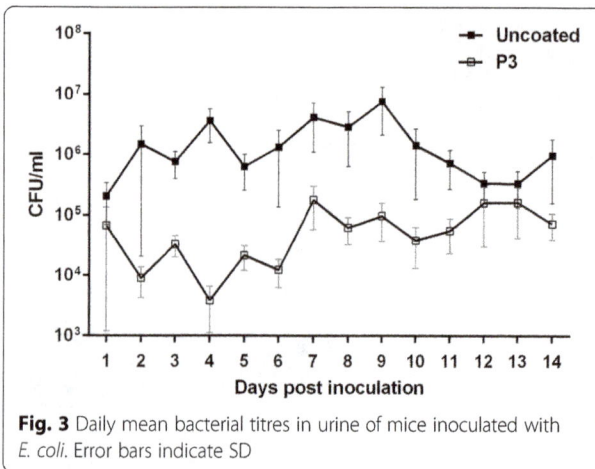

Fig. 3 Daily mean bacterial titres in urine of mice inoculated with *E. coli*. Error bars indicate SD

efficacy of our coating to a clinically tested silver coating which is licensed by the major regulatory agencies and in clinical use globally, the results of this proof-of-concept study would be more relevant as various reviews and meta-analyses have demonstrated ability of silver to reduce CAUTI [26–28]. We also do recognise that the proprietary nature of the commercial control catheter limits our ability to compare the details of the different coatings.

These results suggest that the P3 coating could inhibit *E. coli* biofilm formation both on catheter surface and in the bladder effectively in mice and in pigs.

bladder infection with P3 coated catheter as compared to the pig with commercial Dover™ catheter. Similarly, a reduction was also observed in bacterial colonization in the urethra (4 fold) and kidneys (19 fold) (Fig. 2).

Although an uncoated catheter would be an appropriate control to demonstrate efficacy in the pig model, the aim of this study was to develop a catheter which could be marketed for clinical use. However, by comparing the

Antibacterial activity in mice

Daily bacterial load in urine was calculated for 14 dpi in six mice implanted with P3 coated catheters. In the uncoated catheter implanted group, bacteriuria was quantified in 5 mice for 14 dpi and one mouse for 10 dpi. Consistently less bacteriuria (51–99%) was observed in mice with P3 coated catheters as compared to mice with uncoated catheters for up to 14 days (Fig. 3).

The higher values of IL6 in uncoated group (Additional file 1: Figure S2) indicating more inflammation as compared to P3 group supporting the finding of

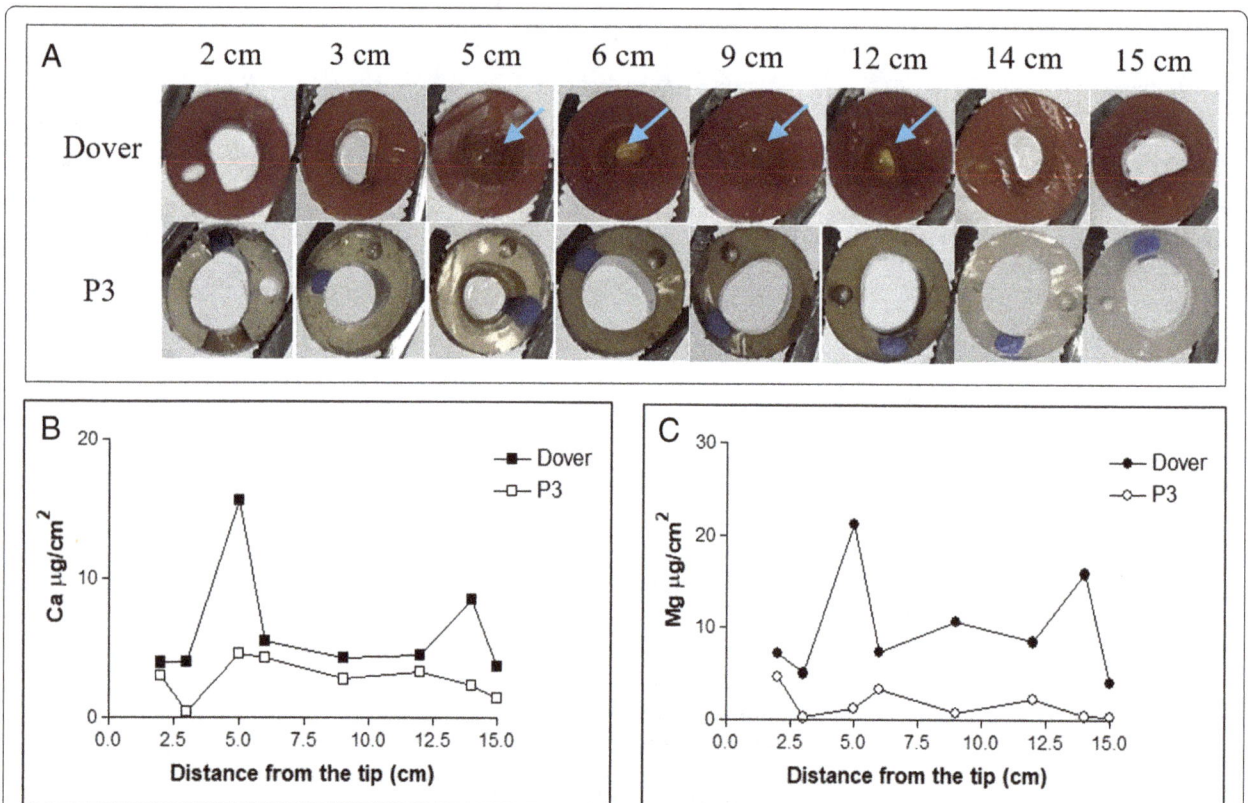

Fig. 4 a) Photos of cross-section of catheter segments collected from pigs implanted with Dover™ catheter and P3 coated catheter, on 21dpi and 20dpi, respectively. Catheter segments at different positions along the length are shown. Arrows indicate catheter lumen was either partially or completely blocked by crystals and/or biofilm. Average amounts of **B)** calcium and **c)** magnesium on the catheter segments

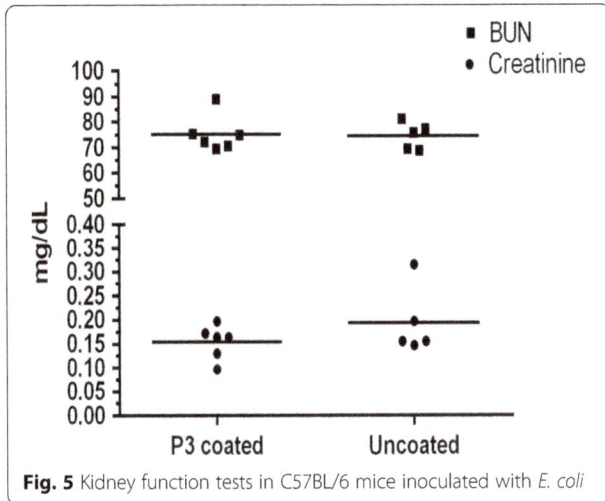

Fig. 5 Kidney function tests in C57BL/6 mice inoculated with *E. coli*

low activity of pathogenic bacteria in P3 group mice compared with controls.

Reduction of encrustation in pigs

Figure 4a shows the cross-sections of the catheters that challenged with *E. coli*. As can be seen, segments of the Dover™ catheter collected 21 dpi were totally or partially blocked, while the P3 coated catheter retrieved 20 dpi remained patent throughout the length assessed (up to 15 cm from the catheter tip, the length inserted in the urethra and bladder). Quantitative results from ICP-OES measurement indicate that both calcium (2.3 times on an average) and magnesium (6 times on an average) amounts were lower on P3 coated catheter as compared to Dover™ catheter (Fig. 4b and c). This indicates that P3 coated catheter inhibited encrustation formation during uropathogenic *E. coli* infection more effectively compared to the commercially available Dover™ catheter.

There were 1.8 times less calcium and magnesium precipitates in the bladder of the pigs with P3 coated catheter as compared to the silver coated Dover™ catheter (Additional file 1: Figure S3).

Toxicity

All mice lost up to 18% body weight in the first two dpi but recovered well 3rd day onwards (Additional file 1: Figure S4). Mice with the P3 coated catheter show slightly lower (~ 5%) weight loss as compared to mice with uncoated catheters indicating that silver does not appear to cause any general harm to the animals over a period of two weeks.

Kidney function was also assessed by measuring levels of creatinine and blood urea nitrogen (BUN) in serum at endpoint. As seen in Fig. 5, no major differences were observed in kidney functions (both parameters) of mice with uncoated catheter and those with P3 coated catheters. BUN readings were higher than normal and creatinine values were slightly lower than normal values [29, 30] in both groups indicating that the increase may not be due to P3 coating, but possibly due to the hydration status or inflammatory state of the animals.

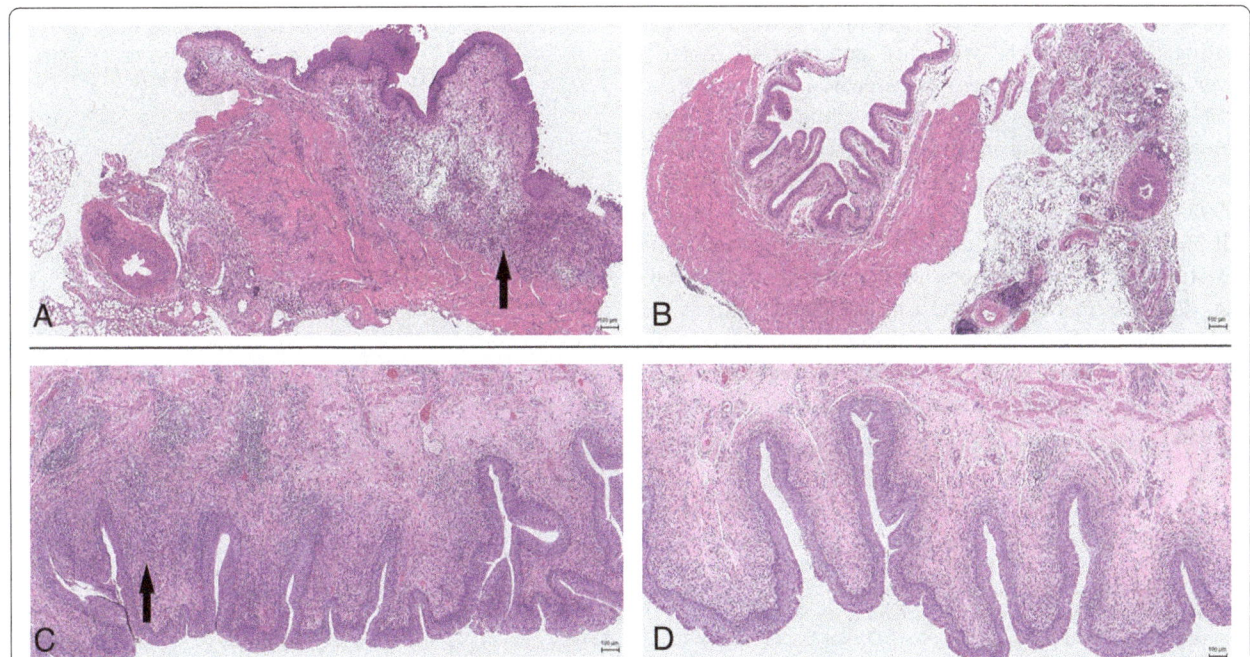

Fig. 6 Representative hematoxylin and eosin staining (scale bars 100 μm) of 5 μm section of urinary bladders of **a**) Mice with uncoated catheter and **b**) Mice with P3 coated catheter **c**) Pigs with silver coated Dover™ catheter and **d**) Pigs with P3 coated catheter. Images suggest a higher granulocyte infiltration in the sub-mucosal layer (indicated by black arrows) in **a** and **c** as compared to that in **b** and **d** respectively

Silver levels could not be measured in urine of mice with P3 catheters due to undetectable (low) levels.

Histopathology

The degree of bladder inflammation appeared more severe in the uncoated group as compared to the P3 group. Moderate to severe pyogranulomatous, lympho-plasmacytic, oedematous cystitis as well as minimal to moderate pyogranulomatous, lymphoplasmacytic sero-sitis was seen in mice implanted with uncoated catheters infected with *E. coli* (Fig. 6a). On the other hand, no sig-nificant findings were observed in mice with P3-coated catheter and *E. coli* except in one mouse with moderate pyogranulomatous, lymphoplasmacytic serositis (Fig. 6b). Similar results were observed with pig bladders wherein moderate cystitis was seen in animal with the silver coated Dover™ catheter (Fig. 6c) whereas mild cystitis was observed in animal with P3 catheter (Fig. 6d). This indicates that the P3 coating is not harmful to the bladder compared to uncoated catheter (in mice) or silver coated Dover™ catheter (in pigs); it may even have an anti-inflammatory effect.

Conclusion

In this study, we have demonstrated, using a murine model and a novel porcine model the safety, and anti-microbial effect of the P3 coating. The results also sug-gest an anti-encrustation capability of P3 coating. In the porcine model, using a proof of concept with a single animal, we demonstrated the potential efficacy of P3 coating in comparison with the commercial Dover™ silver coating. The P3 coated catheter was safe for use as indicated by the absence of systemic clinical and labora-tory signs in both animal models. This suggests low tox-icity from the catheter coating material in line with ISO 10993–11:2006.

It should be noted that due to the small group size in the study and the limitations of the current pig model (e.g. difficulty in retaining the catheter), more extensive evaluations of the efficacy and safety of the P3 coated catheter are needed before proceeding for regulatory ap-proval, human studies and widespread clinical use of the catheter.

Abbreviations

[poly(SBMA-*co*-AAm)]: poly(sulfobetaine methacrylate-*co*-acrylamide); AgNPs: Silver nanoparticles; BSC: Biosafety cabinet; BUN: Blood urea nitrogen; CAUTI: Catheter Associated Urinary Tract Infections; CFU: Colony forming unit; dpi: day(s) post inoculation; IACUC: Institutional Animal Care and Use Committee; ICP-OES: Inductive Coupled Plasma-Optical Emission Spectrom-etry; LB: Lysogeny broth; P3: Anti-fouling coating prepared by coating PDA-AgNP-PDA-AgNP-PDA-poly(SBMA-*co*-AAm) layers on the inside as well as outside surfaces of the silicone tubing; PBR: Prestige BioResearch Pte Ltd., Singapore; PDA: Polydopamine; SEM: Scanning electron microscopy; UPEC: Uropathogenic *Escherichia coli*

Acknowledgement

This work was partly presented at Urofair 2017, Singapore (Oral presentation), at the 15th International Congress of Bacteriology and Applied Microbiology 2017, Singapore (Poster presentation) and at the 33rd Annual European Association of Urology Congress 2018, Copenhagen, Denmark (Moderated poster presentation). Abstracts were published in BJU International 119 (S4); 42, and in European Urology Supplements 17 (2); e481.

Funding

This work was supported by Technology Enterprise Commercialisation Scheme-Proof-Of-Concept grant of SPRING Singapore (TI/TECS/POC/14/10). The funding organization played a role in design of the study.

Authors' contributions

KGN, EC and PAT designed and supervised the experiments. KDM, RW and JNR performed the experiments and analysed the results. KDM and RW drafted the manuscript. KGN, EC and PAT critically reviewed the manuscript. All authors have read and approved the final manuscript.

Consent for publication

Not applicable.

Competing interests

Paul A Tambyah has received research grants from Sanofi-Pasteur, Fabentech and GSK and honoraria from Johnson and Johnson. All other authors declare that they have no competing interest.

Author details

[1]Department of Medicine, Yong Loo Lin School of Medicine, National University of Singapore, 1E, Kent Ridge Road, NUHS Tower Block, Level 10, Singapore 119228, Singapore. [2]ACI Medical Pte Ltd, Singapore 069534, Singapore. [3]Department of Surgery, Yong Loo Lin School of Medicine, National University of Singapore, Singapore 119228, Singapore. [4]Department of Chemical and Biomolecular Engineering, National University of Singapore, Singapore 117585, Singapore.

References

1. Dudeck MA, Edwards JR, Allen-Bridson K, Gross C, Malpiedi PJ, Peterson KD, Pollock DA, Weiner LM, Sievert DM. National Healthcare Safety Network report, data summary for 2013, Device-associated module. Am J Infect Control. 2015(43):206–21.
2. Nicolle LE. Catheter associated urinary tract infections. Antimicrob Resist Infect Control. 2014;3:23.
3. Tambyah PA, Oon J. Catheter-associated urinary tract infection. Curr Opin Infect Dis. 2012;25:365–70.
4. CDC: Urinary Tract Infection (Catheter-Associated Urinary Tract Infection [CAUTI] and Non-Catheter-Associated Urinary Tract Infection [UTI]) and Other Urinary System Infection [USI]) Events. In: Device-associated Module CAUTI. 2015. http://www.cdc.gov/nhsn/PDFs/pscManual/7pscCAUTIcurrent. pdf Accessed 25 June 2015.
5. Maki DG, Tambyah PA. Engineering out the risk for infection with urinary catheters. Emerg Infect Dis. 2001;7:342–7.
6. Flores-Mireles AL, Walker JN, Caparon M, Hultgren SJ. Urinary tract infections: epidemiology, mechanisms of infection and treatment options. Nat Rev Microbiol. 2015;13:269–84.
7. Spaulding CN, Kau AL, Klein RD, Janetka JW, Gordon JI, Hultgren SJ. Small-molecule inhibitors against type 1 pili selectively target uropathogenic *E. coli* in the gut and bladder. FASEB J. 2017;31:939.939.
8. Pitout JDD, DeVinney R: *Escherichia coli* ST131: a multidrug-resistant clone primed for global domination. *F1000Research* 2017, 6:F1000 Faculty Rev-1195.

9. Mobley HL, Donnenberg MS, Hagan EC. Uropathogenic Escherichia coli. EcoSal Plus. 2009;3

10. Stickler DJ. Proteus mirabilis biofilm formation and catheter design. In: Denstedt J, Atala A, editors. *Biomaterials and Tissue Engineering in Urology.* Cambridge: Woodhead Publishing; 2009. p. 157–90.

11. Amalaradjou M, A R, Venkitanarayanan K. Role of Bacterial Biofilms in Catheter-Associated Urinary Tract Infections (CAUTI) and Strategies for Their Control. In: Nelius T, editor. *Recent Advances in the Field of Urinary Tract Infections.* London: IntechOpen; 2013.

12. Choong S, Wood S, Fry C, Whitfield H. Catheter associated urinary tract infection and encrustation. Int J Antimicrob Agents. 2001;17:305–10.

13. Stickler D, Morris N, Moreno MC, Sabbuba N. Studies on the formation of crystalline bacterial biofilms on urethral catheters. Eur J Clin Microbiol Infect Dis. 1998;17:649–52.

14. Trautner BW, Darouiche RO. Role of biofilm in catheter-associated urinary tract infection. Am J Infect Control. 2004;32:177–83.

15. Donelli G. Biofilm-based healthcare-associated infections : volume I. New York: Springer; 2014.

16. Mandakhalikar KD, Chua RR, Tambyah PA. New Technologies for Prevention of catheter associated urinary tract infection. Current Treatment Options in Infectious Diseases. 2016;8:24–41.

17. Wang R, Neoh KG, Kang ET, Tambyah PA, Chiong E. Antifouling coating with controllable and sustained silver release for long-term inhibition of infection and encrustation in urinary catheters. J Biomed Mater Res B Appl Biomater. 2015;103:519–28.

18. Kadurugamuwa JL, Modi K, Yu J, Francis KP, Purchio T, Contag PR. Noninvasive biophotonic imaging for monitoring of catheter-associated urinary tract infections and therapy in mice. Infect Immun. 2005;73:3878–87.

19. Guiton PS, Hung CS, Hancock LE, Caparon MG, Hultgren SJ. Enterococcal biofilm formation and virulence in an optimized murine model of foreign body-associated urinary tract infections. Infect Immun. 2010;78:4166–75.

20. Swindle MM, Makin A, Herron AJ, Clubb FJ Jr, Frazier KS. Swine as models in biomedical research and toxicology testing. Vet Pathol. 2012;49:344–56.

21. Chen SL, Hung CS, Xu J, Reigstad CS, Magrini V, Sabo A, Blasiar D, Bieri T, Meyer RR, Ozersky P, et al. Identification of genes subject to positive selection in uropathogenic strains of Escherichia coli: a comparative genomics approach. Proc Natl Acad Sci U S A. 2006;103:5977–82.

22. Mandakhalikar KD, Rahmat JN, Chiong E, Neoh KG, Shen L, Tambyah PA. Extraction and quantification of biofilm bacteria: method optimized for urinary catheters. Sci Rep. 2018;8:8069.

23. ISO. Biological evaluation of medical devices -- Part 11: Tests for systemic toxicity. In: *Biological evaluation of medical devices,* vol. ISO 10993–11: 2006: International Organization for Standardization. Geneva: ISO; 2006.

24. Miles AA, Misra SS, Irwin JO. The estimation of the bactericidal power of the blood. J Hyg (Lond). 1938;38:732–49.

25. Mukherjee D, Zou H, Liu S, Beuerman R, Dick T. Membrane-targeting AM-0016 kills mycobacterial persisters and shows low propensity for resistance development. Future Microbiol. 2016;11:643–50.

26. Beattie M, Taylor J. Silver alloy vs. uncoated urinary catheters: a systematic review of the literature. J Clin Nurs. 2011;20:2098–108.

27. Saint S, Veenstra DL, Sullivan SD, Chenoweth C, Fendrick AM. The potential clinical and economic benefits of silver alloy urinary catheters in preventing urinary tract infection. Arch Intern Med. 2000;160:2670–5.

28. Saint S, Elmore JG, Sullivan SD, Emerson SS, Koepsell TD. The efficacy of silver alloy-coated urinary catheters in preventing urinary tract infection: a meta-analysis. Am J Med. 1998;105:236–41.

29. Fernandez I, Pena A, Del Teso N, Perez V, Rodriguez-Cuesta J. Clinical biochemistry parameters in C57BL/6J mice after blood collection from the submandibular vein and retroorbital plexus. J Am Assoc Lab Anim Sci. 2010;49:202–6.

30. Serfilippi LM, Pallman DR, Russell B. Serum clinical chemistry and hematology reference values in outbred stocks of albino mice from three commonly used vendors and two inbred strains of albino mice. Contemp Top Lab Anim Sci. 2003;42:46–52.

Species distribution and antibiotic susceptibility profile of bacterial uropathogens among patients complaining urinary tract infections

Adane Bitew[1*], Tamirat Molalign[2] and Meseret Chanie[3]

Abstract

Background: Urinary tract infection is the second most common type of infection and the problem is further compounded by the emergence of drug resistance in bacterial uropathogens. The aim of this study was to determine the spectrum of bacterial uropathogens and their drug resistant pattern.

Methods: A single institutional cross-sectional study was carried out at Arsho Advanced Medical laboratory from September 2015 to May 2016. A total of 712 urine samples were collected, inoculated onto primary isolation culture media, incubated at 37 °C for 18–24 h, and significant bacteriuria was determined. Identification and the antimicrobial susceptibility testing of bacteria were determined by using the automated VITEK 2 compact system.

Results: Out of 712 urine samples processed, 256 (36%) yielded significant bacteriuria of which 208 (81.25%) were obtained from female and 48 (18.75%) from male patients. Age group of 25–44 were more affected with the infection. Of 256 bacterial isolates recovered, *Escherichia coli,* was the dominant bacterium. Ampicillin and trimethoprim/sulfamethoxazole were the least effective drugs while piperacillin/tazobactam was the most effective drug against Gram-negative bacteria. Erythromycin was the least effective drug while vancomycin was the most active drug against Gram-positive bacteria.

Conclusions: Observation of many bacterial species causing UTI in this study warrants, a continuous epidemiological survey of UTI in health institutions across the country. High level of drug resistance to the commonly prescribed drugs necessitates a search for other options.

Keywords: UTIs, Drug resistance, Species distribution, Ethiopia

Background

Urinary tract infection (UTI) is an infection of the bladder (cystitis) or the kidneys (pyelonephritis). It is the second most common type of infection accounting for about 8.1 million visits to health care providers each year [1]. Women are more are more susceptible to UTI than men. Over 50% of all women will experience at least one UTI during their life-time, with 20–30% experiencing recurrent UTI [2, 3].

Urinary tract infection is a morbid disease in terms of loss of working days and treatment cost [4]. In the United States alone, UTI has been reported to cause > 6 million outpatient visits [5] and 479,000 hospitalizations annually [6]. Furthermore, the annual treatment cost of UTI in this part of the world has been estimated to be greater than 2.47 billion USD [2]. They are also important cause of sepsis resulting in high mortality rates [7].

Infants, pregnant women, patients with spinal cord injuries, diabetes, multiple sclerosis, acquired immunodeficiency disease syndrome or underlying urologic abnormalities are subjects that are at increased risk for UTI. In addition, catheter-associated UTI is the most common nosocomial infection [7].

* Correspondence: Adane.Bitew@aau.edu.et
[1]Department of Medical Laboratory Sciences, College of Health Sciences, Addis Ababa University, Addis Ababa, Ethiopia
Full list of author information is available at the end of the article

Many previous studies have shown that *E. coli* is the most common etiological agent of UTI in both hospital and community acquired infections. Hospital acquired UTI has also been characteristically associated with a higher prevalence of enterococci and Coagulase- Negative Staphylococci [8–13]. In addition, *Klebsiella pneumonia, Streptococcus agalactiae, Proteus mirabilis,* viridans streptococci, *Klebsiella oxytoca, Pseudomonas aeruginosa, Citrobacter freundii, Enterobacter cloacae,* and *Staphylococcus aureus* have been identified as etiologic agents of UTI [7].

Due to the rapidly evolving adaptive strategies of bacteria, the etiology of UTI and antibiotic resistance profile of bacterial uropathogens have changed considerably over the past years, both in community and nosocomial infections [13]. Many studies conducted from the USA and Europe have revealed increasing antibiotic resistance among uropathogenic *E. coli* to ampicillin, trimethoprim, and sulfonamides [9, 10, 12]. Apparent shift in the etiological agents of urinary tract infection and associated problem of antibiotic resistance amongst bacterial uropathogens from time to time and from one institution to another have initiated health institution to carry out continuous evaluation of UTI from the view point of their spectrum and drug susceptibility testing.

Accurate identification of bacterial uropathogens and determining their drug susceptibility pattern are critical for efficient management of patients with UTI. They are also associated with significant clinical and financial benefits, via the reduction of mortality rates and overall hospitalization costs [14]. In view of this, identification and antimicrobial susceptibility testing of clinical isolates by means of fully automated systems have become a common practice in many laboratories. The VITEK 2 compact system is a new automated system designed to provide accurate identification and susceptibility testing results for most clinical isolates of both Gram-positive and Gram-negative bacteria. Apart from accurate identification and susceptibility testing shortened turnaround times, improved specimen handling, enhanced quality control, reproducibility and the ability to track results are further advantages of the system [15].

Unfortunately, in Ethiopian health care providing institutions, identification and drug susceptibility profile of bacterial uropathognes have been carried by conventional methods that appeared to be inferior to the fully automated systems. Against this background, the present study was designed to determine the spectrum of bacterial uropathogens and their antimicrobial susceptibility profile by employing the VITEK 2 compact system among patients referred to Arsho advanced medical laboratory private limited company with a complain of UTI.

Methods

Study site, period and socio-demographic data

The present study was a single institutional cross-sectional study carried out at Arsho Advanced Medical laboratory, Addis Ababa, Ethiopia from June 2015 to May 2016. Willingness to participate in the study, presumptive diagnosis of urinary tract infection and no history of antibacterial therapy within 2 weeks prior to their attendance were the inclusion criteria. The requisition form filled up by physicians was used as standard proforma to document socio-demographic information of study subjects. Age groups of patients were classified following WHO guideline [16].

Sample collection and inoculation of primary isolation culture media

Clean-catch midstream urine was collected from patients complaining of UTI; referred from different health institutions in the city with sterile wide-mouthed urine cup. Urine samples were inoculated onto Blood Agar base (Oxoid, Basingstoke, Hampaire, UK) to which 10% sheep blood is incorporated and Cysteine Lactose Electrolyte Deficient medium (Oxoid, Basingstoke, Hampaire, UK) using a calibrated loop with a capacity of 1 μl in safety cabinet. All inoculated plates were incubated at 37 °C for 18–24 h aerobically and the number of colonies was counted. Colony counts yielding bacterial growth of $>10^5/$ ml of urine ($\geq$100,000 colonies) were regarded as significant for bacteriuria. Urine samples yielded three and more bacterial species were not considered for further investigation. Pure isolates of bacterial pathogen were preliminary characterized by colony morphology, Gram-stain, and catalase test before inoculating them into AST-GN72 and AST-GP71 cards.

Inoculum size determination

Quality control bacteria and pure cultures of bacterial isolates were suspended in 3 ml of sterile saline (aqueous 0.45 to 0.50% NaCl, pH 4.5 to 7.0) in a 12 × 75 mm clear plastic (polystyrene) test tube to achieve a turbidity equivalent to that of a McFarland 0.50 standard (range, 0.50 to 0.63), as measured by the DensiChek (bioMe'rieux) turbidity meter. These suspensions were used for the inoculation of GN72 and GP71 identification cards while AST cards were inoculated after bacterial suspensions were further diluted following the instruction of the manufacture.

Identification and determination of antimicrobial susceptibility

Species identification and antimicrobial susceptibility testing of Gram-positive and Gram-negative bacteria were determined with the automated VITEK 2 compact system (bioMérieux, France) using AST, GN72 and GP71 cards. The VITEK 2 compact system (bioMe'rieux) is an integrated modular system that consists of a filling-sealer unit, a reader-incubator, a computer control module, a data terminal, and a multicopy printer. The system detects bacterial growth and metabolic changes in the microwells of thin plastic cards using a fluorescence-based technology.

AST-GN72 cards were used for the identification and susceptibility testing of none-spore-forming, fermenting, and non-fermenting Gram-negative bacilli while the AST-GP71 cards were used for the automated identification and susceptibility testing of non-spore-forming Gram-positive bacteria. The cards were automatically filled by a vacuum device and were automatically sealed and subjected to a kinetic fluorescence measurement in accordance with the manufacturer's instructions. Brief, identification cards were inoculated with quality control bacteria and pure cultures of bacterial isolate suspensions using an integrated vacuum apparatus. A test tube containing the bacterial suspension was placed into a special rack (cassette) and the identification card was placed in the neighboring slot while inserting the transfer tube into the corresponding suspension tube. The filled cassette was inserted manually into the VITEK 2 compact reader-incubator module. After the vacuum was applied and air was re-introduced into the station, the bacterial suspension was forced through the transfer tube into micro-channels that fill all the test wells and inoculated cards were automatically sealed prior to loading into the carousel incubator. All card types were incubated automatically incubated 35.5 ± 1.0 °C. Each card was removed from the carousel incubator once every 15 min, transported to the optical system for reaction readings, and then returned to the incubator until the next read time. Data were collected at 15-min intervals during the entire incubation period and final identification results were obtained in approximately 18 h or less. All cards used were automatically discarded in a waste container.

AST-GN72 cards consists of 64 biochemical method and substrates for identification and a panel of 19 antibiotics for drug susceptibility testing. Antibiotics with their different concentration used for the determination of drug susceptibility profile of Gram-negative bacteria in this investigation were: ampicillin (4,8,32), amoxicilin/clavulanic acid (4/2,16/8,32/16), cefalotin (2,8,32), cefazolin (4, 16, 64), cefepime (2,8,16,32), cefoxitin (8,16,32), cefpodoxime (0.5, 1, 4), ceftazidime (1,2,8,32), ceftriaxone (1,2,8,32), cefuroxime (2,8,32), ciprofloxacin (0.5,2,4), gentamicin (4,16,32), levofloxacin (0.25,0.5,2,8), nitrofurantoin (16,32,64), piperacillin/tazobactam (2/4,8/4,24/4,32/4,32/8), tetracycline (2,4,8), tobramycin (8,16,64), trimethoprim/sulfamethoxazole (1/19,4/76,16/304).

Similarly, the AST-GP71 card consists of an array of biochemical tests for species characterization and antibiotics for drug susceptibility testing of Gram-positive

bacteria. Antibiotics with their different concentration used for the determination of drug susceptibility pattern of Gram-positive bacteria in this investigation were:- cefoxitin screen (6), ciprofloxacin (1, 2, 4), clindamycin(0.5,1,2), daptomycin (0.5, 1, 2, 4, 16), erythromycin (0.25,0.5,2), gentamicin (8,16,64), inducible clindamycin resistance (CM 0.5, CM/E 0.25/0.5), levofloxacin (0.25,2,8), linezolid (0.5,2,8), minocycline (0.12,0.5,1), moxifloxacin (0.25,2,8), nitrofurantoin (16,32,64), oxacillin (0.5,1,2), quinupristin/dalfopristin (0.25,0.5,2), rifampicin (0.25,0.5,2), tetracycline (0.5,1,2), tigecycline (0.25,0.5,1), trimethoprim/sulfamethoxazole (2/38,8/152,16/304), and vancomycin (1,2,4,8,16).

Quality control
For quality control of susceptibility tests *E. coli* ATCC 25922, *P. aeruginosa* ATCC 27853, *S. aureus* ATCC 25923 and *E. faecalis* ATCC929212 strains were used.

Ethical clearance
All ethical considerations and obligations were duly addressed and the study was conducted after the approval of the Department Research and Ethical Review Committee (DRERC) of the Department of Medical Laboratory Sciences, College of Health Sciences, and Addis Ababa University. Informed written consent was obtained from participants before data collection. The respondent was given the right to refuse to take part in the study and to withdraw at any time during the study period. All the information obtained from the study subjects were coded to maintain confidentially. When the participants were found to be positive for bacterial pathogen, they were informed by the hospital clinician and received proper treatment. Assent form was completed and signed by family member and/or adult guardian for participants under the age of 16 years.

Results
Of a total of 712 urine samples processed during the study period, 519 (72.9%) were collected from female patients and 193 (27.1%) from male patients. Two hundred fifty six (36%) urine samples yielded significant bacteriuria of which 208 (81.2%) were obtained from female patients and 48 (18.8%) from male patients. Cases of 75% UTI were recorded among young and middle age patients with an age group of 15–64 years. Pediatric patients (0–14 years) and elderly patients (≥65 years) accounted for 11.3 and 13.7% of the total number of UTI, respectively (Table 1). Urinary tract infection was the highest (43.8%) in patients of age group 25–44 followed by age groups of 45–64 (20%).

A total 256 (27 species) bacterial isolates belonging to 14 genera were recovered, of which 175 (68.4%) of the isolates (15 species) were Gram-negative and 81 (31.6%) isolates (12 species) were Gram-positive bacteria. *E. coli* and *K. pneumoniae*, were the two predominant Gram-negative

Table 1 Gender and age distribution of study participants

Variable	Categories	Samples collected n = 712	Sample s collected n = 712	
			UTI yes = 256	UTI no = 456
Gender	Female	519 (72.9)	208(81.2)	311(68.2)
	Male	193 (27.1)	48(18.8)	145 (31.8)
	Total	712 (100)	256(100)	456 (100)
Age group	<1	28 (3.9)	18(7.0)	10 (2.2)
	1–14	55 (7.7)	11(4.3)	44 (9.6)
	15–24	74 (10.4)	29(11.3)	45(9.9)
	25–44	330 (46.3)	112(43.8)	218(47.8)
	45–64	152 (21.3)	51(19.9)	101 (22.1)
	65+	73 (10.3)	35(13.7)	38 (8.3)
	Total	712 (100)	256(100)	456 (100)

Table 3 Distribution and frequency of Gram positive bacterial isolates

Genus	Species	n (%) of the total isolates
Staphylococcus	S. saprophytics	18 (7.0)
	S. aureus	9 (3.5)
	S. warneri	9 (3.5)
	S. epidermidis	8 (3.1)
	S. hominis	6 (2.3)
	S. lentus	3 (1.2)
	S. haemolyticus	2 (0.8)
Streptococcus	S. agalactiae	8 (3.1)
	S. porcinus	1 (0.4)
Enterococcus	E. faecalis	14 (5.5)
	E. gallinarum	1 (0.4)
Kocuria	K. kristinae	2 (0.8)
Total (4)	12	81 (31.6)

bacteria consisting of (52.7%) and 7% of the total isolates, respectively. *S. sapropyticus* and *E. faecalis* were the first and the second predominant Gram positive bacteria, respectively (Tables 2 and 3).

The overall drug susceptibility profile of Gram-negative bacteria for the 19 antibacterial drugs tested is summarized in Table 4. Ampicillin had the highest overall resistance rate (78.3%) for Gram negative bacteria followed by trimethoprim/sulfamethoxazole (66.3) and tetracycline (62.3%). Gram-negative bacteria showed better sensitivity towards piperacillin/tazobactam combination, cefoxitin, gentamicin, and nitrofurantoin with the overall resistance rates of 17.7, 24, 25.7, and 29.1%, respectively. *E. coli*, the most frequently isolated bacterium, showed 77.8, 70.4 and 69.6% resistance

rates to ampicillin, trimethoprim/sulfamethoxazole, and tetracycline, respectively. The least resistance rate (20%) of the bacterium was observed for nitrofurantoin. *K. pneumoniae*, the second most commonly isolated Gram- negative bacterium exhibited a resistance rate of 100% for ampicillin and 66.7% for trimethoprim/ sulfamethoxazole. The least resistance rate (5.6%) of this bacterium was observed for piperacillin/tazobactam combination. *Moraxella nonliquefiens* and *P. aeruginosa* the 3rd most frequently isolated Gram-negative bacteria were 100% resistant to 15 and nine drugs, respectively. *Acinetobacter baumannii* the 4th most frequently isolated bacteria was 100% resistant to ten drugs. Out of 175 isolates of Gram-negative bacteria, 2 (1.14%) isolates were resistant to all the antibiotics tested and 15 (8.6%) of the isolates were pandrug-resistant to cephalosporins.

The most common bacterial isolates found to be pandrug-resistant to cephalosporins were *E. coli, K. pneumoniae,* and *P. aeruginosa*.

Table 5 summarizes, the overall drug resistant pattern of Gram-positive bacteria for a panel of 16 antibacterial drugs tested. The highest overall resistance rate of Gram-positive bacteria was observed for erythromycin (82.2%), followed by tetracycline (75.6%) and clindamycin (68.4%) but, all Gram-positive bacterial isolates showed better sensitivity towards vancomycine with a sensitivity rate of 100% followed by daptomycin (98.1%), nitrofurantoin (97.1%), gentamicin (93%), and linezolid (92.1%). *S. saprophyticus*, the most frequently isolated Gram-positive bacterium, was 100% sensitive to vancomycine, minocycline and tigocycline. As depicted in Table 5, *E. faecalis,* the 2nd most frequently isolated Gram-positive bacterium was 100% susceptible to seven drugs.

Table 2 Distribution and frequency of Gram negative bacterial isolates

Genus	Species	n (%) of the total isolates
Escherichia	E. coli	135 (52.7)
Klebsiella	K. pneumonia	18 (7.0)
	K. oxytoca	1 (0.4)
Pseudomonas	P. aeruginosa	3 (1.2)
	P. fluorescens	1 (0.4)
	P. luteola	2 (0.8)
Moraxella	M. nonliquefiens	3 (1.2)
Citrobacter	C. diversus	2 (0.8)
	C. freundii	1 (0.4)
Acinetobacter	A.baumannii	2 (0.8)
Providencia	P. alcalifaciens	1 (0.4)
	P. rettgeri	1 (0.4)
Francisella	F. tularensis	1 (0.4)
Morganella	M. morganii	1(0.4)
Sphingomonas	S. paucimobilis	3(1.2)
Total (10)	15	175 (68.4)

Table 4 Percentage antimicrobial resistance profile of Gram-negative bacterial isolates (n = 175)

Species	AM	AMC	CF	CZ	CXM	CXMA	FOX	CPD	CAZ	CRO	FEP	CIP	GM	LEV	FT	TM	TE	SXT	TZP
E. Coli (135)	77.8	45.2	59.3	42.2	43.7	45.2	22.9	37.8	35.6	34.8	43.7	50.4	28.1	55.6	20.0	39.3	69.6	70.4	21.5
K. pneumoniae (18).	100	22.2	55.6	50	44.4	44.4	5.6	44.4	44.4	44.4	50	16.7	22.2	11.1	61.1	38.9	44.4	66.7	5.6
P. aeruginosa(3)	100	100	100	100	100	100	100	100	33.3	100	33.3	33.3	0	0	100	0	100	100	33.3
M. nonliquefaciensm(3)	100	0	100	100	100	100	0	100	0	100	100	100	100	100	100	100	100	100	0
C. diversus (2)	100	100	100	100	50	100	100	50	50	50	50	50	0	0	0	0	0	100	0
A.baumannii (2)	100	100	100	100	100	100	100	100	0	100	0	50	0	0	100	0	0	0	0
P. luteola (2)	50	0	50	50	50	50	50	50	0	0	0	0	0	0	50	0	0	0	0
K. oxytoca (1)	100	0	0	0	0	0	0	0	0	0	0	0	0	0	100	0	0	0	0
P.fluoresces (1)	100	100	0	0	0	0	0	0	0	0	0	0	0	0	0	0	100	0	0
M. morganii (1)	100	100	100	100	100	100	100	100	100	0	0	100	0	0	100	0	0	100	0
C. freundii (1)	0	100	100	100	100	100	100	100	0	0	0	100	0	100	100	0	100	100	0
P.alcalifaciens (1)	0	0	0	0	0	0	0	0	0	0	0	0	0	0	0	100	0	0	0
P.rettgeri (1)	0	0	0	0	100	0	0	0	0	100	0	100	0	0	0	0	0	0	0
S.Paucimobilis (3)	0	0	0	0	0	0	0	0	0	0	0	0	0	0	0	0	0	0	0
F. tularensis (1)	0	0	0	0	0	0	0	0	0	0	0	0	0	0	0	0	0	0	0
All isolates	78.3	42.9	58.9	45.1	45.7	46.9	24	40.6	33.7	37.1	41.7	45.7	25.7	46.3	29.1	36	62.9	66.9	17.7

AM ampicillin, AMC amoxicillin/clavulanic acid, CF cefalotin, CZ cefazolin, FEP cefepime, FOX cefoxitin, CPD cefpodoxime, CAZ ceftazidime, CRO ceftriaxone, CXM cefuroxime, CXMA cefroxime axetil, CIP ciprofloxacin, GM gentamicin, LEV levofloxacin, FT nitrofurantoin, TZP piperacillin/tazobactam, TE tetracycline, TM tobramycin, SXT trimethoprim/sulfamethoxazole, S sensitive, R resistance, P pattern

Discussion

Urinary tract infection is caused by both Gram-negative and Gram-positive bacteria. However, the most commonly encountered bacteria are Gram negative in which E. coli consisting of the largest proportion of bacterial uropathogen worldwide [7, 17]. This is evident by the present study in which, out of 256 (27 species) bacterial isolates recovered, 175 (68.4%) were Gram- negative bacteria. Our finding of Gram-negative bacteria as the predominant species in patients with UTI was consistent

Table 5 Percentage antimicrobial resistance profile of Gram-positive bacterial isolate (n = 81)

Species	CIP	CM	E	GM	LEV	MNO	MXF	FT	QDA	RA	TE	TGC	SXT	LIN	VA	DAP
E. faecalis (14)	7.1	7.1	85.8	0	0	85.8	0	0	100	0	78.6	7.1	7.1	7.1	0	0
S. aureus (9)	33.3	66.7	66.7	22.2	22.2	11.1	0	0	22.2	33.3	66.7	33.3	55.6	0	0	0
S. epidermidis (8)	62.5	100	75	0	62.5	12.5	0	0	50	50	62.5	25	25	37.5	0	–
S.saprophyticus (18)	27.8	88.9	94.4	16.7	38.9	0	38.9	5.6	38.9	50	72.2	0	55.6	5.6	0	5.6
S. agalactiae (8)	0	100	–	–	0	–	–	–	0	–	100	25	–	0	0	–
S. haemolyticus (2)	0	50	0	0	0	0	0	0	0	50	0	0	0	–	0	0
S. lentus (3)	100	33.3	66.7	0	66.7	66.7	33.3	0	66.7	33.3	100	0	100	0	0	0
S. hominis (6)	66.7	100	100	0	66.7	50	0	0	66.7	66.7	83.3	0	50	0	0	0
S. warneri (9)	44.4	66.7	77.8	0	22.2	22.2	11.1	11.1	11.1	44.4	77.8	0	55.6	0	0	–
K. kristinae (2)	100	50	100	0	–	–	–	–	–	–	–	–	–	–	–	–
S. porcinus (1)	0	–	100		–	–	–	–	–	–	–	–	–	–	–	–
E. gallinarum (1)	100	–	100	–	100	100	–	0	–	–	100	–	–	100	0	–
All isolates	34.6	68.4	82.2	7.0	29.5	31.4	13.1	2.9	44.2	37.7	75.6	10.4	42	7.9	0	1.9

CIP ciprofloxacin, CM clindamycin, E erythromycin, GM gentamicin, LEV levofloxacin, MN0 minocycline, MXF moxifloxacin, FT nitrofurantoin, QDA ouinupristin/ dalfopristin, RA rifampicin, TE tetracycline, TGC tigecycline, LIN linezolid, SXT trimethoprim/sulfamethoxazole, VA vancomycin, DAP daptomycin, S sensitive, R resistance
P = Pattern
MIC of K. kristinae, S. porcinus and S. agalactiae was carried out by disc diffusion assay method
- = Not tested

with similar studies conducted locally [18–23] and internationally [7]. In the present study, 77.1% of the Gram negative bacterial isolates and 52% of the total bacterial isolates were strains of *E. coli*. *E. coli* has been reported as the main bacterial uropathogen accounting for 75 to 90% of bacterial isolates among patients with UTI [24, 25]. *E. coli* as the predominant bacterial uropathogen in the present study was consistent with similar studies conducted locally [18–23]. The prevalence of other predictable bacterial uropathogens varies from region to regions and from one study to another study [26, 27]. In this study, *S. saprophyticus and K. pneumonia* were the 2nd predominate isolates each consisting of 7% of the total bacterial isolates.

Of the 712 clinical samples collected from patients with cases of UTI, bacteria were isolated in 256 (36%) clinical samples. Urinary tract infection in the present study was relatively higher than similar local studies [18–23]. Local studies reported UTI in the range of 9 to 22.7%. Disparity in the rates of UTI in different studies could result from difference in the definition of bacteriuria, methodology, the length of the study period, size and type of study population.

In our study, the majority of UTI was recorded from females indicating that women are more likely to develop UTI than men. Our result, in this regard was in concordance with the findings of similar studies [28–31]. Women are more prone to develop UTI than men probably due to their anatomical and physiological changes [28, 32, 33]. Age groups of 25–44 and 45–64 were more affected with the infection than other age groups. Our finding in this regard was in agreement with the results of a studies done locally [23] and internationally [34].

In the current study, drug susceptibility testing of Gram negative and Gram- positive bacteria was performed against a panel of 19 and 16 antibacterial drugs, respectively. The number of drugs tested against urinary isolates in the present study was far greater than the number of drugs tested in previous studies in Ethiopia [18–23] and this may increase the option for the selection of drugs for the treatment of urinary tract infections.

The overall drug resistance rates of the Gram-negative bacterial isolates ranged from 17.7% for piperacillin/tazobactam combination and 78.3% for ampicillin. Lower resistance rates of Gram- negative bacteria for ampicillin than our study have been reported in studies conducted in Italy (36%) [35], UK (23%) [36], USA (43%) [37], Canada (33%) [11] and Norway (25%) [38]. However, a resistance rate of 87%, which is higher than ours, has been reported in India [39]. The resistance rates of bacterial uropathogens for ampicillin have also been found out to be 45, 50 and 100% in children from Canada, Europe and Africa, respectively [40–42]. High resistance rates of bacterial uropathogens for trimethoprim/

sulfamethoxazole combination (66.3), in which the first choice of drug for the empirical treatment of UTI in Ethiopia and tetracycline (62.3%) was also observed in the present study. Our result was concurrent with similar study conducted in Ethiopia [23]. A notable observation was that the majority of Gram negative bacteria showed higher sensitivity pattern towards nitrofurantoin, gentamicin, cefoxitin and piperacillin/tazobactam with a sensitivity of 70.1, 74.3, 76 and 82.3%, respectively. As far as species specific antimicrobial resistance rates are concerned, *E. coli* the first more frequently isolated bacterium, showed high level of resistance (70–79%) for trimethoprim/sulfamethoxazole and ampicillin respectively. Similarly, *K. pneumoniae* the 2nd most frequently isolated Gram- negative bacterium demonstrated high level of resistance (66.7–100%) for trimethoprim/sulfamethoxazole and ampicillin, respectively. Similar result was obtained in a study conducted by Lu et al. [43, 44]. However, *E. coli* and *K. pneumoniae* revealed low level of resistance for nitrofurantoin (20%) and piperacillin/tazobactam (5.6%), respectively.

The overall drug resistance rates of Gram-positive bacterial isolates ranged from 0% for vancomycine and 82.2% for erythromycin followed by tetracycline (75.6%) and clindamycin (68.4%). An overall resistance rate of 85.6 and 76.7% of uropathognes for erythromycin and tetracycline, respectively has been reported in a similar study conducted in Ethiopia [23]. However, the majority of Gram-positive bacterial isolates showed higher sensitivity pattern towards vancomycine, daptomycin, nitrofurantoin, gentamicin, and linezolid with a sensitivity rates of 100, 98.1, 97.1, 93.0 and 92.1% respectively. As far as species specific antimicrobial resistance rates are concerned, *S. saprophytics*, the first more frequently isolated Gram-positive bacterium, showed high level of resistance (88.9–94.4%) for clindamycin and erythromycin, respectively. However, the bacterium was 100% sensitive to vancomycine, minocycline, tigocycline and 94.4% to linozilid and daptomycin. Contrary to our finding, a study conducted in Ethiopia by Amare et al. [45] documented 4.5% prevalence rate of vancomycin resistant Coagulase -Negative Staphylococci.

Our result revealed that Gram-positive and Gram-negative bacteria isolated in this study were more resistant to the commonly prescribed drugs in Ethiopia such as erythromycin, tetracycline, clindamycin, ampicillin, and trimethoprim/sulfamethoxazole combinations than of the drugs tested. The reason for this might be an irrational usage, easy availability and the over the counter sale of the antimicrobials without a proper prescription and an appropriate dosing schedule.

Conclusion

Observation of many bacterial species implicated in causing UTI in this study warrants, a continuous epidemiological survey of UTI in health institutions across the country. High level of drug resistance against the commonly prescribed drugs necessitates a search for other options.

Limitation of the study

Lack of clinical information to confirm whether urinary tract infections were hospital or community-acquired and complicated or uncomplicated were the major limitations of the present study.

Acknowledgements
The authors would like to acknowledge Arsho Advanced medical Laboratory for the provision of laboratory supplies and allowing to use the vitek 2 compact system for free. The authors are also indebted to the patients and study participants. We are very grateful for Mitwab Hussein for editing the final document.

Funding
No funding agent.

Authors' contributions
TM, has participated in culture media preparation, identification of bacterial pathogens, in drafting the manuscript, have given final approval of the version to be published; analysis and interpretation of data, and agree to be accountable for all aspects of the work in ensuring that questions related to the accuracy or integrity of any part of the work are appropriately investigated and resolved. AB has participated in design, analysis and interpretation of data, bacterial identification, write up of the manuscript, agree to be accountable for all aspects of the work in ensuring that questions related to the accuracy or integrity of any part of the work are appropriately investigated and resolved. MC has participated in specimen collection, collection of socio demographic data, design, analysis and interpretation of data, bacterial identification, agree to be accountable for all aspects of the work in ensuring that questions related to the accuracy or integrity of any part of the work are appropriately investigated and resolved. All authors read and approved the final manuscript.

Authors' information
TM, is a medical laboratory technologist with MSc degree in microbiology, he has been working as a medical laboratory technologist for Saint Peter hospital for many years.
AB is an associate professor of microbiology and consultant health science specialist with a PhD degree. He has been working as a researcher and instructor offering courses to graduate students in the college of health sciences, Addis Ababa University for more than 20 years. He has published many original articles in peer-reviewed international journal.
MC is a medical laboratory technologist with MSc degree in microbiology, he has been working as a laboratory manager for Arsho Advanced Medical laboratory for many years.

Consent for publication
Not applicable as details, images and/or videos related to study subjects were not recorded for this study.

Competing of interests
The authors declare that they have no competing interests.

Author details
[1]Department of Medical Laboratory Sciences, College of Health Sciences, Addis Ababa University, Addis Ababa, Ethiopia. [2]Department of Medical Laboratory, St. Peter Tuberculosis Specialized Hospital, Addis Ababa, Ethiopia. [3]Arsho Advanced Medical Laboratory Private Limited Company, Addis Ababa, Ethiopia.

References
1. Schappert SM, Rechtsteiner EA. Ambulatory medical care utilization estimates for 2006. National health statistics reports; no 8. Hyattsville: National Center for Health Statistics; 2008.
2. Foxman B, Barlow R, D'Arcy H, Gillespie B, Sobel JD. Urinary tract infection: self-reported incidence and associated costs. Ann Epidemiol. 2000;10:509–15.
3. Griebling TL. Urinary tract infection in women. In: Litwin MS, Saigal CS, editors. Urologic Diseases in America. Department of Health and Human Services, Public Health Service, National Institutes of Health, National Institute of Diabetes and Digestive and Kidney Diseases. Washington, D.C.: GPO; 2007. NIH publication 07–5512. p. 587–619.
4. Foxman B, Frerichs RR. Epidemiology of urinary tract infection: I. Diaphragm use and sexual intercourse. Am J Public Health. 1985;75:1308–13.
5. Kozak LJ, DeFrances CJ, Hall MJ. National hospital discharge survey: 2004 annual summary with detailed diagnosis and procedure data. Vital Health Stat 13. 2006(Oct):1–209.
6. Kidney N, Clearinghouse UDI. Kidney and urologic diseases statistics for the United States. Bethesda: National Institute of Diabetes and Digestive and Kidney Diseases; 2010.
7. Foxman B. Epidemiology of urinary tract infections: incidence, morbidity, and economic costs. Am J Med. 2002;113(suppl 1A):5–13.
8. Vorland LH, Carlson K, Aalen O. An epidemiological survey of urinary tract infections among outpatients in Northern Norway. Scand J Infect Dis. 1985;17: 277–83.
9. Gupta K, Hooton TM, Wobbe CL, Stamm WE. The prevalence of antimicrobial resistance among uropathogens causing acute uncomplicated cystitis in young women. Int J Antimicrob Agents. 1999;11:305–8.
10. Barrett SP, Savage MA, Rebec MP, Guyot A, Andrews N, Shrimpton SM. Antibiotic sensitivity of bacteria associated with community acquired urinary tract infections in Britain. J Antimicrob Chemother. 1999;44:359–65.
11. Jones RN, Kugler KC, Pfaller MA, Winokur PL. SENTRY Surveillance Group: Characteristics of pathogens causing urinary tract infections in hospitals in North America: results from the SENTRY Antimicrobial Surveillance Program, 1997. Diagn Microbiol Infect Dis. 1999;35:55–63.
12. Vromen M, van der Ven AJ, Knols A, Stobberingh EE. Antimicrobial resistance patterns in urinary tract isolates from nursing home residents. Fifteen years of data reviewed. J Antimicrob Chemother. 1999;44:113–6.
13. Manges AR, Natarajan P, Solberg OD, Dietrich PS, Riley LW. The changing prevalence of drug-resistant *Escherichia coli* clonal groups in a community: evidence for community outbreaks of urinary tract infections. Epidemiol Infect. 2006;134:425–31.
14. Doern GV, Vautour R, Gaudet M, Levy B. Clinical impact of rapid in vitro susceptibility testing and bacterial identification. J Clin Microbiol. 1994;32:1757–62.
15. Donay JL, Mathieu D, Fernandes P, Pregermain C, Bruel P, Wargnier A, et al. Evaluation of the automated phoenix system for potential routine use in the clinical microbiology laboratory. J Clin Microbiol. 2004;42:1542–6.
16. Series M, WHO. Provisional Guidelines on Standard International Age Classifications: Statistical Papers, vol. 74. New York: United Nations; 1982. p. 4–11.
17. Davoodian P, Nematee M, Sheikhvatan M. The inappropriate use of urinary catheters and its common complications in different hospital wards. Saudi Journal of Kidney Diseases and Transplantation. 2012;23:63–7.
18. Assefa A, Asrat D, Woldeamanuel Y, G/Hiwot Y, Abdella A, Melesse T. Bacterial profile and drug susceptibility pattern of urinary tract infection in pregnant women at Tikur Anbessa Specialized Hospital Addis Ababa, Ethiopia. Ethiop Med J. 2008;46:227–35.
19. Beyene G, Tsegaye W. Bacterial uropathogens in urinary tract infection and antibiotic susceptibility pattern in Jimma University specialized hospital, Southwest Ethiopia. Ethiop J Health Sci. 2011;21:141–6.
20. Alemu A, Moges F, Shiferaw Y, Tafess K, Kassu A, Anagaw B, et al. Bacterial profile and drug susceptibility pattern of urinary tract infection in pregnant women at University of Gondar Teaching Hospital, Northwest Ethiopia. BMC Research Notes. 2012;5:4–7.
21. Ferede G, Yismaw G, Wondimeneh Y, Sisay Z. The Prevalence and Antimicrobial Susceptibility pattern of Bacterial Uropathogens Isolated from pregnant women. Euro J Exp Biol. 2012;2:1497–502.

22. Demilie T, Beyene G, Melaku S, Tsegaye W. Urinary bacterial profile and antibiotic susceptibility pattern among pregnant women in North West Ethiopia. Ethiop J Health Sci. 2012;22:121–8.

23. Kibret M, Abera B. Prevalence and antibiogram of bacterial isolates from urinary tract infections at Dessie Health Research Laboratory, Ethiopia. Asian Pac J Trop Biomed. 2014;4:164–8.

24. Gupta K, Hooten TM, Stamm WE. Increasing antimicrobial resistance and the management of uncomplicated community-acquired urinary tract infections. Ann Intern Med. 2001;135:41–50.

25. Nicolle E. Epidemiology of urinary tract infection. Infect Med. 2001;18:153–62.

26. Bean D, Krahe D, Wareham DW. Antimicrobial resistance in community and nosocomial Escherichia coli urinary tract isolates, London 2005–2006. Ann Clin Microbiol Antimicrob. 2008;7:13.

27. Akram M, Shahid M, Khan AU. Etiology and antibiotic resistance patterns of community acquired urinary tract infections in JNMC Hospital Aligarh, India. Ann Clin Microbiol Antimicrob. 2007;6:4.

28. Oladeinde BH, Omoregie R, Olley M, Anunibe JA. Urinary tract infections in a rural community of Nigeria. N Am J Med Sci. 2011;3(2):75.

29. Manjunath G, Prakash R, Vamseedhar Annam KS. The changing trends in the spectrum of the antimicrobial drug resistance pattern of the uropathogens which were isolated from hospitals and community patients with urinary tract infections in Tumkur and Bangalore. Int J Biol Med Res. 2011;2:504–7.

30. Akram M, Shahid M, Khan AU. The aetiology and the antibiotic resistance patterns of community-acquired urinary tract infections in the JNMC Hospital Aligarh, India. Ann Clin Microbial Antimicrob. 2007;6:4–11.

31. Barate DL, Ukesh C. The bacterial profile and the antibiotic resistance pattern of urinary tract infections. DAV Inter J f Sci. 2012;1:21–4.

32. Hooton TM. Pathogenesis of urinary tract infections: an update. J Antimicrob Chemother. 2000;46(Suppl 1):1–17.

33. Kolawale AS, Kolawole OM, Kandaki-Olukemi YT, Babatunde SK, Durowade KA, Kolawole CF. Prevalence of urinary tract infections (UTI) among patients attending Dalhatu Araf Specialist Hospital, Lafia, Nasarawa State, Nigeria. Int J Med Sci. 2009;1:163–7.

34. Desai P, Ukey PM, Chauhan AR, Malik S, Mathur M. Etiology and antimicrobial resistance patterns of uriopathogens in a hospital from suburb of Mumbai. Int J Biol Med Res 2012; 3: 2007–2012.

35. Bonadio M, Meini M, Spetaleri P, Gilgi C. Current microbiological and clinical aspects of urinary tract infections. Eur J Urol. 2001;40:439–45.

36. Farrell DJ, Morrissey I, De Robeis D, Robbins M, Felmingham D. UK multicenter study of the antimicrobial susceptibility of bacterial pathogens causing urinary tract infection. J Inf Secur. 2003;46:94–100.

37. Mathai D, Jones RN, Pfaller MA. SENTRY Participant Group of North America Epidemiology and frequency of resistance among pathogens causing urinary tract infections in 1,510 hospitalized patients: a report from the SENTRY Antimicrobial Surveillance program (North America). Diag Microbiol Infect Dis. 2001;40:129–36.

38. Grude N, Tveten Y, Kristiansen B-E. Urinary tract infections in Norway: bacterial aetiology and susceptibility. A retrospective study of clinical isolates. Clin Microbiol Infect. 2001;7:543–7.

39. Navaneeth BV, Belwadi S, Sughanthi N. Urinary pathogens' resistance to common antibiotics: a retrospective analysis. Trop Dr. 2002;32:20–2.

40. Adjei O, Opoku C. Urinary tract infections in African infants. Int J Antimicrob Agents. 2004;24(Suppl. 1):S32–4.

41. Haller M, Brandis M, Berner R. Antibiotic resistance of urinary tract pathogens and rationale for empirical intravenous therapy. Pediatr Nephrol. 2004;19:982–6.

42. Prais D, Straussberg R, Avitzur Y, Nussinovitch M, Harel L, Amir J. Bacterial susceptibility to oral antibiotics in community acquired urinary tract infection. Arch Dis Child. 2003;88:215–8.

43. Yismaw G, Asrat D, Woldeamanuel Y, Unakal CG. Urinary tract infection: Bacterial etiologies, drug resistance profile and associated risk factors in diabetic patients attending Gondar University Hospital, Gondar, Ethiopia. Eur J Exp Biol. 2012;2:889–98.

44. Lu PL, Liu YC, Toh HS, Lee YL, Liu YM, Ho CM, et al. Epidemiology and antimicrobial susceptibility profiles of Gram-negative bacteria causing urinary tract infections in the Asia-Pacific region: 2009–2010 results from the Study for Monitoring Antimicrobial Resistance Trends (SMART). Int J Antimicrob Agents. 2012;40S1:S37–43.

45. Amare B, Abdurrahman Z, Moges B, Ali J, Muluken L, Alemayehu M, et al. Postoperative Surgical Site Bacterial Infections and Drug Susceptibility Patterns at Gondar University Teaching Hospital, Northwest Ethiopia. J, Bacteriol Parasitol. 2011:2–8. http://dx.doi.org/10.4172/2155-9597.1000126

The impact of cathelicidin, the human antimicrobial peptide LL-37 in urinary tract infections

Ibrahim H. Babikir[1,4*], Elsir A. Abugroun[2], Naser Eldin Bilal[3], Abdullah Ali Alghasham[4], Elmuataz Elmansi Abdalla[4] and Ishag Adam[4]

Abstract

Background: The defense mechanisms of the urinary tract are attributed mainly to the innate immune system and the urinary tract urothelium which represent the first line of defense against invading pathogens and maintaining sterility of the urinary tract. There are only a few publications regarding cathelicidin (LL-37) and a urinary tract infection (UTI). This study was done to investigate the plasma and urine levels of human LL-37 in patients with UTI.

Methods: A case-control study was conducted at Omdurman Hospital, Sudan during the period from August 2014 to May 2017. The cases were patients with confirmed UTI and the controls were healthy volunteers without UTI. Sociodemographic and clinical data were obtained from each participant using questionnaires. Urine cultures and antimicrobial susceptibility were tested. Plasma and urine levels of LL-37 were determined using an enzyme-linked immunosorbent assay (ELISA) kit. SPSS (version 16.0) was used for analyses.

Results: Cases and controls (87 in each arm) were matched according to their basic characteristics. Compared with controls, the median (inter-quartile) LL-37 level in plasma [2.100 (1.700–2.700) vs. 1.800 (1.000–2.200) ng/ml, $P = 0.002$] and in urine [0.900 (0.300–1.600) vs. 0.000 (0.000–1.000) ng/mg creatinine, $P < 0.001$] was significantly higher in cases. There was no significant difference in the median plasma [2.1 (1.7–2.9) vs. 2.000 (1.700–2.400) ng/ml, $P = 0.561$] and urine [0.850 (0.275–2.025) vs. 0.900 (0.250–1.350) ng/mg creatinine, $P = 0.124$]. The uropathogenic *Escherichia coli* (UPEC) was the predominant isolate, $n = 38$ (43.7%). LL-37 levels between the *E. coli* isolates and the other isolated organisms. There was no significant correlation between plasma and urine LL-37 levels ($r = 0.221$), even when the data of the cases were analyzed separately.

Conclusion: LL-37 is notably increased among patients with UTI compared with normal control subjects. Severity of UTI increases the levels of LL-37. The increased level was not only in the patient's urine, but has also been observed in the patient's plasma. Detection of increased levels of LL-37 could help to differentiate subjects with suspected UTI. Accordingly, LL-37 could act as a good marker for diagnosing UTIs.

Keywords: Urinary tract infections, Cathelicidin, LL-37, Antimicrobial peptide, Vitek 2 System, Uropathogenic *E. coli*, Sudan

* Correspondence: almakibrahim@hotmail.com
[1]College of Medical Laboratory Sciences, Microbiology Department, University of Khartoum, Khartoum, Sudan
[4]College of Medicine, Qassim University, Buraydah, Qassim, Kingdom of Saudi Arabia
Full list of author information is available at the end of the article

Background

Urinary tract infection (UTI) is a major health problem as it is one of the most common bacterial infections. The predominant causal organism is *Escherichia coli* (*E. coli*). The innate immune response to urinary pathogens can both control and predispose to subsequent recurrence of UTIs, at least for a significant proportion of patients [1, 2].

Increasing bacterial resistance to common antibiotics has been a growing public health concern [2, 3]. Emergence of multi-drug resistant microbes was seen as early as the 1950s as the result of antibiotic misuse or overuse [4, 5].

Although, there are many routes by which microbes can reach the urinary tract and the kidneys [6, 7], the defensive mechanisms of the innate immune system, in addition to the urinary tract urothelium, represent the first line of defense against these invading pathogens helping the urinary tract to remain sterile [1]. Dysfunction in these immune mechanisms may lead to acute disease, massive infection and tissue destruction, which may turn the 'friendly' host defense into troublesome and disturbing enemies and give rise to disease, in addition to long-term complications such as hypertension and chronic kidney disease [1, 8]. Progression to renal scarring and permanent impairment of renal function and tissue destruction may occur [9, 10].

In mammals, several defense mechanisms guard against the threat of infection, including the innate immune response and physical factors, such as urine flow, pH, and ionic composition together with expression of natural antimicrobial peptides (AMPs) [1, 8]. AMPs are considered the first line of innate immune defense against invading pathogens as they play a fundamental role in protection from prokaryotes [11]. At least two distinct groups of AMPs have been reported; the defensins and cathelicidin. In contrast to the multiple defensins (alpha, beta, and gamma), to date, only one cathelicidin has been found in humans [11–13]. The gene product is synthesized as a propeptide and is referred to as human cationic antimicrobial peptide-18 (hCAP-18/LL-37). hCAP-18 is the precursor molecule and its molecular weight is 18 Kd. In various tissues, hCAP-18 is cleaved by proteases to form two parts; the N-terminal (cathelin) and C-terminal part. The latter is further cleaved enzymatically to produce a 37 amino acid peptide which starts with two leucines, hence the name LL-37; LL-37 is considered the main biologically active broad spectrum antimicrobial agent [14, 15].

Due to the cationic nature of LL-37, an amphipathic α-helical peptide, it has broad spectrum antimicrobial activity against bacteria, fungi, viruses, and parasites, but notably, shows low toxicity to human cells. During inflammation, it has been identified as a potent chemoattractant for innate and adaptive immune cells [9, 16]. LL-37 has been shown to neutralize lipopolysaccharides (LPS), which are endotoxins of Gram-negative bacteria that are released upon cell death, by binding to them with high affinity [17, 18]. Additionally, LL-37 has been shown to inhibit the association of LPS with its receptor, suppressing LPS-induced apoptosis of endothelial cells [19], and to block the effects of flagellin and lipoteichoic acid on dendritic cells [20].

Attention and interest concerning endogenous defense has been stimulated by increasing concern regarding antimicrobial overuse. Enhancement of natural mechanisms will be an exciting novel therapeutic avenue in the management of UTIs [1, 21]. LL-37 has potent, direct antimicrobial activity at minimum inhibitory concentrations (MIC) than synthetically and traditionally used antimicrobial agents [22, 23]. Moreover, these peptides have potential activity against multiple drug-resistant microbes [23, 24]. Thus, AMPs or their derivatives potentially represent a new category of antimicrobial agents [23, 24].

Production of cathelicidin peptides by blood cells [4] and by the epithelial cells in the urothelium mucous membranes has been proposed as a natural innate immune response to maintain a normal sterile urinary tract and represents a candidate for a novel class of antimicrobials [25, 26]. Despite the mechanisms of the innate immune response, bacteria still cause UTIs. In contrast, involvement of the adaptive immune response to UTIs is poorly understood. However, it has been suggested that secretory immunoglobulin A (sIgA) antibodies inhibit bacterial colonization by lowering bacterial adherence to the mucosa antibodies during UTIs, even though serum production of antibodies is characteristically difficult to detect in UTIs [27].

To our knowledge, this is the first study on cathelicidin in Sudan. However, there are a few globally published data on LL-37 and UTI [2, 8, 21, 26]. The current study was conducted to investigate plasma and urinary levels of LL-37 in patients with (culture positive) UTI compared with healthy volunteers, and to add to the previous research on UTI in Sudan [28, 29].

Methods

This is a case-control study was conducted at Omdurman Hospital, Sudan, during the period June–September 2014. Institutional review board approval was obtained from the Faculty of Medical Laboratory Sciences Research Ethics Review Board, University of Khartoum, Sudan. A signed written informed consent was obtained from all subjects or from the parents or guardians in case of the participants under the 16 years of age. Sociodemographic and clinical data were obtained from each participant using structured pre-tested questionnaires.

Study setting and population

Consecutive patients with UTI symptoms who attended the referral clinic were approached to participate in the study. Cases were (males and females) those who met the inclusion criteria; signs and symptoms of UTI, willingness (the participant agreed to participate), and no other health problem or underlying disease. The controls were apparently healthy volunteers with no current or previous history of UTIs. Diabetic patients, pregnant women or subjects with anatomical or functional abnormalities of the urinary tract or subjects with underlying diseases were excluded from both the case and control groups.

For cases, an initial survey covered medical history, demographics and symptoms (dysuria, frequency, urgency, lower abdominal or suprapubic pain, fever, costovertebral tenderness [flank pain], nausea and vomiting), in addition to their culture positive results.

Collection and processing specimens

Paired Blood and urine samples were collected from each participant. Under a septic technique, 5 ml of blood was withdrawn in Ethylene-diamine-tetra-acetic acid (EDTA) anticoagulant tube. The blood samples were directly tested for complete blood count (CBC) using Sysmex KX-21 N, and then carefully centrifuged (1500×g at 4 °C for 15 min) to separate plasma. Plasma specimens were stored at −80 °C. For urine specimens all participants were asked to provide a midstream urine sample according to the clean-catch procedure. Urine Samples were collected using a sterile screw capped wide mouth container and processed immediately. In the medical laboratory each urine sample was divided into two; the first half was stored at −80 °C and the second half was immediately inoculated on standard culture media. A standard quantitative (1 μL and 10 μL) loop was used to inoculate urine samples on to Cysteine Lactose Electrolyte Deficient (CLED) agar, MacConkey's and Blood Agar (Oxoid, Basingstoke, UK). Plates were incubated aerobically at 35–37 °C for 24 h and the outcome was judged as significant/non-significant growth, or contaminated (discarded). The rest of urine was centrifuged (1500×g for 5 min) to prepare urine debris for direct microscopic examination for Red Blood Cells (RBCs), pus cells (leukocyturia), epithelial cell count, casts, crystals and parasitic infection if present. In the normal urine sediment a few count of RBCs, pus cells (0–5 per high power field, HPF) and epithelial cells may present. Epithelial cell count reported as "few," "moderate," or "many" per low power field (LPF).

A portion of the urine specimens was used for dipstick test rapid response urinalysis Reagent Strips (Combi-Screen PLUS, Roche, USA). For the control participants, nitrite and leukocyte esterase positivity were considered as a positive indicator for active infection and those were excluded from the study. When the patient had a nitrite and leukocyte esterase dipstick negative results, UTI confirmed by urine culture examination.

LL-37 analysis for both plasma and urine samples was performed using ELISA kit (HK321–02 HycultBiotech, Gmbh, Germany) as described elsewhere [30–32].

The bacterial identification and the antimicrobial susceptibility were done by using the fully automated VITEK-2 Compact System (see below).

Measurements

Colony counting is the numerical cut-off estimation for the number of viable bacteria in a milliliter of uncentrifuged urine; it is a quantitative estimation that enables us to differentiate the true bacteriuria from urethral or vulval contamination, which may occur during collection of mid-stream or "clean-catch" urine [26, 28, 29]. Multiplication of microbes in the urinary system is defined by the presence of more than 10^5 CFU/ml of urine, which is significantly diagnostic of UTI [26, 28, 30]. Significant UTI was defined as urine culture plates showing $\geq 10^5$ colony-forming units (CFU)/mL freshly voided urine. Referring to the cut-off of 10^5 CFU/ml, a positive urine culture was identified as $\geq 10^5$ CFU/ml of one to two organisms from a clean-catch specimen [28, 29].

The bacterial identification and the antimicrobial susceptibility were done by using the fully automated VITEK-2 Compact System. Prior application of Vitek system clinically significant isolates were sub-cultured for purity and inoculated on specific plates (nutrient agar or blood agar), then incubated aerobically at 35–37 °C in 5% CO_2. Isolated bacteria were differentiated according to their colonial morphology and gram stain. After overnight incubation, the bacterial colonies were used to prepare a standardized saline inoculum for the appropriate VITEK identification (ID) card. For identification of bacteria, special ID and sensitivity (AST) cards (BioMérieux) were used. Gram positive ID card: [GP Reference 21 342], gram Positive sensitivity card: [GP/AST-580 Reference 22 233], gram negative ID card: [GN Reference 21 341], and gram negative sensitivity card: [AST-N291 Reference 415 062]. All methods and techniques were conducted as described by the manufacturer. The VITEK-2 ID and AST cards were logged and loaded into the VITEK-2 Compact system. The VITEK-2 Compact system automatically reported and printed the results through software 06.01.

A total sample size of 87 participants in each arm of the study was calculated using a formula for the difference in the mean of the proposed variables (plasma and urine LL-37) that would provide 80% power to detect a 5% difference at $\alpha = 0.05$ and which assumed that 10% of participants might not have complete data.

The urinary LL-37 levels was performed using [human LL-37 ELISA Kit (Hycult ®)] according to the manufacturer procedure. Final concentrations were based on a standard curve and are shown in ng/ml.

For normalization we divided a urine LL-37 concentration in "ng/ml" by creatinine in "mg/ml" to determine normalized LL-37 in "ng/mg creatinine" i.e. "ng LL-37/mg creatinine".

The urinary creatinine (Ucr) levels were analyzed as described previously (32), briefly, we measured urinary creatinine colorimetrically by diluting urine samples 1:20

in dilution buffer from the Creatinine Assay Kit (Creatinine-J. REF. 100,111, SPINREACT, S.A./SAU-Ctra. Santa Coloma, 7 E-17176 SANT ESTEVE DE BAS-Girona, Spain). Urinary creatinine calculated in mg/ml based on a standard curve. The normalized levels of LL-37 were expressed as "ng LL-37/mg creatinine" ratios. Creatinine equation formula [LL-37/UCrX100].

Statistics

SPSS for window (version 16.0) was used for analyses. Students'-test and χ^2 were used to compare the continuous variables (when normally distributed) and proportions between the cases and controls, respectively. The levels of LL-37 were not normally distributed and were compared between the cases and controls by Mann-Whitney U test. Logistic and linear regression was performed with UTI (logistic) and log of LL-37 level (linear); these were the dependent variables. Spearman correlation (non-parametric) was performed between the plasma and urine levels. $P < 0.05$ was considered statistically significant.

Results

During the study period, 197 subjects were initially screened, among these 23 (11.7%) were excluded because they had incomplete data, or, not enough samples. The two groups (87 in each arm) which were enrolled were matched in their basic characteristics, as shown in Table 1. There were 38 (43.7%) and 46 (52.9%), $P = 0.288$ males in the case and control groups, respectively.

The common organisms isolated from the 87 cases were *Escherichia coli* (38, 43.7%), *Klebsiella pneumoniae* (16, 18.4%), *Enterobacter cloacae* (4, 4.6%), *Pseudomonas aeruginosa* (4, 4.6%), *Proteus mirabilis* (3, 3.4%), *Acinetobacter baumannii* (3, 3.4%), *Acinetobacter lwoffii* (3, 3.4%), *Klebsiella oxytoca* (2, 2.3%), *Morganella morganii* (2, 2.3%), *Pantoea agglomerans* (3, 3.4%), *Pseudomonas luteola* (2, 2.3%), *Enterococcus faecalis* (2, 2.3%), *Enterococcus faecium* (2, 2.3%), *Staphylococcus aureus* (2. 2.3%), *Staphylococcus saprophyticus* (1, 1.1%).

Compared with the control group, median (inter-quartile) plasma [2.100 (1.700–2.700) vs. 1.800 (1.000–2.200) ng/ml,

$P = 0.002$] and in urine [0.900 (0.300–1.600) vs. 0.000 (0.000–1.000) ng/mg creatinine, $P < 0.001$] LL-37 levels were significantly higher for the cases group (Fig. 1a and b).

There was a significant difference in the plasma and urine levels of LL-37 between males and females when the data for cases and controls were analyzed as a whole or when the data of the controls were analyzed separately. Moreover, in the male cases group, the LL-37 plasma [2.000 (1.675–2.325) vs. 1.800 (0.600–2.200) ng/ml, $P < 0.001$] and urine [0.650 (0.100–1.250) vs. 0.000 (0.000–0.250) ng/mg creatinine, $P < 0.001$], However, the females had significantly higher median (inter-quartile) plasma LL-37 levels [2.2 (1.800–3.050 vs. 1.900 (1.350–2.200) ng/ml, $P = 0.001$] and urine [0.900 (0.7000–2.050) vs. 0.000 (0.000–0.600) ng/mg creatinine, $P < 0.001$] LL-37 levels were significantly higher for the female cases group (Fig. 1a and b).

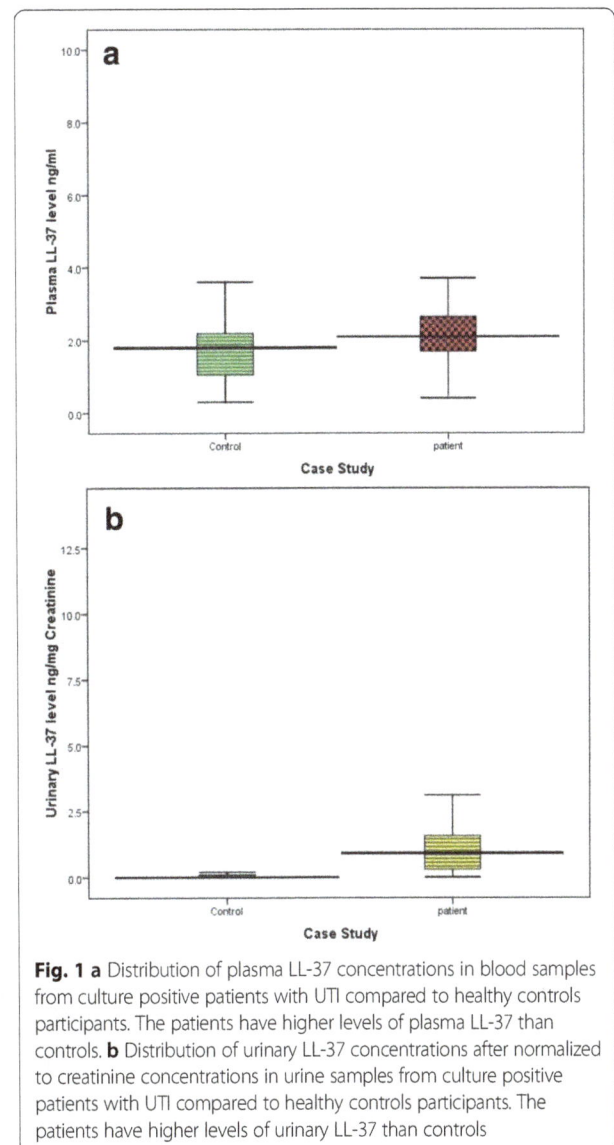

Fig. 1 a Distribution of plasma LL-37 concentrations in blood samples from culture positive patients with UTI compared to healthy controls participants. The patients have higher levels of plasma LL-37 than controls. b Distribution of urinary LL-37 concentrations after normalized to creatinine concentrations in urine samples from culture positive patients with UTI compared to healthy controls participants. The patients have higher levels of urinary LL-37 than controls

Table 1 Comparing number (%) of age and gender between controls and cases with urinary tract infection

Gender	Cases	Controls	P. value
Male	46 (52.9)	38 (43.7)	0.225
Female	41 (47.1)	49 (56.3)	
Age groups			
Children	18 (20.7)	15 (17.3)	0.856
Adults	43 (49.4)	45 (51.7)	
Elderly	26 (29.9)	27 (31.0)	

Compared plasma and urine levels of LL-37 between males and females group, in consideration to the severity of (upper and lower) UTI, median (inter-quartile) plasma [2.000 (1.675–2.325) vs. 2.200 (1.800–3.050) ng/ml, $P = 0.002$] and urine [0.650 (0.100–1.250) vs. 0.900 (0.7000–2.050)] ng/mg creatinine, However, there were no significant difference between males and females in urinary LL-37 levels, a considerable increase of plasma LL-37 was detected among the females (Fig. 2).

There was no significant difference in the median (inter-quartile) plasma [2.1 (1.7–2.9) vs. 2.000 (1.700–2.400) ng/ml, $P = 0.561$] and urine [0.850 (0.275–2.025) vs. 0.900 (0.250–1.350) ng/mg creatinine, $P = 0.102$] LL-37 levels between the *E. coli* isolates and the other isolated organisms.

There was no significant correlation between the plasma and urine level ($r = 0.221$), even when the data of the cases were analyzed separately. According to linear regression analysis, UTI was significantly associated with high plasma and urinary levels of LL-37 Table 2.

Discussion

The main findings of the current study were the significantly higher levels of both plasma and urinary LL-37 levels among patients with UTI compared with those of controls. Our findings are in agreement with recent reports [8, 33]. Nielsen et al., reported that, the urinary LL-37 levels were significantly higher during infection than post infection, yet the post infection

LL-37 levels were significantly lower in patients with UTI than those of controls [32]. In another setting, Ovunç Hacıhamdioglu D. et al., showed no significant differences in the levels of urinary LL-37 between the children with UTI and the control groups [34].

In previous reports, the activity and functions of some other biomarker compounds have been mentioned, as for example, the antibacterial properties of the epithelial cells plays a role in the innate immunity of the urinary tract [35]. Moreover, it has been shown that some factors of innate immunity (Tamm-Horsfall protein) interfere with bacterial adherence [36], sIgA antibodies inhibit bacterial colonization [37], and inhibit bacterial growth [38] or directly kill uropathogens [39, 40]; the bacterial attachment results in exfoliation of host bladder epithelial cells [41].

Similar results were shown by Chromek et al. who studied urinary cathelicidin from both healthy children and children with UTIs and observed that cathelicidin is constitutively expressed in the urinary tract. Milan Chromek and his colleges mentioned that, the direct contact with microbes induces urinary epithelial cells to substantially increase production and secretion of cathelicidin, protecting the urinary tract from microbial adherence. Cathelicidin deficiency predisposes to urinary infections as it has been shown that mice which are CRAMP-deficient (Camp–/–) are more susceptible to UTI than CRAMP-producing (Camp+/+) mice [31].

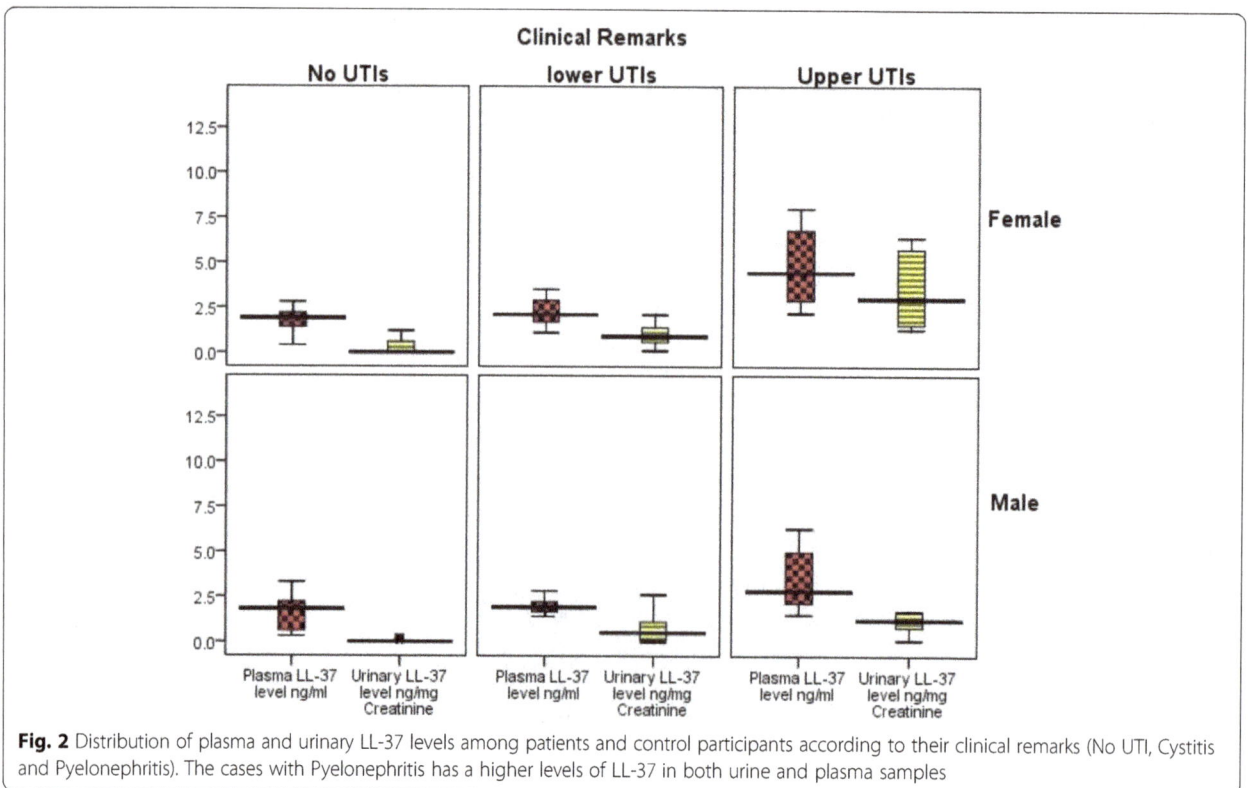

Fig. 2 Distribution of plasma and urinary LL-37 levels among patients and control participants according to their clinical remarks (No UTI, Cystitis and Pyelonephritis). The cases with Pyelonephritis has a higher levels of LL-37 in both urine and plasma samples

ml: Nanograms per milliliter; *P. aeruginosa*: *Pseudomonas aeruginosa*; *P. mirabilis*: *Proteus mirabilis*; SPSS: Statistical package for the social sciences; Ucr: urinary creatinine; UPEC: Uropathogenic *E. coli*; UTI: Urinary tract infection; V2C: VITEK-2 Compact System; WBC: White blood cell; χ^2: Chi-Square

Acknowledgements
The authors are very grateful to all the patients and healthy control participants for their participation in the study.

Funding
We would like to confirm that there was no funding for this study.

Authors' contributions
IB and EAA carried out the study and participated in drafting the manuscript. NB, AA, and EEA participated in designing the study and participated in drafting the manuscript. IB carried out the laboratory work. IA coordinated and participated in designing the study, statistical analysis and drafting the manuscript. All the authors read and approved the final version.

Consent for publication
Not applicable.

Competing interests
The authors declare that they have no competing interests.

Author details
[1]College of Medical Laboratory Sciences, Microbiology Department, University of Khartoum, Khartoum, Sudan. [2]Faculty of Medical Laboratory Sciences, University of Science and Technology, Omdurman, Sudan. [3]Khartoum University Central Research Laboratory, University of Khartoum, PO Box 321, Khartoum, Sudan. [4]College of Medicine, Qassim University, Buraydah, Qassim, Kingdom of Saudi Arabia.

References
1. Spencer JD, Schwaderer AL, Becknell B, Watson J, Hains DS. The innate immune response during urinary tract infection and pyelonephritis. Pediatr Nephrol. 2014;29(7):1139–49.
2. Kucheria R, Dasgupta P, Sacks S, Khan M, Sheerin N. Urinary tract infections: new insights into a common problem. Postgrad Med J. 2005;81(952):83.
3. Stapleton A. Prevention of recurrent urinary-tract infections in women. Lancet. 1999;353(9146):7–8.
4. Zanetti M, Gennaro R, Skerlavaj B, Tomasinsig L, Circo R. Cathelicidin peptides as candidates for a novel class of antimicrobials. Curr Pharm Des. 2002;8(9):779–93.
5. Matejuk A, Leng Q, Begum M, Woodle M, Scaria P, Chou S, et al. Peptide-based antifungal therapies against emerging infections. Drugs Future. 2010; 35(3):197.
6. Minardi D, d'Anzeo G, Cantoro D, Conti A, Muzzonigro G. Urinary tract infections in women: etiology and treatment options. Int J Gen Med. 2011;4:333–43.
7. Kumar V, Abbas AK, Aster JC. Robbins basic pathology: Elsevier health sciences; 2012.
8. Ragnarsdóttir B, Lutay N, Grönberg-Hernandez J, Köves B, Svanborg C. Genetics of innate immunity and UTI susceptibility. Nat Rev Urol. 2011;8(8): 449–68.
9. Song J, Abraham S. Innate and adaptive immune responses in the urinary tract. Eur J Clin Investig. 2008;38(s2):21–8.
10. Foxman B. The epidemiology of urinary tract infection. Nat Rev Urol. 2010; 7(12):653–60.
11. Zasloff M. Antimicrobial peptides of multicellular organisms. Nature. 2002; 415(6870):389–95.
12. Ganz T. Defensins: antimicrobial peptides of innate immunity. Nat Rev Immunol. 2003;3(9):710–20.
13. Tomasinsig L, Zanetti M. The cathelicidins-structure, function and evolution. Curr Protein Pept Sci. 2005;6(1):23–34.
14. Sorensen OE, Follin P, Johnsen AH, Calafat J, Tjabringa GS, Hiemstra PS, et al. Human cathelicidin, hCAP-18, is processed to the antimicrobial peptide LL-37 by extracellular cleavage with proteinase 3. Blood. 2001;97(12):3951–9.
15. Zaiou M, Nizet V, Gallo RL. Antimicrobial and protease inhibitory functions of the human cathelicidin (hCAP18/LL-37) prosequence. J Investig Dermatol. 2003;120(5):810–6.
16. Agerberth B, Charo J, Werr J, Olsson B, Idali F, Lindbom L, et al. The human antimicrobial and chemotactic peptides LL-37 and α-defensins are expressed by specific lymphocyte and monocyte populations. Blood. 2000; 96(9):3086–93.
17. Larrick JW, Hirata M, Balint RF, Lee J, Zhong J, Wright SC. Human CAP18: a novel antimicrobial lipopolysaccharide-binding protein. Infect Immun. 1995; 63(4):1291–7.
18. Nagaoka I, Hirota S, Niyonsaba F, Hirata M, Adachi Y, Tamura H, et al. Augmentation of the lipopolysaccharide-neutralizing activities of human cathelicidin CAP18/LL-37-derived antimicrobial peptides by replacement with hydrophobic and cationic amino acid residues. Clin Diagn Lab Immunol. 2002;9(5):972–82.
19. Suzuki K, Murakami T, Kuwahara-Arai K, Tamura H, Hiramatsu K, Nagaoka I. Human anti-microbial cathelicidin peptide LL-37 suppresses the LPS-induced apoptosis of endothelial cells. Int Immunol. 2011;23(3):185–93.
20. Kandler K, Shaykhiev R, Kleemann P, Klescz F, Lohoff M, Vogelmeier C, et al. The anti-microbial peptide LL-37 inhibits the activation of dendritic cells by TLR ligands. Int Immunol. 2006;18(12):1729–36.
21. Becknell B, Schwaderer A, Hains DS, Spencer JD. Amplifying renal immunity: the role of antimicrobial peptides in pyelonephritis. Nat Rev Nephrol. 2015; 11(11):642–55.
22. Zanetti M. Cathelicidins, multifunctional peptides of the innate immunity. J Leukoc Biol. 2004;75(1):39–48.
23. Zanetti M. The role of cathelicidins in the innate host defenses of mammals. Curr Issues Mol Biol. 2005;7(2):179–96.
24. Reddy K, Yedery R, Aranha C. Antimicrobial peptides: premises and promises. Int J Antimicrob Agents. 2004;24(6):536–47.
25. Andres E, Dimarcq J. Cationic anti-microbial peptides: from innate immunity study to drug development. Rev Med Interne. 2004;25(9):629–35.
26. Zasloff M. Antimicrobial peptides, innate immunity, and the normally sterile urinary tract. J Am Soc Nephrol. 2007;18(11):2810–6.
27. Underdown BJ, Schiff JM. Immunoglobulin A: strategic defense initiative at the mucosal surface. Annu Rev Immunol. 1986;4(1):389–417.
28. Hamdan HZ, Ziad AHM, Ali SK, Adam I. Epidemiology of urinary tract infections and antibiotics sensitivity among pregnant women at Khartoum North Hospital. Ann Clin Microbiol Antimicrob. 2011;10(1):2.
29. Hamdan HZ, Kubbara E, Adam AM, Hassan OS, Suliman SO, Adam I. Urinary tract infections and antimicrobial sensitivity among diabetic patients at Khartoum, Sudan. Ann Clin Microbiol Antimicrob. 2015;14(1):26.
30. Chromek M, Slamova Z, Bergman P, Kovacs L, Podracka L, Ehren I, et al. The antimicrobial peptide cathelicidin protects the urinary tract against invasive bacterial infection. Nat Med. 2006;12(6):636–41.
31. Chromek M, Brauner A. Antimicrobial mechanisms of the urinary tract. J Mol Med. 2008;86(1):37–47.
32. Nielsen KL, Dynesen P, Larsen P, Jakobsen L, Andersen PS, Frimodt-Møller N. Role of urinary cathelicidin LL-37 and human β-defensin 1 in uncomplicated Escherichia coli urinary tract infections. Infect Immun. 2014; 82(4):1572–8.
33. Ali AS, Townes CL, Hall J, Pickard RS. Maintaining a sterile urinary tract: the role of antimicrobial peptides. J Urol. 2009;182(1):21–8.
34. Övünç HD, Altun D, Hacıhamdioğlu B, Çekmez F, Aydemir G, Kul M, et al. The association between serum 25-Hydroxy vitamin D level and urine cathelicidin in children with a urinary tract infection. J Clin Res Pediatr Endocrinol. 2016;8:325.
35. Norden CW, Green GM, Kass EH. Antibacterial mechanisms of the urinary bladder. J Clin Investig. 1968;47(12):2689.
36. Bates JM, Raffi HM, Prasadan K, Mascarenhas R, Laszik Z, Maeda N, et al. Tamm-Horsfall protein knockout mice are more prone to urinary tract infection rapid communication. Kidney Int. 2004;65(3):791–7.

Table 2 Linear regression analysis of associated factors, log of plasma and urine LL-37 levels

Variable	Log of plasma LL-37 (ng/ml)			Log of urine LL-37 ng/mg creatinine		
	Coefficient	SE	P	Coefficient	SE	P
Age	−0.002	0.001	0.113	0.000	0.002	0.986
Male gender	−0.093	0.040	0.022	−0.109	0.059	0.066
TWBCs	0.018	0.008	0.038	−0.012	0.013	0.358
Neutrophils	−0.001	0.006	0.893	−0.001	0.007	0.913
Lymphocytes	−0.001	0.006	0.812	−0.004	0.007	0.596
Basophiles	0.001	0.008	0.933	−0.007	0.010	0.513
Urinary tract infections	0.153	0.045	0.001	0.162	0.077	0.038
Plasma LL-37 ng/ml	–	–	–	0.238	0.019	< 0.001

Our findings provide the first evidence in adult and young children of both genders that the level of LL-37 correlates with positive urine culture in cases of urinary infections. Furthermore, LL-37 levels can be used as a marker of infection and could save time in confirming an accurate diagnosis of UTI in the acute phase. The ability to make an early decision about whether there is an infection or not and would be helpful in limiting unnecessary antimicrobial administration for suspected urinary infections, see Fig. 2. In turn, this would decrease health care costs and the problems associated with inappropriate use of antibiotics. Our results demonstrated differences in plasma and urinary levels of LL-37 between subjects with and without UTIs. To the best of our knowledge, this is the first study performed in apparently healthy and non-hospitalized controls that compares their plasma and urine LL-37 levels with patients (both genders) with UTIs. Additionally, this is the first study to compare inter-individual baseline plasma and urine LL-37 levels for patients and for controls. Table 2, Figs. 1a and b and 3.

In the current study there was no significant difference in both plasma and urine LL-37 levels when comparing isolates of *E. coli* and other uropathogens. This indicates that the microbial infection increases the levels of LL-37 in both plasma and urine concurrently.

To determine the exact circulating level of LL-37 in plasma in relation to UTIs further research needs to be conducted. Studies with much larger subject numbers are required. The limitation of the current study; there was no follow-up sampling to detect LL-37 level after clearance of infection.

Conclusion

Infection of the urinary tract increases the levels of LL-37. The observed increased level was not only in the patient's urine, but has also been observed in the plasma of patients during the period of infection of the urinary tract. Detection of increased levels of LL-37 could help to differentiate subjects with suspected UTI. Accordingly, LL-37 could act as a good marker for diagnosing UTIs.

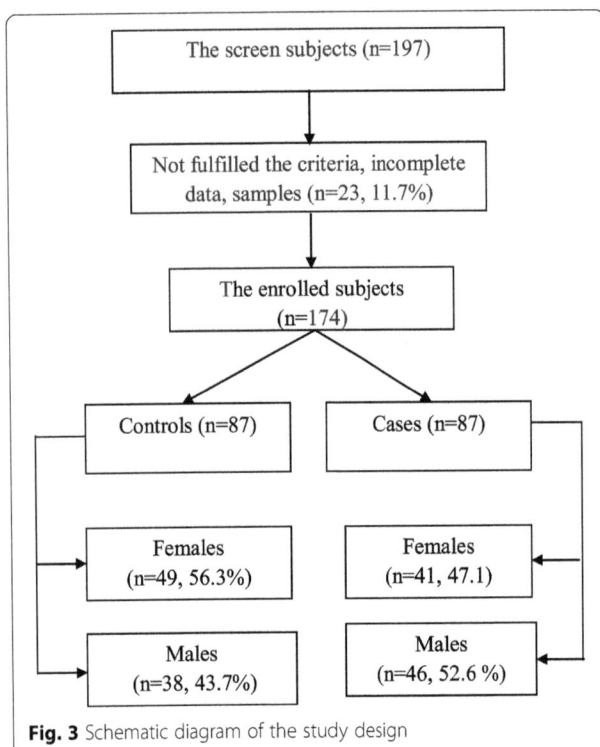

Fig. 3 Schematic diagram of the study design

Abbreviations
(>): Greater than; (≥): Greater than or equal; (°C): Degrees Celsius; (Camp−/−): CRAMP-deficient; (Camp+/+): CRAMP-producing; (P=): P-value; (r =): Correlation; (sIgA): Secretory IgA antibodies; (vs): Versus; AMPs: Antimicrobial peptides; AST: Antibiotic sensitivity test; AST-N: Gram negative antibiotic sensitivity card; CAMP: Cathelicidin gene; CBC: Complete blood count; CFU/ml: Colony-forming unit per milliliter; CLED: Cysteine lactose electrolyte deficient; CRAMP: Cathelin-related antimicrobial peptide; *E. coli*: *Escherichia coli*; *E. faecalis*: *Enterococcus faecalis*; EDTA: Ethylene-diamine-tetra-acetic acid; ELISA: Enzyme-linked immunosorbent assay; GN card: Gram negative identification card; GP card: Gram positive ID card; GP/AST: Gram positive antibiotic sensitivity card; Greater than; hCAP-18: Human cationic antimicrobial peptide-18; ID card: Identification card; *K. pneumoniae*: *Klebsiella pneumoniae*; kD: Kilodalton; LL-37: Cathelicidin; LPS: Lipopolysaccharides; *M. morganii*: *Morganella morganii*; MIC: Minimum inhibitory concentrations; ng/

37. Fliedner M, Mehls O, Rauterberg E-W, Ritz E. Urinary sIgA in children with urinary tract infection. J Pediatr. 1986;109(3):416–21.
38. Abrink M, Larsson E, Gobl A, Hellman L. Expression of lactoferrin in the kidney: implications for innate immunity and iron metabolism. Kidney Int. 2000;57(5):2004–10.
39. Morrison G, Kilanowski F, Davidson D, Dorin J. Characterization of the mouse beta defensin 1, Defb1, mutant mouse model. Infect Immun. 2002; 70(6):3053–60.
40. Valore EV, Park CH, Quayle AJ, Wiles KR, McCray PB Jr, Ganz T. Human beta-defensin-1: an antimicrobial peptide of urogenital tissues. J Clin Investig. 1998;101(8):1633.
41. Mulvey MA, Lopez-Boado YS, Wilson CL, Roth R, Parks WC, Heuser J, et al. Induction and evasion of host defenses by type 1-piliated uropathogenic Escherichia coli. Science. 1998;282(5393):1494–7.

Empiric antibiotic therapy in urinary tract infection in patients with risk factors for antibiotic resistance in a German emergency department

Sebastian Bischoff[1], Thomas Walter[2], Marlis Gerigk[3], Matthias Ebert[1] and Roger Vogelmann[1*] (iD)

Abstract

Background: The aim of this study was to identify clinical risk factors for antimicrobial resistances and multidrug resistance (MDR) in urinary tract infections (UTI) in an emergency department in order to improve empirical therapy.

Methods: UTI cases from an emergency department (ED) during January 2013 and June 2015 were analyzed. Differences between patients with and without resistances towards Ciprofloxacin, Piperacillin with Tazobactam (Pip/taz), Gentamicin, Cefuroxime, Cefpodoxime and Ceftazidime were analyzed with Fisher's exact tests. Results were used to identify risk factors with logistic regression modelling. Susceptibility rates were analyzed in relation to risk factors.

Results: One hundred thirty-seven of four hundred sixty-nine patients who met the criteria of UTI had a positive urine culture. An MDR pathogen was found in 36.5% of these. Overall susceptibility was less than 85% for standard antimicrobial agents. Logistic regression identified residence in nursing homes, male gender, hospitalization within the last 30 days, renal transplantation, antibiotic treatment within the last 30 days, indwelling urinary catheter and recurrent UTI as risk factors for MDR or any of these resistances. For patients with no risk factors Ciprofloxacin had 90%, Pip/taz 88%, Gentamicin 95%, Cefuroxime 98%, Cefpodoxime 98% and Ceftazidime 100% susceptibility. For patients with 1 risk factor Ciprofloxacin had 80%, Pip/taz 80%, Gentamicin 88%, Cefuroxime 78%, Cefpodoxime 78% and Ceftazidime 83% susceptibility. For 2 or more risk factors Ciprofloxacin drops its susceptibility to 52%, Cefuroxime to 54% and Cefpodoxime to 61%. Pip/taz, Gentamicin and Ceftazidime remain at 75% and 77%, respectively.

Conclusions: We identified several risk factors for resistances and MDR in UTI. Susceptibility towards antimicrobials depends on these risk factors. With no risk factor cephalosporins seem to be the best choice for empiric therapy, but in patients with risk factors the beta-lactam penicillin Piperacillin with Tazobactam is an equal or better choice compared to fluoroquinolones, cephalosporins or gentamicin. This study highlights the importance of monitoring local resistance rates and its risk factors in order to improve empiric therapy in a local environment.

Keywords: Antimicrobial resistance, Emergency medicine, Infectious disease, Multidrug resistance, Risk factors, Urinary tract infection, Antibiotic therapy

* Correspondence: Roger.vogelmann@medma.uni-heidelberg.de
[1]Second Department of Internal Medicine, University Medical Center
Mannheim, Medical Faculty Mannheim, Heidelberg University,
Theodor-Kutzer Ufer 1-3, D-68167 Mannheim, Germany
Full list of author information is available at the end of the article

Background

Urinary tract infections (UTI) are among the most common bacterial infections worldwide. Their therapy is becoming more challenging as resistance rates for standard antibiotics are increasing [1]. The increase of antibiotic resistances and multi-drug resistance (MDR) pathogens in UTI is associated with higher rates of inadequate empirical therapy due to impaired antibiotic coverage [2].

Therefore, early identification of patients at risk for antibiotic resistances is an important aspect for effective treatment. Preceding studies identified a variety of risk factors mainly for treatment failure for either fluoroquinolones or trimethoprim-sulfamethaxol or for UTI with MDR pathogens. Rarely did they quantify the impact of risk factors on overall susceptibility to standard empirical therapy choices [3–8].

The goal of our study was to identify risk factors associated with several antibiotic resistances and MDR pathogens in patients presenting with UTI, mainly pyelonephritis or urosepsis, to the emergency department (ED) of a German academic tertiary care facility. We hypothesized that the identification of risk factors will improve empiric antibiotic therapy in the ED.

Methods

The study was retrospectively conducted with anonymized patient data from the ED of an academic tertiary care facility. The local ethics committee of the Medical Faculty of Mannheim has approved the study. Cases were eligible for the study, if they were diagnosed with lower or upper UTI in the ED between January 2013 and June 2015. Lower UTI was defined as dysuria, pollakisuria or positive leucocyte and nitrite in urine in patients with reduced vigilance. Upper UTI was defined by additional flank pain, fever, positive systemic inflammation serum parameters or perinephritic abscess in sonography [9].

Patient information included the following: demographic parameters (gender, age, residence), laboratory analysis (C-reactive protein, leucocyte count, serum creatinine and glomerular filtration rate (GFR) calculated after Modification of Diet in Renal Disease formula), physical condition at admission (signs of exsiccosis, symptoms at presentation), urine analysis (isolated pathogen, pathogen count, antimicrobial susceptibility testing), comorbidities (diabetes mellitus, indwelling urinary catheter, renal transplantation, dialysis), pre-ED antibiotic treatment within the last 30 days, prior hospitalization within the last 30 days and UTI within the last 12 months.

We assessed patients with clinical symptoms consistent with UTI and positive urine culture. A positive result was defined as colony-forming unit $> 10^4$/ml for catheter- or midstream-urine and $> 10^3$/ml for single-use-

catheter. Urine cultures labeled by the microbiology laboratory as "contamination" or "mixed flora" were excluded.

MDR and extensively drug-resistant (XDR) pathogens were defined according to the European Centre for Disease Prevention and Control [10]: MDR describes pathogens non-susceptible to at least one agent in three or more antimicrobial categories. XDR describes pathogens fully susceptibly to only two or less antimicrobial categories.

Data were grouped by presence of antibiotic resistances towards antimicrobial substances frequently used in the treatment of UTIs. We chose Ciprofloxacin (Cip), Ceftazidime, Cefpodoxime, Gentamicin, Piperacillin with Tazobactam (Pip/taz) and Cefuroxime for further analysis. Risk factors for carbapenem non-susceptibility were not analyzed as overall non-susceptibility was low. Differences in parameters between groups with or without resistances towards a certain antibiotic were tested for significance with Fisher's exact testing.

Logistic regression was then performed to identify risk factors for resistances toward antimicrobial substances mainly used in upper UTI treatment, MDR pathogens and pathogens simultaneously resistant to Ciprofloxacin, Pip/taz and Ceftazidime (sCPC). The results were presented with odds ratios and their corresponding 95% confidence interval (CI). The area under the curve (AUC)/c-statistic of a Receiver Operating Characteristic (ROC) analysis was calculated and used to estimate the accuracy of fit of our model. The AUC measures the accuracy for the prediction with an AUC = 1.0 representing perfect prediction.

Susceptibility data were calculated for Ciprofloxacin, Ceftazidime, Cefpodoxime, Cefuroxime, Pip/taz, Gentamicin and Imipenem. Susceptibility was analyzed for the whole patient collective as well as subgroups defined by the number of risk factors present.

All analyses were performed using SAS system for Microsoft version 9.4. (SAS Institute Inc., Cary, North Carolina, USA).

Results

Demographics and pathogen distribution

Between January 2013 and June 2015, the ED treated and admitted 469 cases, who met the criteria of UTI. In 184 cases no urine culture was performed, 143 urine cultures had a negative result or were contaminated. In 5 cases the initial diagnosis of upper UTI could not be confirmed during hospital stay. One hundred thirty-seven had an uncontaminated urine culture with a positive result, of which 130 (94.9%) met the criteria for upper UTI. These patients were mostly female (80/137, 58.4%) with a median age of 76.0y (average 72.1y, range 17-97y). Twenty-seven patients resided in nursing homes (19.7%), 22 had indwelling urinary catheters (16.1%), 33 were admitted to a hospital within the last 30 days (24.1%) and 20 received antibiotic treatment within 30 days prior to their ED visit (14.6%; Table 1). In all patients, symptoms of infection started before admission, thus presenting either community acquired UTI or community-onset healthcare-associated urinary tract infections.

Table 1 Demographic parameters of patients with a positive urine culture

	All (n = 137)	
	n	Percentage
Age		
Mean	72.1	(18.2)
< 65 years	30	(21.9)
65–80 years	55	(40.1)
> 80 years	52	(38.0)
Gender		
female	80	(58.4)
Nursing home		
yes	27	(19.7)
Hospitalization within 30 days		
yes	33	(24.1)
Antibiotic treatment within 30 days		
yes	20	(14.6)
Recent UTI		
yes	30	(21.9)
Diabetes		
yes	47	(34.3)
Renal transplantation		
yes	4	(2.9)
Indwelling urinary catheter		
yes	22	(16.1)
Hemodialysis		
yes	4	(2.9)
Exsiccosis		
yes	40	(29.2)
Fever		
yes	50	(36.5)
leucocyte count		
> 12 /nl	56	(40.9)
GFR (from serum creatinine)		
< 15 ml/min	5	(3.7)
< 60 ml/min	79	(57.7)
C-reactive protein		
> 100 mg/l	64	(46.7)

GFR glomerular filtration rate

Of 137 urine cultures, main pathogens were *Escherichia coli* in 64.2% (n = 88), *Klebsiella pneumoniae* or *oxytoca* in 12.4% (n = 17), *Enterococci spp.* in 5.1% (n = 7), *Pseudomonas aeruginosa* in 5.1% (n = 7), *Proteus mirabilis* in 4.4% (n = 6), *Staphylococcus aureus* in 3.7% (n = 5) and *Citrobacter spp.* in 2.2% (n = 3) of cases.

All samples were tested for susceptibility towards Ciprofloxacin (Cip), Piperacillin with Tazobactam (Pip/taz), Gentamicin, Cefuroxime, Cefpodoxime and Ceftazidime and Imipenem. In our study 36.5% (50/137) of pathogens can be classified as MDR. Most MDR pathogens were *E. coli* (62.7%) followed by *K. pneumonia* (13.7%). XDR pathogens were detected in 3.7% (5/137). Non-susceptibility to all three antibiotics Ciprofloxacin, Pip/taz and Ceftazidime (sCPC), which are commonly used for the empiric therapy of severe pyelonephritis, was detected in 5.1% (7/137).

Risk factors for antibiotic non-susceptibility
An analysis of patient characteristics revealed residence in nursing homes, prior hospitalization within 30 days, usage of antibiotics 30 days prior to admission, indwelling urinary catheter, recent or recurrent UTI, gender, renal transplantation and serum leucocyte count > 12.0/ nl as significantly different between patients with and without non-susceptibility ($p < 0.05$ in Fisher's exact testing; data not shown). Logistic regression was performed to allocate risk factors to non-susceptibility to a certain antibiotic, MDR pathogen or to simultaneous non-susceptibility towards Ciprofloxacin, Pip/taz and Ceftazidime (sCPC). Seven factors showed a significant association (Table 2). ROC analysis yielded AUC values of 0.650 to 0.868 indicating an overall good fit of our models.

Antimicrobial susceptibility in relation to risk factors
Overall susceptibility for commonly used antibiotics in upper UTI was low with 71.5% for Cip, 80.3% for Pip/taz, 84.6% for Gentamicin, 73.7% for Cefuroxime, 76.6% for Cefpodoxime and 85.4% for Ceftazidime (Table 3). Ampicillin with Sulbactam had an overall susceptibility of 54.7% and was therefore not further analyzed. Only Imipenem showed an acceptable susceptibility rate of 96.4%.

In order to recommend non-carbapenem antibiotics for the treatment of upper UTI in the ED we analyzed susceptibility rates by previously identified risk factors. Without a risk factor present all antibiotics had a susceptibility rate of around 90% and above (n = 41). If one of seven risk factors were present, susceptibility for all antibiotics except for Imipenem dropped to around 80% (n = 40) (Fig. 1). For 2 or more risk factors Cip, Cefuroxime and Cefpodoxime dropped to 60% and below, while Pip/taz, Gentamicin and Ceftazidime remained at around 75% (n = 56). In this case, the

Table 2 Logistic regression modelling presented as Odds Ratio with 95% confidence interval and corresponding AUC

Target	Nursing home residence	Hospitalization within 30 days	Male sex	Renal transplantation	Indwelling urinary catheter	Use of antibiotics within 30 days	Recurrent UTI	AUC
Pip/taz	n.s.	3.7 (1.4–9.5)**	n.s.	15.4 (1.4–172.1)*	n.s.	n.s.	n.s.	0.699
Ciprofloxacin	n.s.	4.4 (1.8–10.6)**	n.s.	n.s.	5.2 (1.8–14.7)**	n.s.	n.s.	0.749
Gentamicin	n.s.	n.s.	n.s.	24.8 (2.4–257.2)**	3.1 (1.0–9.4)*	n.s.	n.s.	0.650
Cefuroxime	n.s.	n.s.	7.3 (2.9–18.5)***	n.s.	n.s.	5.7 (1.8–17.7)**	n.s.	0.792
Cefpodoxime	n.s.	n.s.	6.5 (2.5–17.0)***	n.s.	n.s.	5.3 (1.7–16.3)**	n.s.	0.788
Ceftazidime	n.s.	n.s.	3.7 (1.3–10.6)*	16.4 (1..5–182.1)*	n.s.	n.s.	n.s.	0.715
MDR	n.s.	3.6 (1.5–8.5)**	n.s.	n.s.	n.s.	n.s.	4.0 (1.7–9.8)**	0.707
sCPC	22.8 (3.4–151.2)**	n.s.	9.5 (1.4–62.5)*	n.s.	n.s.	n.s.	n.s.	0.868

$* p < 0.05$; $** P < 0.01$; $*** p < 0.001$; n.s. not significant, UTI urinary tract infection, AUC Area under the curve, Pip/taz Piperacillin/Tazobactam, MDR multidrug resistance, sCPC simultaneous non-susceptibility for Pip/taz, Ciprofloxacin and Ceftazidime

susceptibility rate of Imipenem also dropped to 91.1% (Table 3). Whereas cephalosporins and Gentamicin seem to be preferable in patients with no risk factors in regard to susceptibility, their susceptibility rates were similar to Pip/taz and Cip in patients with one risk factor. Interestingly, Pip/taz, Gentamicin and Ceftazidime kept their susceptibility rate relatively stable with more risk factors whereas Cip, Cefuroxime and Cefpodoxime dropped their susceptibility rates to a greater extent.

The logistic regression modelling showed that not all antibiotics share the same risk factor profile (Table 2), therefore sub analysis was performed. In our population, patients, who have been admitted to a hospital within the previous 30 days and resided in a nursing home ($n = 9$), showed a much better susceptibility rate for cephalosporins (77.8%) compared to Gentamicin (55.6%), Pip/taz (33%) or Ciprofloxacin (11%). In contrast, patients with antibiotic therapy 30 days prior to admission ($n = 20$) had a high susceptibility rate for Pip/taz 95% compared to

Gentamicin (80.0%), Cefuroxime 45.0%, Cefpodoxime 50.0%, Ceftazidime 75.0% and Ciprofloxacin 60.0%. Our data suggest that patients with previous antibiotic therapy may be better treated with Pip/taz as empiric therapy.

Therapy algorithm

From our data we concluded for our ED that for patients without a risk factor a cephalosporin-based empiric treatment or Gentamicin has the lowest rate of non-susceptibility (Fig. 2). However, with one or more risk factors Pip/taz is equal to or better as cephalosporins or Ciprofloxacin, particularly in case of prior antibiotic therapy. An exception could be patients residing in a nursing home and who have been admitted to a hospital

Table 3 Susceptibility in % in relationship to number of risk factors (RF)

	Overall ($n = 137$)	0 RF ($n = 41$)	1 RF ($n = 40$)	>= 2 RF ($n = 56$)
Ciprofloxacin	71.5%	90.2%	80.0%	51.8%
Pip/taz	80.3%	87.8%	80.0%	75.0%
Gentamicin	84.7%	95.1%	87.5%	75.0%
Ceftazidime	85.4%	100%	82.5%	76.8%
Cefpodoxime	76.6%	97.6%	77.5%	60.7%
Cefuroxime	73.7%	97.6%	77.5%	53.7%
Imipenem	96.4%	100%	100%	91.1%

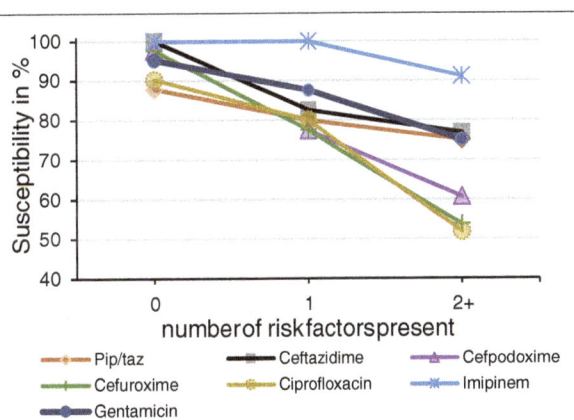

Fig. 1 Susceptibility in relationship to number of risk factors - Susceptibility in % for Piperacillin/Tazobactam (red), Ceftazidime (grey), Cefpodoxime (violet), Cefuroxime (green), Ciprofloxacin (yellow), Imipenem (light blue) and Gentamicin (dark blue) are plotted for 0, 1 and 2 and more (2+) risk factors present

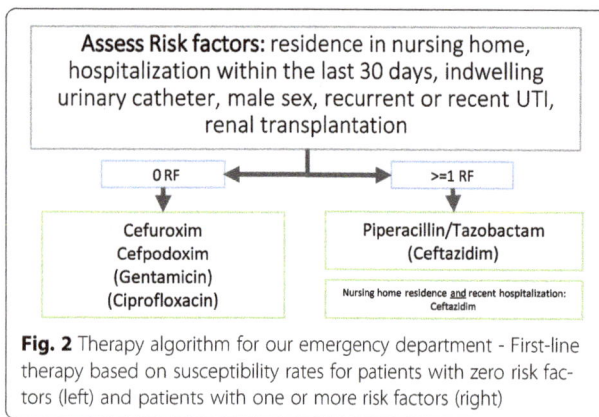

Assess Risk factors: residence in nursing home, hospitalization within the last 30 days, indwelling urinary catheter, male sex, recurrent or recent UTI, renal transplantation

0 RF   >=1 RF

Cefuroxim
Cefpodoxim
(Gentamicin)
(Ciprofloxacin)

Piperacillin/Tazobactam
(Ceftazidim)

Nursing home residence and recent hospitalization:
Ceftazidim

Fig. 2 Therapy algorithm for our emergency department - First-line therapy based on susceptibility rates for patients with zero risk factors (left) and patients with one or more risk factors (right)

in the previous 30 days. They could benefit from Cefpodoxime or Cefuroxime as an initial treatment choice.

In our study, only 80 of 124 patients (64.5%) received an empiric therapy that showed susceptibility to its causing pathogen in urine culture testing. Thirty-three patients received a cephalosporin as empiric therapy, 10 Pip/taz, 15 Ciprofloxacin, but 54 Ampicillin/Sulbactam. An empiric therapy based on common guidelines for upper UTI such as ciprofloxacin would have an overall susceptibility of 71, 5% (Table 3). Following our risk factor based decision algorithm, 86.1% (107/124) would have received a susceptible antibiotic treatment. In this algorithm, patients with one or more risk factors would have been treated with Pip/taz except for patients, who had been admitted to the hospital within the last 30 days prior to admission and reside in a nursing home, which would have received a cephalosporine. All patients without a risk factor would have received Cefpodoxime or Cefuroxime as first line therapy (Fig. 2).

Discussion

With the increase of microbial resistance, empiric therapy recommendations without taking local resistance data into account can lead to inferior treatment results. In our data set treating patients with upper UTI per current treatment guidelines would have led to incorrect antibiotic coverage in nearly 30% of cases [9]. Early identification of patients at risk of antibiotic resistances and thus therapy failure is an important part of an effective empiric therapy.

In the past risk factors for extended-spectrum-betalactamase producing bacteria in non-hospitalized patients with UTI have for example been identified as recent hospitalizations within 3 months, previous antibiotic usage, age > 60 years, diabetes mellitus, male gender, previous UTI with *Klebsiella spp.*, residence in long-term care facilities, indwelling urinary catheters, recurrent UTIs and previous fluoroquinolone use [11, 12]. Analogous results were obtained for fluoroquinolones [3, 6–8, 13]. In a similar setting to ours, Faine et al. evaluated risk factors

for MDR pathogens in UTI in the United States [14]. Their overall MDR rate was only 6.7% in contrast to 36.5% in our population. Faine et al. used a more restrictive MDR definition, which may explains the observed difference in MDR rates and they identified male gender, chronic hemodialysis and nursing home residence as risk factors [14].

We identified several risk factors for UTI with non-susceptible pathogens in our study. They are similar to those previous identified risk factors such as prior hospitalization within 30 days, residence in nursing homes, recurrent UTI, male gender, renal transplantation, permanently indwelling urinary catheter and prior usage of antibiotics within the last 30 days. Our analysis considered several antibiotics and demonstrates that not all risk factors are associated with non-susceptibility to all antimicrobial categories. For example, residing in a nursing home was the only significant risk factor for infection with MDR pathogens, whereas hospitalization within 30 days and indwelling urinary catheter were significant for Ciprofloxacin resistance. This seems consistent with published data that showed various risk factors associated with different antimicrobial categories in different studies [3, 13, 15]. A large multicenter, prospective study would be necessary to further explore, which risk factors cause non-susceptibility to certain antimicrobial categories.

Stratification of empiric antibiotic therapy by risk factors can improve pathogen coverage significantly. In our study, susceptibility to standard antibiotics was overall less than 85%. However, when analyzed by presence of risk factors our data showed that patients with no risk factors had > 85% susceptibility for all standard antibiotics. Patients with one risk factor present had still a susceptibility rate of 77.5 to 82.5% for cephalosporins and 80.0% for Pip/taz. Patients with two or more risk factors remained only susceptible to Imipenem, but its susceptibility for Pip/taz, Gentamicin and Ceftazidime was reasonable with 75.0% or 76.8%, respectively.

Interestingly, in our study antibiotic use within the last 30 days was associated with a higher resistance rate in cephalosporins and Ciprofloxacin compared to the beta-lactam penicillin Pip/taz consisted with observations that cephalosporins and fluoroquinolones may increase the resistance rates of bacteria [16]. Our data suggest that patients with previous antibiotic therapy may be better treated with Pip/taz empirically although the number of patients in this sub-analysis was low in order to draw a statistical sound conclusion.

There are several important limitations to consider in our study. It was a single-center, retrospective data analysis, which depended on the accuracy of history taking by the health care provider on call. Certain published risk factors, such as employment in health care, exposure to farming, family members with multidrug resistant pathogens, ambulant chemotherapy and wound care, had to be excluded from our study as they have not been recorded consistently in all cases. A selection bias towards antibiotic resistance cannot be excluded as not all patients presenting with UTI received a urine culture or had a positive urine culture result. Overall, the rate of antibiotic resistance or MDR pathogens was high compared to similar studies.

However, our results are among the first to show risk factors for antibiotic resistances and MDR pathogens in UTI patients in Germany. In contrast to most studies, we analyzed patients admitted to an emergency department in a large tertiary care hospital and did not solely focus on a single antibiotic substance or on MDR pathogens. Our results show that implementation of risk factors can lead to significant improvement in susceptibility in empirical therapy.

Our study revealed also another important aspect as patients diagnosed with upper UTI in the ED were admitted to the ward with an empiric antibiotic therapy, but the sampling of urine cultures was often referred to the ward nursing team due to logistical reasons. This led to a high number of negative urine cultures as the antibiotic treatment was applied before urine cultures were taken. Studies like these can help not only to identify local resistant patterns or risk factors for resistant bacteria, it also helped us to identify serious organizational problems in the daily routine.

Current treatment guidelines often recommend fluoroquinolones and cephalosporins as treatment options in uncomplicated upper UTI. Both antimicrobial categories should be viewed critical, because they lead to a significant increase of *Clostridium difficile* colitis and may further increase the rate to MDR pathogens [16, 17]. Piperacillin/Tazobactam is less prone to induce antibiotic resistance [18]. It also inhibits *C. difficile* colonization during therapy [19]. In this regard, Pip/Taz is the better antibiotic choice. Gentamicin can cause severe side effects, such as kidney and inner ear damage and needs extended monitoring in comparison to other antibiotics especially in elderly patients. Therefore, in our institution we do not recommend Gentamicin for empiric therapy in upper UTI infections.

β-Lactamase inhibitors (BLIs) such as Tazobactam play an important role in overcoming β-lactam resistance in Gram-negative bacteria. Because of the emergence of varieties of β-lactamases, their effectiveness has diminished over time. New BLI combinations with broad-spectrum antibiotics are promising for increasing the effectiveness of empiric antibiotic therapy in UTI [20]. Ceftolozane/tazobactam and ceftazidime/avibactam have been approved for UTI treatment and increase the overall susceptibility to gram-negative bacteria. In particular, ceftazidime/avibactam has been shown to be effective in

isolates from UTI patients resistant to Pip/Taz, Cephalosporins and Carbapenems [21, 22]. In our study, bacteria were not routinely tested for these new ß-lactamase inhibitor combinations as they are regarded as last line therapies in severely ill patients due to highly resistant bacteria.

In our setting, all standard antibiotics had a relatively low overall susceptibility. A simple risk factor based treatment algorithm using cephalosporins in patients without risk factors and Pip/taz in all other patients except for patients residing in nursing homes with recent hospitalization in the previous 30 days increases the antibiotic coverage rate to 86.1%. It can be debated whether the use of Pip/taz in all cases as a broad-spectrum beta-lactam penicillin derivative with an overall susceptibility rate of 80.3% would be much different in its clinical outcome. With its advantages regarding *C. difficile* colonization and induction of resistances Pip/taz could be the better choice compared to cephalosporins and fluoroquinolones for urinary tract infections.

Conclusions

We retrospectively identified seven independent risk factors for antimicrobial resistances in UTI patients in the local emergency department: prior hospitalization within 30 days, residence in nursing homes, recurrent UTI, male gender, renal transplantation, permanently indwelling urinary catheter and prior usage of antibiotics within the last 30 days. Antibiotic susceptibility changes significantly in regard to risk factors present in a patient population. These results can be used to improve empirical antibiotic therapy in emergency departments with high rates of resistances. The beta-lactam penicillin-derivate piperacillin/tazobactam is likely the better choice compared to fluoroquinolones and cephalosporins as susceptibility in patients with risk factors is comparable or better. Whether the incidence of *C. difficile* colitis and the increase of multi-resistant bacteria can be reduced by treatment with piperacillin/tazobactam should be explored in further randomized, prospective multi-center studies. We encourage readers to monitor their local susceptibility rates to choose appropriate empirical therapy, as the local situation may significantly differ from guideline and literature results.

Abbreviations

AUC: Area under the curve; BLI: β-Lactamase inhibitor; Cip: Ciprofloxacin; ED: Emergency department; GFR: Glomerular filtration rate; MDR: Multidrug-resistant; Pip/taz: Piperacillin/tazobactam; sCPC: Simultaneous resistance towards Ciprofloxacin, Piperacillin/tazobactam and Ceftazidime; UTI: Urinary tract infection; XDR: Extensively drug-resistant

Acknowledgements

We thank the ED team and all its health care providers of the University hospital Mannheim for their dedication to their patients, the microbiology department for their diagnostic routine in providing antibiotic resistance data. We acknowledge that we used the data information system of the hospital EPOS system (SAP, Germany) and i/med-info (Dorner Health IT solutions, Germany) for data collection.

Funding
We acknowledge the financial support of the Deutsche Forschungsgemeinschaft and Ruprecht-Karls-Universität Heidelberg within the funding program Open Access Publishing.

Authors' contributions
SB, ME, RV conceptualized the study. SB, TW, MG collected the data. SB, MG, RV analyzed the data set. SB, TW, MG, ME, RV wrote the manuscript. All authors read and approved the final manuscript.

Consent for publication
Data were collected by chart review. The local ethics committee waived the necessity for individual informed consent.

Competing interests
Roger Vogelmann, Sebastian Bischoff, Thomas Walter, Marlis Gerigk and Matthias Ebert declare that they have no conflict of interest.

Author details
[1]Second Department of Internal Medicine, University Medical Center Mannheim, Medical Faculty Mannheim, Heidelberg University, Theodor-Kutzer Ufer 1-3, D-68167 Mannheim, Germany. [2]Emergency Department, University Medical Center Mannheim, Medical Faculty Mannheim, Heidelberg University, Theodor-Kutzer Ufer 1-3, D-68167 Mannheim, Germany. [3]Department of Microbiology, University Medical Center Mannheim, Medical Faculty Mannheim, Heidelberg University, Theodor-Kutzer Ufer 1-3, D-68167 Mannheim, Germany.

References
1. Wagenlehner F, Tandogdu Z, Bartoletti R, Cai T, Cek M, Kulchavenya E, Koves B, Naber K, Perepanova T, Tenke P, et al. The global prevalence of infections in urology study: a long-term, worldwide surveillance study on urological infections. Pathogens. 2016;5(1)
2. Horcajada JP, Shaw E, Padilla B, Pintado V, Calbo E, Benito N, Gamallo R, Gozalo M, Rodriguez-Bano J, group I et al: Healthcare-associated, community-acquired and hospital-acquired bacteraemic urinary tract infections in hospitalized patients: a prospective multicentre cohort study in the era of antimicrobial resistance. Clin. Microbiol. Infect 2013, 19(10):962-968.
3. Khawcharoenporn T, Vasoo S, Ward E, Singh K. High rates of quinolone resistance among urinary tract infections in the ED. Am. J. Emerg. Med. 2012;30(1):68–74.
4. Rosa R, Abbo LM, Raney K, Tookes HE 3rd, Supino M. Antimicrobial resistance in urinary tract infections at a large urban ED: factors contributing to empiric treatment failure. Am. J. Emerg. Med. 2017;35(3):397–401.
5. Zatorski C, Jordan JA, Cosgrove SE, Zocchi M, May L. Comparison of antibiotic susceptibility of Escherichia Coli in urinary isolates from an emergency department with other institutional susceptibility data. Am. J. Health Syst. Pharm. 2015;72(24):2176–80.
6. Kratochwill L, Powers M, MA MG, King L, O'Neill JM, Venkat A. Factors associated with ciprofloxacin-resistant Escherichia Coli urinary tract infections in discharged ED patients. Am. J. Emerg. Med. 2015;33(10):1473–6.
7. Filiatrault L, RM MK, Patrick DM, Roscoe DL, Quan G, Brubacher J, Collins KM. Antibiotic resistance in isolates recovered from women with community-acquired urinary tract infections presenting to a tertiary care emergency department. Cjem. 2012;14(5):295–305.
8. Smithson A, Chico C, Ramos J, Netto C, Sanchez M, Ruiz J, Porron R, Bastida MT. Prevalence and risk factors for quinolone resistance among Escherichia

Coli strains isolated from males with community febrile urinary tract infection. European journal of clinical microbiology & infectious diseases : official publication of the European Society of Clinical Microbiology. 2012; 31(4):423–30.
9. Wagenlehner FM, Schmiemann G, Hoyme U, Funfstuck R, Hummers-Pradier E, Kaase M, Kniehl E, Selbach I, Sester U, Vahlensieck W, et al. National S3 guideline on uncomplicated urinary tract infection: recommendations for treatment and management of uncomplicated community-acquired bacterial urinary tract infections in adult patients. Der Urologe Ausg A. 2011; 50(2):153–69.
10. Magiorakos AP, Srinivasan A, Carey RB, Carmeli Y, Falagas ME, Giske CG, Harbarth S, Hindler JF, Kahlmeter G, Olsson-Liljequist B, et al. Multidrug-resistant, extensively drug-resistant and pandrug-resistant bacteria: an international expert proposal for interim standard definitions for acquired resistance. Clin. Microbiol. Infect. 2012;18(3):268–81.
11. Colodner R, Rock W, Chazan B, Keller N, Guy N, Sakran W, Raz R. Risk factors for the development of extended-spectrum beta-lactamase-producing bacteria in nonhospitalized patients. Eur. J. Clin. Microbiol. Infect. Dis. 2004; 23(3):163–7.
12. Vardi M, Kochavi T, Denekamp Y, Bitterman H. Risk factors for urinary tract infection caused by Enterobacteriaceae with extended-spectrum beta-lactamase resistance in patients admitted to internal medicine departments. The Israel Medical Association journal : IMAJ. 2012;14(2):115–8.
13. Talan DA, Krishnadasan A, Abrahamian FM, Stamm WE, Moran GJ, Group EMINS. Prevalence and risk factor analysis of trimethoprim-sulfamethoxazole- and fluoroquinolone-resistant Escherichia Coli infection among emergency department patients with pyelonephritis. Clin. Infect. Dis. 2008;47(9):1150–8.
14. Faine BA, Harland KK, Porter B, Liang SY, Mohr N. A clinical decision rule identifies risk factors associated with antimicrobial-resistant urinary pathogens in the emergency department: a retrospective validation study. Ann Pharmacother. 2015;49(6):649–55.
15. Sotto A, De Boever CM, Fabbro-Peray P, Gouby A, Sirot D, Jourdan J. Risk factors for antibiotic-resistant Escherichia Coli isolated from hospitalized patients with urinary tract infections: a prospective study. J Clin Microbiol. 2001;39(2):438–44.
16. Gutkind GO, Di Conza J, Power P, Radice M. Beta-lactamase-mediated resistance: a biochemical, epidemiological and genetic overview. Curr Pharm Des. 2013;19(2):164–208.
17. de With K, Allerberger F, Amann S, Apfalter P, Brodt HR, Eckmanns T, Fellhauer M, Geiss HK, Janata O, Krause R, et al. Strategies to enhance rational use of antibiotics in hospital: a guideline by the German Society for Infectious Diseases. Infection. 2016;
18. Lee J, Oh CE, Choi EH, Lee HJ. The impact of the increased use of piperacillin/tazobactam on the selection of antibiotic resistance among invasive Escherichia Coli and Klebsiella Pneumoniae isolates. Int. J. Infect. Dis. 2013;17(8):e638–43.
19. Kundrapu S, Sunkesula VC, Jury LA, Cadnum JL, Nerandzic MM, Musuuza JS, Sethi AK, Donskey CJ. Do piperacillin/tazobactam and other antibiotics with inhibitory activity against Clostridium Difficile reduce the risk for acquisition of C. Difficile colonization? BMC Infect Dis. 2016;16:159.
20. Bush K. A resurgence of beta-lactamase inhibitor combinations effective against multidrug-resistant gram-negative pathogens. Int J Antimicrob Agents. 2015;46(5):483–93.
21. Sader HS, Castanheira M, Flamm RK, Jones RN. Antimicrobial activities of Ceftazidime-Avibactam and comparator agents against gram-negative organisms isolated from patients with urinary tract infections in U.S. medical centers, 2012 to 2014. Antimicrob Agents Chemother. 2016;60(7):4355–60.
22. Flamm RK, Sader HS, Farrell DJ, Jones RN. Ceftazidime-avibactam and comparator agents tested against urinary tract isolates from a global surveillance program (2011). Diagnostic microbiology and infectious disease. 2014;80(3):233–8.

Hospitalization for community-acquired febrile urinary tract infection: validation and impact assessment of a clinical prediction rule

Janneke E. Stalenhoef[1]* ⓘ, Willize E. van der Starre[1], Albert M. Vollaard[1], Ewout W. Steyerberg[2], Nathalie M. Delfos[3], Eliane M.S. Leyten[4], Ted Koster[5], Hans C. Ablij[6], Jan W. van 't Wout[4], Jaap T. van Dissel[4†] and Cees van Nieuwkoop[7†]

Abstract

Background: There is a lack of severity assessment tools to identify adults presenting with febrile urinary tract infection (FUTI) at risk for complicated outcome and guide admission policy. We aimed to validate the Prediction Rule for Admission policy in Complicated urinary Tract InfeCtion LEiden (PRACTICE), a modified form of the *pneumonia severity index*, and to subsequentially assess its use in clinical practice.

Methods: A prospective observational multicenter study for model validation (2004–2009), followed by a multicenter controlled clinical trial with stepped wedge cluster-randomization for impact assessment (2010–2014), with a follow up of 3 months. Paricipants were 1157 consecutive patients with a presumptive diagnosis of acute febrile UTI (787 in validation cohort and 370 in the randomized trial), enrolled at emergency departments of 7 hospitals and 35 primary care centers in the Netherlands.
The clinical prediction rule contained 12 predictors of complicated course. In the randomized trial the PRACTICE included guidance on hospitalization for high risk (>100 points) and home discharge for low risk patients (<75 points), in the control period the standard policy regarding hospital admission was applied. Main outcomes were effectiveness of the clinical prediction rule, as measured by primary hospital admission rate, and its safety, as measured by the rate of low-risk patients who needed to be hospitalized for FUTI after initial home-based treatment, and 30-day mortality.

Results: A total of 370 patients were included in the randomized trial, 237 in the control period and 133 in the intervention period. Use of PRACTICE significantly reduced the primary hospitalization rate (from 219/237, 92%, in the control group to 96/133, 72%, in the intervention group, $p < 0.01$). The secondary hospital admission rate after initial outpatient treatment was 6% in control patients and 27% in intervention patients (1/17 and 10/37; $p < 0.001$).

Conclusions: Although the proposed PRACTICE prediction rule is associated with a lower number of hospital admissions of patients presenting to the ED with presumptive febrile urinary tract infection, futher improvement is necessary to reduce the occurrence of secondary hospital admissions.

Keywords: Community-acquired febrile urinary tract infection, Severity assessment, Prediction tool, Hospitalization

* Correspondence: J.E.Stalenhoef@lumc.nl
†Equal contributors
[1]Department of Infectious Diseases, Leiden University Medical Center, C5-P,
PO Box 96002300 RC Leiden, the Netherlands
Full list of author information is available at the end of the article

Background

The majority of adults presenting to hospital with an acute febrile illness suffer from respiratory or urinary tract infections [1, 2]. The course of infection may be unpredictable and fever may reflect the onset of sepsis with potential progression to septic shock and multi organ failure. However, adults with fever of bacterial origin usually present with a mild illness at emergency departments (ED) and respond favourably to antibiotic treatment. It thus appears that the vast majority of these patients can be managed safely as outpatients. In daily clinical practice the need for hospital-based treatment for febrile urinary tract infection (FUTI) is assessed on basis of history, comorbidity and on severity of local and vital signs.

For respiratory tract infection there are validated clinical rules to calculate the mortality risk, such as the *Pneumonia Severity Index* (PSI), which is used to provide guidance on decisions regarding treatment and hospital admission [3–5]. To date, there are no such rules to assess the risk of poor outcome in patients presenting with FUTI.

The risk of complicated course of FUTI increases with age and comorbidity, but the event rate of life-threatening complications is low [6–8]. Physicians tend to apply low thresholds for hospitalization, which suggests that many admissions may be avoidable [9, 10]. Therefore, clinical tools that predict prognosis in patients with FUTI are needed to identify those who benefit from hospital admission, and those who may safely be managed as outpatients.

The main predicting factors of mortality in the PSI are not specific for pneumonia such as age, co-morbidity and physical or laboratory signs of sepsis [3]. We therefore considered that this risk assessment might also apply for community-acquired infections other than pneumonia. As our focus was on the evaluation of a practical and bedside available prediction tool, we modified the PSI by erasing all the laboratory variables (Table 1) and changed the name in the *Prediction Rule for Admission policy in Complicated urinary Tract InfeCtion LEiden* (PRACTICE). We used data from a prospective observational multi-center cohort study that included 787 consecutive adults with febrile UTI between 2004 and 2009 to validate this PSI-derived prediction rule for complicated course in patients with FUTI (all details and methods are described in the Additional file 1). In this validation cohort, the PRACTICE score identified those at very low risk for 30-day mortality and ICU admission; the area under the curve (AUC) of the receiver operating characteristic curve for these outcomes indicated a good discriminatory power (AUC 30-day mortality: 0.91; AUC 30-day mortality or ICU admission: 0.84). The PRACTICE score was devided in 5 risk categories (see Additional file 1: Table S1), showing that patients with a PRACTICE score < 100 points (*n* = 636) had a very low risk (<2%) of adverse outcomes; yet 380 (60%) of those were hospitalized. Using a cut-off

Table 1 Prediction Rule for Admission policy in Complicated urinary Tract InfeCtion LEiden (PRACTICE)

Characteristic	Allocated points[a]
Demographic	
Age (men)	Age (years)
Age (women)	Age (years) - 10
Nursing home resident	+10
Comorbidity[b]	
Malignancy	+30
Congestive heart failure	+10
Cerebrovascular disease	+10
Liver cirrhosis	+20
Renal disease	+10
Signs & Symptoms	
Altered mental status	+20
Respiratory rate ≥ 30/min	+20
Systolic blood pressure < 90 mmHg	+20
Pulse ≥125/min	+10
Temperature ≥ 40 °C	+15

[a]A total score individual patient score is obtained by summing the points for each characteristic
[b]Malignancy is defined as any cancer except basal- or squamous-cell cancer of the skin that was active within the previous year of presentation. Congestive heart failure is defined as ventricular dysfunction for which the patient is prescribed medication and/or consults a hospital-based medical specialist. Cerebrovascular disease is defined as a history of stroke or transient ischemic attack. Liver disease is defined as a clinical diagnosis of cirrhosis. Renal disease is defined as a history of chronic renal disease
According to risk class the following recommendations will apply:
< 75 points strong recommendation towards home-based management
75–100 points consider home-based management
>100 points strong recommendation towards hospital admission

value of the PRACTICE score ≥ 100 resulted in a negative predictive value for 30-day mortality of 1.00 and for the composite endpoint 'complicated course' (30-day mortality, ICU admission or hospitalization >10 days) of 0.90. Because the cut-off point was chosen to identify low-risk patients, the positive predictive values (PPV) were low (PVV 0.12 and 0.39, respectively). We assumed that the PRACTICE is a good bedside clinical tool to distinguish patients with FUTI at low risk of complicated course who can be managed as outpatients.

The aim of the present study is to validate the PRACTICE in a new prospective cohort to guide the need for hospitalization in patients with FUTI presenting at EDs, with the aim to reduce hospitalization rates without compromising clinical outcome.

Methods
Trial design

We performed a stepped wedge cluster-randomized trial involving consecutive patients presenting with a presumptive diagnosis of FUTI, at the EDs of 7 hospitals in the Netherlands, between January 2010 and June 2014 [11].

These centers also participated in the validation cohort study (see Additional file 1). All participating centers started with a control period, in which routine clinical practice with regard to hospitalization policy was applied. The intervention (use of the PRACTICE) was introduced at the participating centers sequentially, in random order. By the end of the allocation all sites, except one, used the PRACTICE to guide admission policy.

Inclusion criteria were age ≥ 18 years, fever (≥38.0 °C) and/or a history of fever or shaking chills within 24 h before presentation, at least one symptom of UTI (dysuria, perineal pain or flank pain) and a positive nitrite dipstick test or leucocyturia. Exclusion criteria were pregnancy, hemodialysis or peritoneal dialysis, a history of kidney transplantation or polycystic kidney disease. The study protocol was approved by the local Ethics Committee, and all participants signed an informed consent form prior to enrollment.

Intervention and treatment

The PRACTICE score ranges from 8 to >125. Based on the validation cohort it was divided into three risk classes (low <75 points; intermediate 75–100 points; high >100 points) with corresponding recommendations regarding hospitalization policy (Table 1). During the control period, the decision to treat the patient at home or admission to hospital was made at the discretion of the ED physician. At the start of the intervention period the ED physicians were instructed to calculate the PRACTICE score and on that basis decide on hospital-based or home-based treatment. Preferably admission policy was done according to the guidance as described in Table 1, however, the attending physician was responsible for the final decision on treatment location.

Throughout the whole study period the antibiotic therapy was left at the discretion of the treating physician. According to local guidelines, outpatient treatment for FUTI consisted of a 10–14 day course of oral antimicrobials (first choice ciprofloxacin 500 mg b.i.d.) [12]. In case of risk factors for quinolone resistance a single dose of a long-acting parental antimicrobial, e.g. ceftriaxone or an aminoglycoside, at the initiation of therapy was advised while culture results were pending [13].

Admitted patients started with empirical antimicrobials intravenously according to local policy and were switched to an oral antibiotic based on antimicrobial sensitivity testing of the uropathogen cultured.

Study procedures

Within 24–48 h of notification, qualified research nurses collected demographic and clinical data by reviewing the medical record completed with an interview by telephone or in person, using a standardized questionnaire. A midstream-catch urine culture and a set of blood cultures were taken before commencement of antimicrobial therapy. All patients were contacted in person 3–4 days and 28–32 days after enrollment, and contacted by phone at day 13–15 and day 84–92, to assess clinical outcome. Urine culture was repeated at the 28–32 day follow-up visit. In case of (re) admission during the study period, related data were obtained from the medical record and interview. In case a patient was lost to follow up, survival and readmission were assessed by inquiry with the patient's primary care physicians, hospital chart and/or local governmental mortality registries.

Urine and blood cultures were performed using standard microbiological methods at local certified laboratories. Data collection of patients included during the validation period was identical (see Additional file 1).

Endpoints

The primary endpoints were primary hospital admission rate (the percentage of patients who were directly admitted to hospital) and secondary hospital admission rate (the percentage of patients who needed to be hospitalized for FUTI after initial home-based treatment). Secondary outcome measures were 30- and 90-day all-cause mortality rate, ICU admission rate, the total number of hospitalization days over a 3-month follow-up and clinical- and microbiological cure rate through the 10- to 18-day post-treatment visit. Clinical cure was defined as being alive with absence of fever and resolution of UTI symptoms (either absence of symptoms or at least 2 points improvement on a 0 through 5 points severity score), without additional antimicrobial therapy for relapse of UTI [14]. Bacteriologic cure was defined as eradication of the study entry uropathogen with no recurrence of bacteriuria (pathogen growth $<10^4$ cfu/mL in women or $<10^3$ cfu/mL in men combined with disappearance of leucocyturia) [15].

A Data Safety Monitoring Board (DSMB) monitored the study and prescheduled interim analyses were performed according to predefined stopping rules. For the analysis of secondary hospital admission only low risk patients PRACTICE-score = < 100 points were considered.

Definitions

UTI in men, postmenopausal women and in women with any structural or functional abnormality of the urinary tract were considered 'complicated' whereas in all others it was considered 'uncomplicated' UTI [13, 15]. Comorbidity was defined as the presence of any urinary tract disorder, heart failure, cerebrovascular disease, renal insufficiency, diabetes mellitus, malignancy or chronic obstructive pulmonary disease.

Statistical analysis

The primary endpoints were analyzed on the intention-to-treat (ITT) and per-protocol (PP) population.

Evaluable patients for ITT analysis included all patients who met the inclusion criteria and had at least 1 follow up visit. The PP population consisted of cases in which PRACTICE-hospitalization recommendations were actually followed in the intervention period and all cases in the control period. Binomial or categorical outcome measures were analyzed using Chi-square tests (Pearson's or Fisher's). Risk difference with 95% confidence interval (CI) was used to compare the differences of categorical outcomes. Tests of significance were at 0.05 level, two-tailed, for primary hospital admission rate.

A study sample size of 326 patients in both arms was calculated on the basis of secondary hospital admission rate, which was estimated to be approximately 5%, based on our previous study on FUTI [16], to have a power of 90% to show that the secondary admission rate in the intervention period (PRACTICE-guided management) is at least as low as the control period. As we were only interested for non-inferiority and not in equivalence in secondary hospital admission rate, the sample size calculation was based on a one-tailed alpha of 0.025. This

implies that the 90% CI of a two-tailed Chi-square test should not cross the predefined risk difference of 2.5% higher secondary admission rates. All analyses were performed using SPSS 20.0 (SPPS Inc., USA).

Results
Study participants
A total of 370 patients was included, 237 in the control period and 133 in the intervention period (see the flowchart in Fig. 1). In the ITT-population, baseline demographic characteristics were similar in the two groups (Table 2), except for a difference in history of cerebrovascular and chronic renal disease. Patients in who PRACTICE recommendations were followed (the PP-analysis) were significantly older, had more comorbidity and more often suffered complicated UTI than control patients (Table 2).

Fifteen patients who were included in the study by ED-physicians did not completely meet the predefined inclusion criteria, but discharge diagnosis as concluded by the attending physician was FUTI in all

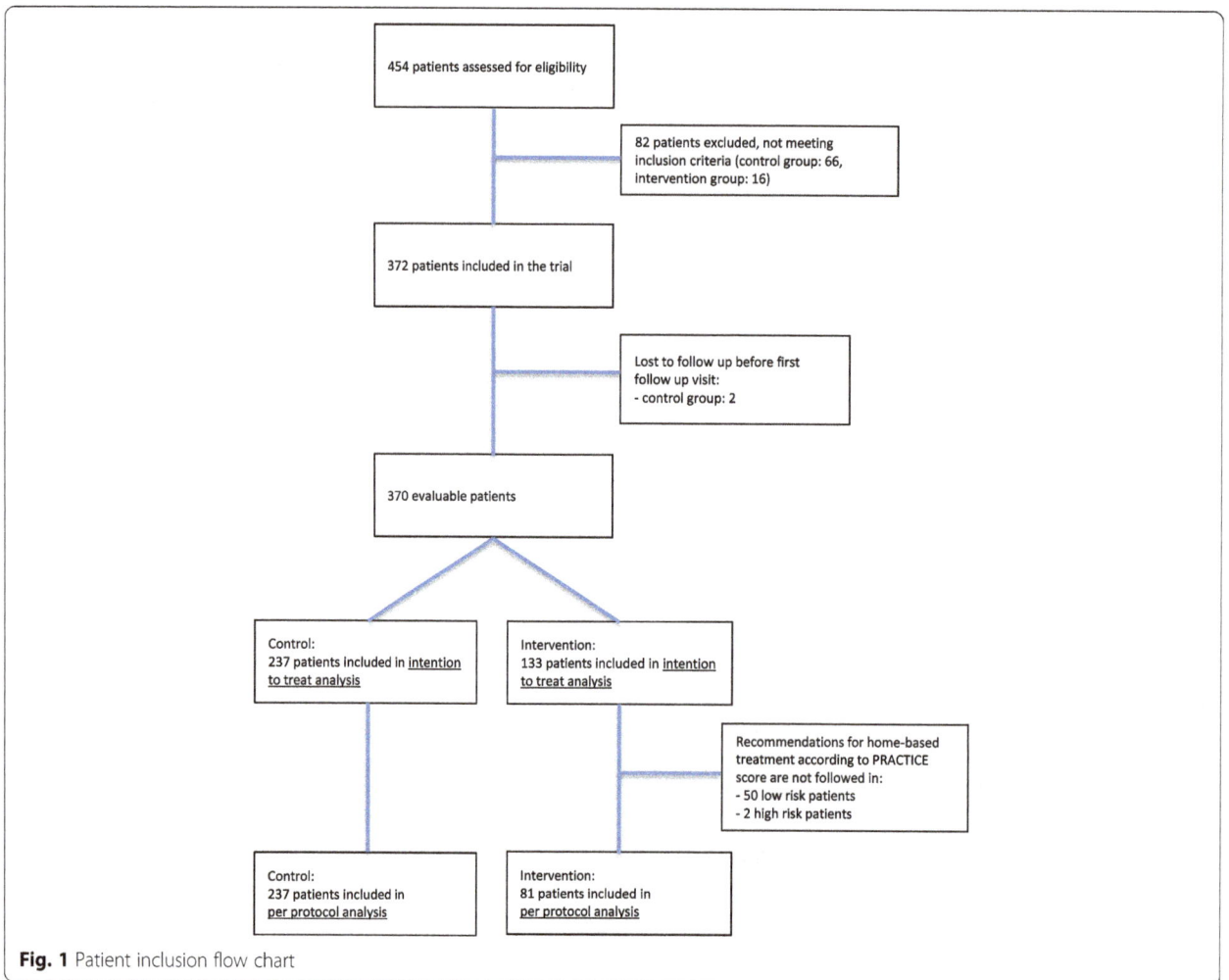

Fig. 1 Patient inclusion flow chart

Table 2 Patients' demographics

	Control group	Intervention group		p	
	ITT = PP	ITT	PP	Control vs ITT	Control vs PP
	n = 237	n = 133	n = 81		
Age in years; median, (IQR)	60 (30)	61 (34)	71 (26)	ns	<0,01
Sex – female	148 (62)	74 (56)	33 (41)	ns	<0,01
Febrile uncomplicated UTI	54 (23)	30 (23)	9 (11)	ns	0,02
Antimicrobial treatment at inclusion	90 (38)[a]	44 (33)	22 (27)	ns	ns
Urologic history					
Present urinary catheter	17 (7)	9 (7)	8 (10)	ns	ns
History of urinary tract disorder[a]	73 (31)	33 (25)	29 (36)	ns	ns
Recurrent UTI[b]	30 (13)[c]	11 (9)[c]	5 (7)	ns	ns
Comorbidity					
Any	124 (52)	77 (58)	57 (70)	ns	<0,01
Diabetes mellitus	36 (15)	29 (22)	25 (31)	ns	<0,01
Malignancy	13 (5)	11 (8)	10 (12)	ns	ns
Heart failure	32 (13)	12 (9)	11 (14)	ns	ns
Cerebrovascular disease	17 (7)	20 (15)	18 (22)	0.02	<0,01
Cirrhosis	1 (0)	2 (1)	1 (1)	ns	ns
Renal insufficiency	12 (5)	20 (15)	18 (22)	<0.01	<0,01
Immunocompromised	19 (8)	10 (8)	5 (6)	ns	ns

Data are presented as n (%) unless otherwise stated. ITT intention to treat analysis, PP per protocol analysis, IQR interquartile range, ns not significant (at 0,05 level), UTI urinary tract infection. [a]Urinary tract disorder: presence of any functional or anatomical abnormality of the urinary tract excluding the presence of a urinary catheter. [b]Recurrent UTI: two or more episodes in the last 6 months or three or more episodes of UTI in the last year. [c]UTI history was unknown in 13 subjects in control period and 6 subjects in intervention period

cases. On hospital presentation, ten of these patients had no specific symptoms of UTI, 8 of these 10 patients had cultures of blood (3) and/or urine (5) positive with significant growth of an uropathogen, 2 had negative urine cultures, and 1 of them used antibiotics at inclusion. The other 5 patients did not have or report fever at inclusion, 1 of them was on TNFα-inhibitors.

Follow up was not completed in 37 patients in the control group and in 13 patients in the intervention group. Based on review of medical charts and governmental records these patients were all alive and without secondary admission, and included as such in the analysis.

Cultures

The results of urine cultures, performed in 347 (93%) patients are shown in Table 3; 125 (36%) urine cultures were either sterile or contaminated of which 65% were obtained during antibiotic (pre)treatment. Blood cultures, performed in 357 (96%) patients, revealed bacteremia in 97 (27%) cases (Table 3). Rate of bacteremia was similar in intervention and control group.

Outcome

The mean PRACTICE scores in the control and intervention groups (ITT analysis) were 62 (95% CI: 57.7 to 65.4) and 64 (95% CI: 58.3 to 69.7), respectively. Mean PRACTICE score in the PP population was 76 (95% CI: 69.0 to 83.3; $p < 0,01$).

Use of the PRACTICE significantly reduced primary hospitalization rate, 96 (72%) patients in the intervention group were admitted in the hospital versus 219 (92%) in the control period ($p < 0.01$) (Table 4). The hospitalization rate was further reduced to 57% in the PP population.

The attending physician overruled the PRACTICE rule in 50 out of 153 patients categorized as low risk, who were admitted to the hospital because of 'sick appearance' ($n = 9$), severe flank pain ($n = 2$), antibiotic treatment at presentation ($n = 7$), comorbidity ($n = 5$), nausea ($n = 3$), uncertain diagnosis ($n = 4$), unknown ($n = 7$) or other reasons ($n = 13$). On the other hand, two patients categorized as high risk were treated at home because they insisted on home based treatment.

The median number of hospitalization days over a 3-month follow-up was 5 days (95% CI 5.6 to 7.0) vs 4 days (95% CI 4.4 to 6.7) for the control and intervention period, respectively.

Clinical and microbiological cure on day 30 did not differ significantly between both groups (Table 4).

The clinical outcomes according to risk class are outlined in Table 5.

Table 3 Bacteria isolated from baseline cultures

	Control period	Intervention period
	n = 237	n = 133
Urine cultures		
Escherichia coli	126 (56)	51 (42)
Klebsiella spp	12 (5)	7 (6)
Proteus spp	5 (2)	3 (2)
Enterococcus spp	3 (1)	-
Pseudomonas aeruginosa	-	1 (1)
Staphylococcus aureus	1 (0)	1 (1)
Other	7 (3)	6 (5)
Contaminated / mixed flora	26 (12)	24 (20)
Total positive urine cultures	154/225 (68)[a]	69/122 (57)[a]
Blood cultures		
Escherichia coli	56 (25)	21 (68)
Klebsiella spp	4 (6)	4 (13)
Proteus spp	-	1 (3)
Enterobacter spp	1 (1)	-
Pseudomonas aeruginosa	1 (1)	-
Staphylococcus aureus	1 (1)	2 (6)
Beta haemolytic streptococcus	1 (1)	2 (6)
Citrobacter spp	1 (1)	-
Bacteroides fragilis	1 (1)	-
Salmonella paratyphi	-	1 (3)
Total positive blood cultures	66/228 (29)[b]	31/129 (24)[b]

Data are presented as n (%). [a]Urine cultures were not performed in 12 patients in the control period and 11 patients in the intervention period. [b]Blood cultures were not obtained in 9 patients in the control period and 4 patients in the intervention period

Safety

In the control period, 18 patients were treated at home (1 high risk and 17 low risk patients), of which 1 low risk patient was admitted 5 days after start of home treatment because of flank pain shown to be due to renal vein thrombosis.

Of the 37 patients in the intervention group who received initial home-based treatment (29 low risk, 6 intermediate risk and 2 high risk patients), 10 patients (27%) had a secondary hospital admission. These 10 patients (7 females; median age 61, range 18–85 years) had a low or intermediate risk for adverse events according to the PRACTICE-score (6 low, 4 intermediate), and were treated with oral ciprofloxacin (n = 9) or amoxicillin-clavulanic-acid (n = 1). Four out of 10 patients consulted the ED for re-evaluation on their own initiative because of worsening of symptoms such as fever or nausea. Six patients (60%) were contacted by phone by the treating physician to return to the hospital because of positive results of blood cultures, which grew Escherichia coli (n = 2, both ciprofloxacin sensitive), Salmonella paratyphi

(n = 1), Staphylococcus aureus (n = 1) and Streptococcus Lancefield group A (n = 1) and G (n = 1). Median hospital stay was 2 days (range 1–14 days). In none of these secondary admissions intensive care treatment was required, and no complications were noted.

The first interim analysis, that took place after inclusion of 133 patients in the intervention group, showed an absolute risk difference in secondary hospital admission rate between intervention and control cohort of 23% (10/35 (29%) subjects in the intervention cohort, vs 1/17 (6%) in the control group). Because the difference in secondary admission rate exceeded the predefined stopping criterion of 20%, the DSMB advised to stop the trial.

Discussion

We assessed the clinical use of a prediction rule, the PRACTICE, that stratifies patients presenting with FUTI into three risk groups for short-term mortality or admission to the ICU, and is based on bed-side available patient characteristics. Our hypothesis that the use of this prediction rule would reduce hospitalization rate was confirmed in this study, as shown by a 20% absolute reduction. The impact of the PRACTICE on admission policy could have been bigger, because in 33% of low risk patients PRACTICE-recommendations were overruled by the attending physician, possibly because of unfamiliarity with the decision rule. Patients in the PP population were older, had more comorbidity and thus a higher PRACTICE score, reflecting the fact that physicians were more likely to follow PRACTICE guidance when admission was recommended. The secondary admission rate of 29% exceeded the predefined stopping criterion (of a 20% absolute increase over that in the control group), and the study was stopped accordingly.

This real world study underlines the importance of the validation of clinical prediction rules in a new cohort to ensure its predictive value and usefulness in clinical setting, but there are some limitations.

The PRACTICE was adapted from the Pneumonia Severity Index (PSI). Selecting candidate predictors for prognostic modelling is generally done by logistic regression analysis. In order to have sufficient power, as a rule of thumb, we need at least ten outcomes per candidate predictor [17]. Predicting 30-day mortality rate of FUTI, which was estimated to be 2–5%, and considering analysis of 20 candidate predictors this implies a sample size of at least 4000–10,000 patients to obtain sufficient power. Based on previous studies, we realized such a large prospective study would be infeasible. Since the PRACTICE score was validated in a prospectively collected broad population of 787 patients and its impact was subsequently analyzed in a randomized intervention trial, our study was conducted according to guidelines for development of clinical prediction rules [18, 19]. As the PRACTICE predicts the composite outcome of complicated

Table 4 Patients' outcomes

	Control period n = 237	Intervention period ITT n = 133	Intervention period PP n = 81
Hospitalization			
Primary hospitalization	219 (92)*	96 (72)*	46 (57)*
Low risk	136	50	0
Intermediate risk	58	29	29
High risk	25	17	17
Secondary admission (all risk classes)	2/18 (11)	10/37 (27)	10/35 (29)
Low risk	1/17	6/29	6/29
Intermediate risk	0/0	4/6	4/6
High risk	1/1	0/2	0/0
Need for ICU admission	8 (3)	1 (1)	1 (1)
Hospital admission >10 days	15 (6)	10 (8)	9 (11)
Total number of hospitalization days in 90 days of follow up [median, CI]	5 [5,6–7,0]	4 [4,4–6,7]	4 [4,2–7,6]
Bacteremia	66/228 (29)	31/129 (24)	21/77 (27)
Mortality			
30-day all-cause mortality	3 (1)	3 (2)	2 (2)
90-day all-cause mortality	7 (3)	5 (4)	4 (5)
Cure at day 30			
Clinical cure	182/209 (87)	98/121 (80)	59/73 (81)
Microbiological cure	170/190 (89)	107/113 (95)	61/65 (94)

Data are presented as n (%) unless otherwise stated. CI confidence interval, ITT intention to treat analysis, PP per protocol analysis, ICU intensive care unit. *$p = < 0.001$

course (30-day mortality, ICU-admission and prolonged hospitalisation), according to the rule of thumb (one predictor for 10 or more outcomes), the validation cohort has sufficient power for reliable statistical analyses [17].

The trial was stopped because of safety concerns, since secondary hospital admission reached our predefined stopping rule. We note that all secondary admitted patients were discharged after a short and uncomplicated hospital stay. Two readmissions because of *E coli* bacteremia might have been avoided, because ciprofloxacin has been shown to be equally effective orally as intravenously in bacteremic UTI [20]. Among secondary admissions were patients with primary bacteremia caused by salmonella, staphylococci and streptococci, in whom presenting aspecific symptoms, e.g. fever and back pain, were mistaken for pyelonephritis, and sent home. Apparently, these patients were 'misdiagnosed' at first consultation as having FUTI, and subsequently were treated for other diagnoses at secondary admission. We included these patients in our analysis because the attending physicians at the EDs enrolled the

Table 5 Clinical outcome of febrile urinary tract infection according to PRACTICE risk class; control and intervention groups combined

PRACTICE score (points)	Low risk Class I-II (<75)			Intermediate risk Class III (76–100)			High risk Class IV-V (>100)			Total
	Control	Intervention	All	Control	Intervention	All	Control	Intervention	All	
No. of patients	153	79	232	58	35	93	26	19	45	370
Clinical outcome										
30-day mortality, %	0	0	0	3 (5)	1 (3)	4 (4)	3 (11)	2 (10)	5 (11)	9 (2)
90-day mortality, %	0	0	0	3 (5)	3 (9)	6 (6)	4 (15)	2 (10)	6 (13)	12 (3)
ICU admission, %	3 (2)	0	3 (1)	2 (3)	0	2 (2)	3 (11)	1 (5)	4 (9)	9 (2)
Length of hospital stay										
Median no. of days [IQR]	4.0 [2]	3.0 [4]	4.0 [3]	6.0 [4]	4.0 [4]	5.0 [4]	6.5 [4]	6.0 [6]	6.0 [4]	5.0 [3]

Data are presented as n (%) unless otherwise stated, *IQR* interquartile range, *ICU* intensive care unit patients in the current trial on a presumptive diagnosis of FUTI and we believe that these diagnostic errors reflect every day patient care [21].

Acute pyelonephritis and urosepsis are common conditions seen in the ED, and it is of importance to be aware that other unusual diseases can mimic its general symptoms. Other studies support our observation that the accuracy of UTI diagnosis may be suboptimal in the ED [22, 23].

Apparently the diagnosis of FUTI is not as straightforward as the diagnosis of pneumonia, where the presence of an infiltrate on chest X-ray is both definitive and confirmative and clinical decision rules such as the PSI have been implemented successfully in daily practice [3]. The PSI was derived from a large cohort of >14,000 patients and validated in almost 40,000 patients, and studies prospectively addressing its use in clinical practice found secondary admission rates of 4–9% [24–27]. The fact that we found higher secondary admission rates in FUTI, might also be explained by a different pathway leading to failure of home treatment in these two infections. Whereas respiratory distress is probably the main cause of secondary hospitalization of pneumonia patients; unability to take oral medication and need for volume resuscitation is more important for FUTI patients. These factors might be underrepresented in the composite outcome of complicated course of FUTI as predicted by the PRACTICE.

Differences in validation and intervention trial cohorts in this study might have attributed to the difference in secondary admission rate. In the historical cohort patients were recruited not only in EDs, but (a minority) also in the practice of general practitioners. The main difference with the historical cohort is the higher percentage of complicated UTI (or in some cases, an alternative diagnosis made on basis of blood culture findings) in the current cohort, which cannot be explained by a difference in sex or age. Other demographic parameters and outcome such as ICU admissions and mortality were comparable in the historical and current cohort.

Our patient group reflects the daily practice of patients presenting with community acquired FUTI, as both men and women, and patients with comorbidity were included. A previous study on women with acute pyelonephritis identified factors associated with hospital admission using a risk stratification model [28]. Age > 65 years, chills, segmented neutrophils >90%, creatinine >1.5 mg/dL, CRP >10 mg/dL and albumin 3.3 g/dL were independent risk factors for patient admission. Since details on mortality or complications are not given, no conclusion can be made on the actual risk for poor outcome. Furthermore, this model was not validated in a prospective cohort. In contrast, our PSI derived predictor variables can be readily assessed at the bedside level on the basis of history and physical examination.

How can the prediction rule for admission policy be optimized? The cut-off value of 75 points had a negative predictive value for predicting 30-day mortality of 100% in the intervention cohort. Lowering the threshold for admission policy in the intervention phase would hypotheticly have led to a hospitalization rate of 77% (102/133), but would still have resulted in a secondary hospitalization rate of 19% (6/31). The effect of the acute host response might be underrepresented in the PRACTICE, because it is based on the 30-day mortality in the validation cohort. Prognosis of the patient presenting with severe febrile illness consist of two factors. Firstly, the severity of the acute host response to the infection and inflammatory cascade eventually leading to shock and multi organ failure is best reflected by the hyperacute mortality. Secondly, the patients general health condition, mainly defined by age and comorbidity, that determines the 30-day mortality in patients who survive the first days of illness. Addition of a plasma biomarker reflecting the severity of sepsis, such as procalcitonin or midregional pro-adrenomedullin [29], might improve the decision rule in identifying patients who benefit from hospital-based treatment in the acute phase and lower the secondary admission rate. Furthermore, improved diagnosis of UTI is necessary to ensure safe implementation of prediction tools regarding clinical decision making.

Conclusion

Implementation of the PRACTICE rule could decrease the number of hospital admissions of patients presenting to the ED with febrile urinary tract infection by 20%, at the expense of a high secondary admission rate.

Abbreviations
AUC: Area under the curve; CI: Confidence interval; DSMB: Data safety monitoring board; ED: Emergency department; FUTI: Febrile urinary tract infection; ICU: Intensive care unit; ITT: Intention-to-treat; PP: Per-protocol (PP); PRACTICE: Prediction Rule for Admission policy in Complicated urinary Tract InfeCtion Leiden; PSI: Pneumonia Severity Index; UTI: Urinary tract infection

Acknowledgements
We thank the patients, research nurses, emergency room physicians, nurses and laboratory staff for their cooperation. We are indebted to Tanny van der Reijden from the LUMC Department of Infectious Diseases for her assistance at the laboratory.

Funding
This study was supported by unrestricted grands by ZonMW, the Bronovo Research Foundation and the Franje1 Foundation. There was no role of the funding organizations in design and conduct of the study; collection, management, analysis, and interpretation of the data; and preparation, review, or approval of the manuscript; or decision to submit the manuscript for publication.

Authors' contributions

JS, WS, JW, CN and JD were involved in clinical design of the study. JS, WS, CN, ND, EL, TK, HA and JW were involved in execution of the study, including screening and enrollment of patients. ES provided interpretation on the modelling output. JS, AV, CN and JD wrote the first draft of this manuscript, with input from all other authors. All authors contributed to and approved the final manuscript.

Competing interests

The authors declare that they have no competing interests.

Data sharing

The relevant patient level data are available on reasonable request from the corresponding author. Consent for data sharing was not obtained but the presented data are anonymised and risk of identification is low.

Author details

[1]Department of Infectious Diseases, Leiden University Medical Center, C5-P, PO Box 96002300 RC Leiden, the Netherlands. [2]Department of Public Health, Erasmus MC - University Medical Center Rotterdam, Rotterdam, The Netherlands. [3]Dept of Internal Medicine, Alrijne Hospital, Leiderdorp, The Netherlands. [4]Dept of Internal Medicine, MCH-Bronovo, The Hague, The Netherlands. [5]Dept of Internal Medicine, Groene Hart Hospital, Gouda, The Netherlands. [6]Dept of Internal Medicine, Alrijne Hospital, Leiden, The Netherlands. [7]Dept of Internal Medicine, Haga Hospital, The Hague, The Netherlands.

References

1. van Dissel JT, Van LP, Westendorp RG, Kwappenberg K, Frolich M. Anti-inflammatory cytokine profile and mortality in febrile patients. Lancet. 1998; 351(9107):950–3.
2. Marco CA, Schoenfeld CN, Hansen KN, Hexter DA, Stearns DA, Kelen GD. Fever in geriatric emergency patients: clinical features associated with serious illness. Ann Emerg Med. 1995;26(1):18–24.
3. Fine MJ, Auble TE, Yealy DM, Hanusa BH, Weissfeld LA, Singer DE, et al. A prediction rule to identify low-risk patients with community-acquired pneumonia. N Engl J Med. 1997;336(4):243–50.
4. Lim WS, van der Eerden MM, Laing R, Boersma WG, Karalus N, Town GI, et al. Defining community acquired pneumonia severity on presentation to hospital: an international derivation and validation study. Thorax. 2003;58(5):377–82.
5. Charles PG, Wolfe R, Whitby M, Fine MJ, Fuller AJ, Stirling R, et al. SMART-COP: a tool for predicting the need for intensive respiratory or vasopressor support in community-acquired pneumonia. Clin Infect Dis. 2008;47(3):375–84.
6. Foxman B, Klemstine KL, Brown PD. Acute pyelonephritis in US hospitals in 1997: hospitalization and in-hospital mortality. Ann Epidemiol. 2003;13(2): 144–50.
7. Efstathiou SP, Pefanis AV, Tsioulos DI, Zacharos ID, Tsiakou AG, Mitromaras AG, et al. Acute pyelonephritis in adults: prediction of mortality and failure of treatment. Arch Intern Med. 2003;163(10):1206–12.
8. Buonaiuto VA, Marquez I, De TI, Joya C, Ruiz-Mesa JD, Seara R, et al. Clinical and epidemiological features and prognosis of complicated pyelonephritis: a prospective observational single hospital-based study. BMC Infect Dis. 2014;14:639.
9. Ramakrishnan K, Scheid DC. Diagnosis and management of acute pyelonephritis in adults. Am Fam Physician. 2005;71(5):933–42.
10. Rhee JE, Kim K, Lee CC, Kang J, Lee JW, Shin JH, et al. The lack of association between age and diabetes and hospitalization in women with acute pyelonephritis. J Emerg Med. 2011;41(1):29–34.
11. Brown C, Hofer T, Johal A, Thomson R, Nicholl J, Franklin BD, et al. An epistemology of patient safety research: a framework for study design and interpretation. Part 2. Study design. Qual Saf Health Care. 2008;17(3):163–9.
12. van Asselt KM, Prins JM, van der Weele GM, Knottnerus BJ, Van PB GSE. Unambiguous practice guidelines on urinary tract infections in primary and secondary care. Ned Tijdschr Geneeskd. 2013;157(36):A6608.
13. Gupta K, Hooton TM, Naber KG, Wullt B, Colgan R, Miller LG, et al. International clinical practice guidelines for the treatment of acute uncomplicated cystitis and pyelonephritis in women: a 2010 update by the Infectious Diseases Society of America and the European Society for Microbiology and Infectious Diseases. Clin Infect Dis. 2011;52(5): e103–20.
14. van Nieuwkoop C, van't Wout JW, Assendelft WJ, Elzevier HW, Leyten EM, Koster T, et al. Treatment duration of febrile urinary tract infection (FUTIRST trial): a randomized placebo-controlled multicenter trial comparing short (7 days) antibiotic treatment with conventional treatment (14 days). BMC Infect Dis. 2009;9:131.
15. Rubin RH, Shapiro ED, Andriole VT, Davis RJ, Stamm WE. Evaluation of new anti-infective drugs for the treatment of urinary tract infection. Infectious Diseases Society of America and the Food and Drug Administration. Clin Infect Dis. 1992;15(Suppl 1):S216–27.
16. van Nieuwkoop C, van't Wout JW, Spelt IC, Becker M, Kuijper EJ, Blom JW, et al. Prospective cohort study of acute pyelonephritis in adults: safety of triage towards home based oral antimicrobial treatment. J Inf Secur. 2010; 60(2):114–21.
17. Steyerberg EW, Eijkemans MJ, Harrell FE Jr, Habbema JD. Prognostic modeling with logistic regression analysis: in search of a sensible strategy in small data sets. Med Decis Mak. 2001;21(1):45–56.
18. McGinn TG, Guyatt GH, Wyer PC, Naylor CD, Stiell IG, Richardson WS. Users' guides to the medical literature: XXII: how to use articles about clinical decision rules. Evidence-based medicine working group. JAMA. 2000;284(1):79–84.
19. Steyerberg EW, Moons KG, van der Windt DA, Hayden JA, Perel P, Schroter S, et al. Prognosis research strategy (PROGRESS) 3: prognostic model research. PLoS Med. 2013;10(2):e1001381.
20. Mombelli G, Pezzoli R, Pinoja-Lutz G, Monotti R, Marone C, Franciolli M. Oral vs intravenous ciprofloxacin in the initial empirical management of severe pyelonephritis or complicated urinary tract infections: a prospective randomized clinical trial. Arch Intern Med. 1999;159(1):53–8.
21. Graber ML. The incidence of diagnostic error in medicine. BMJ Qual Saf. 2013;22(Suppl 2):ii21–7.
22. Caterino JM, Ting SA, Sisbarro SG, Espinola JA, Camargo CA Jr. Age, nursing home residence, and presentation of urinary tract infection in U.S. emergency departments, 2001-2008. Acad Emerg Med. 2012;19(10):1173–80.
23. Gordon LB, Waxman MJ, Ragsdale L, Mermel LA. Overtreatment of presumed urinary tract infection in older women presenting to the emergency department. J Am Geriatr Soc. 2013;61(5):788–92.
24. Marrie TJ, Lau CY, Wheeler SL, Wong CJ, Vandervoort MK, Feagan BG. A controlled trial of a critical pathway for treatment of community-acquired pneumonia. CAPITAL study investigators. Community-acquired pneumonia intervention trial assessing Levofloxacin. JAMA. 2000;283(6):749–55.
25. Atlas SJ, Benzer TI, Borowsky LH, Chang Y, Burnham DC, Metlay JP, et al. Safely increasing the proportion of patients with community-acquired pneumonia treated as outpatients: an interventional trial. Arch Intern Med. 1998;158(12):1350–6.
26. Renaud B, Coma E, Labarere J, Hayon J, Roy PM, Boureaux H, et al. Routine use of the pneumonia severity index for guiding the site-of-treatment decision of patients with pneumonia in the emergency department: a multicenter, prospective, observational, controlled cohort study. Clin Infect Dis. 2007;44(1):41–9.
27. Jo S, Kim K, Jung K, Rhee JE, Cho IS, Lee CC, et al. The effects of incorporating a pneumonia severity index into the admission protocol for community-acquired pneumonia. J Emerg Med. 2012;42(2):133–8.
28. Kang C, Kim K, Lee SH, Park C, Kim J, Lee JH, et al. A risk stratification model of acute pyelonephritis to indicate hospital admission from the ED. Am J Emerg Med. 2013;31(7):1067–72.
29. van der Starre WE, Zunder SM, Vollaard AM, Van NC SJE, Delfos NM, et al. Prognostic value of pro-adrenomedullin, procalcitonin and C-reactive protein in predicting outcome of febrile urinary tract infection. Clin Microbiol Infect. 2014;20(10):1048–54.

Carbapenem susceptibilities of Gram-negative pathogens in intra-abdominal and urinary tract infections: updated report of SMART 2015 in China

Hui Zhang[1], Haishen Kong[2], Yunsong Yu[3], Anhua Wu[4], Qiong Duan[5], Xiaofeng Jiang[6], Shufang Zhang[7], Ziyong Sun[8], Yuxing Ni[9], Weiping Wang[10], Yong Wang[11], Kang Liao[12], Huayin Li[13], Chunxia Yang[14], Wenxiang Huang[15], Bingdong Gui[16], Bin Shan[17], Robert Badal[18], Qiwen Yang[1*] and Yingchun Xu[1*]

Abstract

Background: To evaluate the susceptibility rates of aerobic and facultative Gram-negative bacterial isolates from Chinese intra-abdominal infections (IAI) and urinary tract infections (UTI) focusing on carbapenems and comparing their effectiveness between 2014 and 2015.

Methods: A total of 2318 strains in 2015 (1483 from IAI and 835 from UTI) and 2374 strains in 2014 (1438 from IAI and 936 from UTI) were included in the analysis. Antimicrobial susceptibilities were determined at a central laboratory using CLSI broth microdilution and interpretive standards. Hospital acquired (HA) IAI and UTI were defined as isolates sampled > 48 h and community acquired (CA) as isolates sampled < 48 h after admission.

Results: The main species derived from IAI and UTI in 2015 were *Escherichia coli* (50.86%) and *Klebsiella pneumoniae* (19.20%). Susceptibilities of *Escherichia coli* IAI and UTI strains to imipenem (IPM) and ertapenem (ETP) were > 90% in 2014 and 2015, while the susceptibilities to IPM and ETP of *Klebsiella pneumoniae* IAI strains were > 80% in 2014 but dropped to ≤80% in 2015 for UTI strains. Susceptibilities of IAI *Enterobacteriaceae* strains to IPM and ETP in 2015 were lowest in the colon and abscesses, and *Enterobacteriaceae* susceptibilities of UTI and IAI isolates to IPM and ETP were lowest in medical, pediatric and surgery intensive care units (ICUs) in 2015.

Conclusions: IPM and ETP were effective in vitro against *Enterobacteriaceae* isolated from IAIs and UTIs in 2014 and 2015, but susceptibility to carbapenems in UTIs markedly decreased in 2015.

Keywords: *Enterobacteriaceae*, Carbapenem; ertapenem, Imipenem, Intra-abdominal infection, Urinary tract infection

Background

The Study for Monitoring Antimicrobial Resistance Trends (SMART)-CHINA is a surveillance program which monitors annually in vitro activities of antimicrobial agents against pathogens that cause intra-abdominal infections (IAI) and urinary tract infections (UTI). In a previous Chinese study it was reported that the incidence of Extended-Spectrum β-Lactamases (ESBL)-producing *Escherichia coli* (*E. coli*) strains derived from IAI had significantly increased between 2002 and 2011, while the percentages of ESBL-producing *Klebsiella pneumoniae* (*K. pneumoniae*) strains isolated from IAI remained relatively constant between 30.1 and 39.3%, but these two species were the major pathogens during the entire period [1]. However, Asia has been reported to have the world's highest incidence of ESBL-producing *E. coli*, *K. pneumoniae*, *Klebsiella oxytoca* and *Proteus mirabilis* strains from IAIs and UTIs in 2011, reaching 40% to 45% [2], and a number of recent publications have noted that cephalosporins and fluoroquinolones were not suitable antibiotics for the empirical treatment of IAI and UTI in China [3, 4],

* Correspondence: yangqiwen81@163.com; xycpumch@139.com
[1]Division of Microbiology, Peking Union Medical College Hospital, Peking Union Medical College, Chinese Academy of Medical Sciences, No. 1 Shuaifuyuan, Wangfujing Street, Beijing 100730, China
Full list of author information is available at the end of the article

underlining the importance of monitoring susceptibilities to alternative antibiotics such as the carbapenems. Epidemiological and individual hospital drug susceptibilities are commonly used as a guide for selecting suitable antibiotics for empirical treatments. However, susceptibility analyses have been extended to weighted-incidence syndromic combination antibiograms (WISCA), which reflects the likelihood that regimens treat all relevant organisms in a patient with a given syndrome [5].

In the present study we developed organ-specific weighted incidence antibiograms (OSWIAs) to estimate the likelihood of an isolate from a specific organ being susceptible to a given antibiotic. IAI and UTI derived isolates and their susceptibilities to carbapenems, cephalosporins, fluoroquinolones, broad-spectrum penicillins combined with β-lactamase inhibitors, and an aminoglycoside were compared in different infected organs. In addition, the distribution of *Enterobacteriaceae* and non-*Enterobacteriaceae* infections isolated from HA and CA IAIs and UTIs in different age subgroups as well as the susceptibility patterns of major pathogens in different medical departments were also analyzed.

Methods

Isolates from IAI and UTI infections

The Human Research Ethics Committee of Peking Union Medical College Hospital approved this study and waived the need for consent (Ethics Approval Number: S-K238). A total of 2318 aerobic and facultative Gram-negative bacterial strains (1483 from IAI and 835 from UTI) in 2015 and 2374 strains in 2014 (1438 from IAI and 936 from UTI) collected from 21 hospitals in 16 Chinese cities were retrospectively analyzed. The majority of the intra-abdominal specimens were obtained during surgery, with some paracentesis specimens. The UTI isolates were obtained from clean catch midstream urine, the urinary bladder, kidney and the prostate gland. All duplicate isolates (the same genus and species from the same patient) were excluded. Bacteria were identified by standard methods used in the participating clinical microbiology laboratories. Isolates were considered to be community-associated (CA) if they were recovered from a specimen taken < 48 h after the patient was admitted to a hospital, or HA if the specimen was taken ≥48 h after admission, as previously described [6].

Antimicrobial susceptibility test methods

Minimum inhibitory concentrations (MIC) were determined by broth microdilution according to the Clinical and Laboratory Standards Institute (CLSI) [7] using panels purchased from ThermoFisher Scientific (Cleveland, OH, USA). Relative susceptibility interpretations were based on CLSI clinical breakpoints [8].

Twelve antimicrobial agents commonly used to treat IAI and UTI were tested: ampicillin-sulbactam (SAM), piperacillin-tazobactam (TZP), ceftriaxone (CRO), cefotaxime (CTX), ceftazidime (CAZ), cefoxitin (FOX), cefepime (FEP), ciprofloxacin (CIP), levofloxacin (LVX), amikacin (AMK), imipenem (IPM) and ertapenem (ETP). Reference strains *E. coli* ATCC (American Type Culture Collection) 25,922, *Pseudomonas aeruginosa* ATCC 27853, and *K. pneumoniae* ATCC 700603 (positive ESBL control), were used as quality control (QC) strains for each batch of MIC tests. Results were only included in the analysis when corresponding quality control isolate test results were in accordance with CLSI guidelines and therefore within an acceptable range.

Organ-specific weighted incidence antibiogram (OSWIA) calculation

In order to calculate bacterial sensitivities in various organs of the abdominal cavity OSWIAs were calculated using the following equation:

Weighted susceptibility of a certain antimicrobial drug in a certain organ = antimicrobial susceptibility of A × the constituent ratio of A in the organ + antimicrobial susceptibility of B × the constituent ratio of B in the organ + antimicrobial susceptibility of C × the constituent ratio of C in the organ +... (where A, B and C represent the pathogenic bacteria in a certain organ).

For example when we calculated the OSWIA susceptibility of gall bladder isolates to ETP in 2015, first we extracted specific bacterial infection rates and then multiplied them by the specific bacterial susceptibilities to ETP in 2015. Isolates in 2015 from gall bladder were 241 *Escherichia coli* (50.1%), 87 *Klebsiella pneumoniae* (18.1%), 36 *Enterobacter cloacae* (7.5%)......until 1 *Serratia odorifera* (0.21%). The corresponding susceptibilities to ETP were 87.55% (*Escherichia coli*), 86.21% (*Klebsiella pneumoniae*), 66.67% (*Enterobacter cloacae*)......and 100% (*Serratia odorifera*). According to the above mentioned equation, the susceptibility of gall bladder to ETP was calculated as 50.1% × 87.55% + 18.1% × 86.21% + 7.5% × 66.67%......0.21% × 100% = 85.79%.

Statistical analysis

The susceptibility of all Gram-negative isolates combined was calculated using breakpoints appropriate for each species and assuming 0% susceptible for species with no breakpoints for any given drug. The 95% confidence intervals (CIs) were calculated using the adjusted Wald method; linear trends of ESBL rates in different years were assessed for statistical significance using the Cochran-Armitage test and comparison of ESBL rates were assessed using a chi-squared test. *P*-values < 0.05 were considered to be statistically significant.

Results

Distribution of Enterobacteriaceae isolates acquired from different organ groups of IAI and UTI in 2015

Enterobacteriaceae strains of IAIs were mainly derived from gall bladder (33%), peritoneal fluid (28%), abscesses (14%) liver (7%), appendix (6%) and other organs (1–3%). Comparing *Enterobacteriaceae* strains acquired from HA (76.3%) and CA (23.6%) IAI, the percentages for peritoneal fluid, abscesses and liver-derived isolates were similar, but in HA-derived IAIs, gall bladder isolates were collected more often (35% vs 26%), whereas appendix isolates were less frequently sampled (2% vs 20%) compared to CA isolates (Fig. 1). Similar distributions were found in 2014 (Additional file 1: Figure S1). From UTI pathogens, 99.4% of the strains were acquired from urine, with only 3 strains from the kidneys, and 1 strain each from the bladder and prostate gland. The distribution of HA and CA UTI isolates was 599 (71.9%) and 234 (28.1%) in 2015, and 58.1% and 40.9% in 2014, respectively.

Distribution of all isolates acquired from HA and CA IAI and UTI in 2015

There were 2318 strains collected in 2015, including 1483 strains from IAIs and 835 strains from UTIs. The majority of infections were caused by *E. coli* and *K. pneumoniae*, accounting for 50.86% and 19.20% in 2015 (Table 1) as well as 46.3% and 17.3% in 2014 (Additional file 2: Table S1).

The distribution analysis of strains acquired from IAIs and UTIs in HA and CA in different age groups revealed that *E. coli* was the major IAI pathogen in CA IAI in the 0–39 year age range (CA: 31.76%; HA: 9.01%) and in HA IAI in the 60–79 years age range (CA: 32.35%; HA: 47.38%), as well as in the HA UTI of > 80 year-old patients (CA: 5.56%; HA: 18.53%) (Fig. 2), which was similar in 2014 (Additional file 3: Figure S2).

Comparison of susceptibilities to 12 common antibiotics for *E. coli* and *K. pneumoniae* isolates (IAI and UTI) in 2014 and 2015

E. coli in IAI were highly susceptible to IPM, AMK and ETP (> 90%) in 2014, but the susceptibility to ETP showed a small decrease in 2015 (Fig. 3a) compared to 2014. *K. pneumoniae* from IAI was also highly sensitive to AMK, IPM and ETP (> 80%) in 2014–2015, but the susceptibility to these three antibiotics in 2015 was generally lower than in 2014 (Fig. 3c). More than 90% *E. coli* isolates from UTI were susceptible to IPM, AMK, ETP and TZP. In contrast, compared to 2014 susceptibilities of *K. pneumoniae* strains from UTIs decreased by 10% to AMK, IPM and ETP in 2015, which was a general trend also for all the other antibiotics tested (Fig. 3d). Susceptibilities to all other antibiotics were between 20 and 70% for *E. coli* and 30–75% for *K. pneumoniae* (Fig. 3). Corresponding MIC_{90} values of 12 antibiotics for *E. coli* and *K. pneumoniae* IAI and UTI isolates are presented in the Additional file 4: Table S2.

Comparison of the Enterobacteriaceae susceptibilities to carbapenem antibiotics (ETP and IPM) based on the OSWIA in different organs of IAI patients as well as isolates derived from IAI and UTI patients in different departments between 2014 and 2015

In general, besides abscesses and colon infections in 2015 as well as small intestine infections in 2014 to ETP, most included *Enterobacteriaceae* IAI isolates showed OSWIA susceptibilities to carbapenems of > 80% in 2014 and 2015 (Fig. 4a, Fig. 4b).

In 2015, carbapenem susceptibility rates of *Enterobacteriaceae* isolated from IAIs and UTIs decreased below 80% in medical and surgery ICUs to ETP as well as in general pediatric departments and surgery ICUs in 2015 to IPM. The greatest decline in susceptibility to IPM and ETP was seen between 2014 and 2015 in pediatric ICUs (Fig. 4c, Fig. 4d). In general there was a trend of susceptibility reductions to ETP and IPM in HA, and susceptibility increases to ETP and IPM in CA-derived *Enterobacteriaceae* caused IAIs between 2014 and 2015 (Fig. 4e, Fig. 4f).

Detailed information of MIC_{90} values from *E. coli* and *K. pneumoniae* for ETP and IMP in different organs, departments and HA vs CA infections in 2014 and 2015 are shown in Table 2 and indicate dramatically increased MIC_{90} values of IPM for *E. coli* isolates only in medicine ICUs in 2015, while the MIC_{90} values

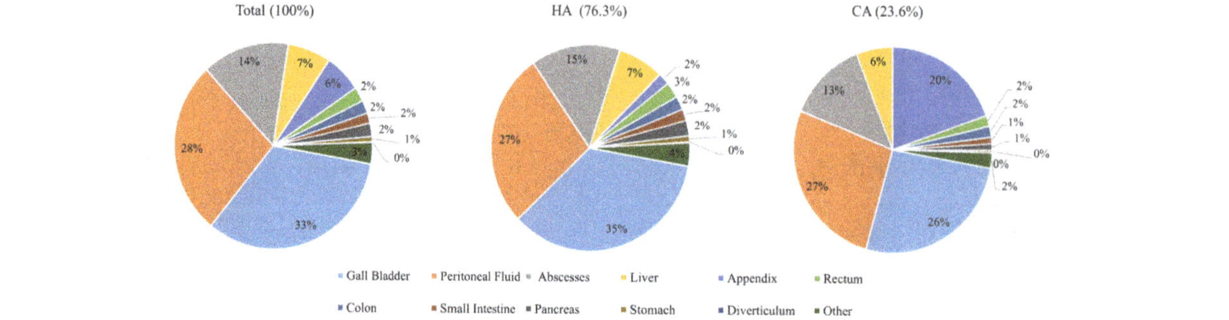

Fig. 1 Distribution of isolates acquired from IAI pathogens in different organ groups in 2015

Table 1 Distribution of the IAI and UTI pathogens in China in 2015

	IAI			UTI			UTI + IAI		
	HA	CA	Total	HA	CA	Total	HA	CA	Total
Enterobacteriaceae	**928 (79.7)**	**287 (90.3)**	**1216 (82.0)**[a]	**523 (87.3)**	**217 (92.7)**	**742 (88.9)**[a]	**1451 (82.3)**	**504 (91.3)**	**1958 (84.5)**[a]
Escherichia coli	477 (41.0)	170 (53.5)	648 (43.7)[a]	367 (61.3)	162 (69.2)	531 (63.6)[a]	844 (47.9)	332 (60.1)	1179 (50.9)[a]
Klebsiella pneumoniae	262 (22.5)	69 (21.7)	331 (22.3)	90 (15.0)	24 (10.3)	114 (13.7)	352 (20.0)	93 (16.9)	445 (19.2)
Enterobacter cloacae	83 (7.1)	17 (5.4)	100 (6.7)	12 (2.0)	4 (1.7)	16 (1.9)	95 (5.4)	21 (3.8)	116 (5.0)
Proteus mirabilis	21 (1.8)	8 (2.5)	29 (2.0)	15 (2.5)	11 (4.7)	26 (3.1)	36 (2.0)	19 (3.4)	55 (2.4)
Citrobacter freundii	16 (1.4)	3 (0.9)	19 (1.3)	12 (2.0)	6 (2.6)	18 (2.2)	28 (1.6)	9 (1.6)	37 (1.6)
Enterobacter aerogenes	24 (2.1)	3 (0.9)	27 (1.8)	8 (1.3)	1 (0.4)	9 (1.1)	32 (1.8)	4 (0.7)	36 (1.6)
Non-*Enterobacteriaceae*	**236 (20.3)**	**31 (9.8)**	**267 (18.0)**	**76 (12.7)**	**17 (7.3)**	**93 (11.2)**	**312 (17.7)**	**48 (8.7)**	**360 (15.5)**
Pseudomonas aeruginosa	104 (8.9)	14 (4.4)	118 (8.0)	44 (7.4)	9 (3.9)	53 (6.4)	148 (8.4)	23 (4.2)	171 (7.4)
Acinetobacter baumannii	103 (8.9)	12 (3.8)	115 (7.8)	20 (3.3)	5 (2.1)	25 (3.0)	123 (7.0)	17 (3.1)	140 (6.0)
Stenotrophomonas maltophilia	16 (1.4)	3 (0.9)	19 (1.3)	4 (0.7)	1 (0.4)	5 (0.6)	20 (1.1)	4 (0.7)	24 (1.0)
Other	58 (5.0)	19 (6.0)	77 (5.2)	27 (4.5)	11 (4.7)	38 (4.6)	85 (4.8)	30 (5.4)	115 (5.0)
All	**1164 (100)**	**318 (100)**	**1483 (100)**	**599 (100)**	**234 (100)**	**835 (100)**	**1763 (100)**	**552 (100)**	**2318 (100)**

[a]32 isolates lacked partial demographic information and could not be identified as CA or HA

for IPM of *K. pneumoniae* IAI isolates from abscesses, colon, peritoneal fluid and others were all > 32 in 2015, pointing out increasing IPM resistance of *K. pneumoniae* infections in 2015. In addition, the MIC_{90} values of IPM for *K. pneumoniae* isolates derived from general surgery departments as well as from ICUs of medicine, pediatric and surgery became > 32 and also reflected in essentially increased HA MIC_{90} values (Table 2), which showed that clinical relevant resistance of IAI derived *K. pneumoniae* isolates to IPM appeared in hospitals in 2015.

Discussion

Enterobacteriaceae were the major pathogens in IAI and UTI, with *E. coli* and *K. pneumoniae* being the most commonly isolated strains, which is in accordance with recent studies in China and abroad [3, 9] [10]. *E. coli* isolated from both UTI and IAI were < 40% susceptible to the tested fluoroquinolones that reflects an overuse of fluoroquinolones in China, which has also been reported for Europe and the US [11, 12]. In addition, in 2015 *E. coli* isolates were < 70% susceptible to all cephalosporins tested including cefoxitin whether they were obtained

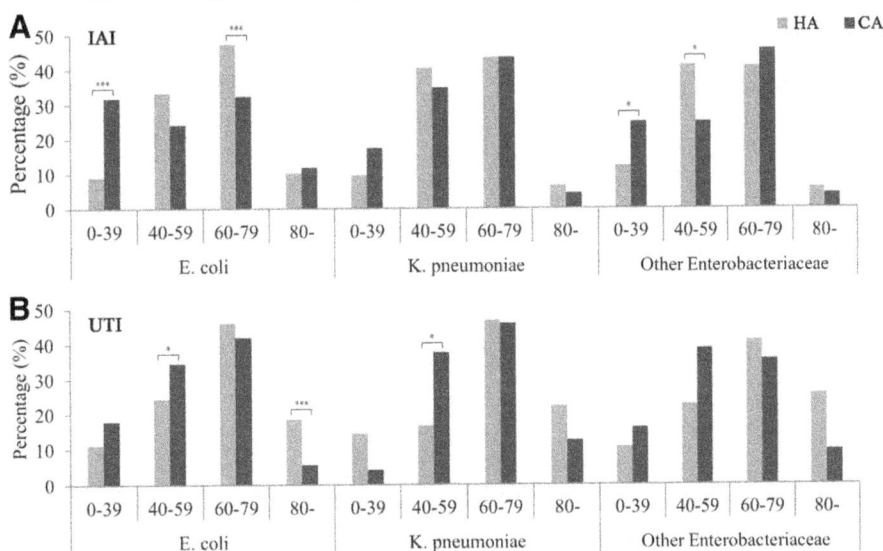

Fig. 2 Distribution of *E. coli*, *K. pneumoniae* and other *Enterobacteriaceae* strains derived from HA and CA **a**) IAIs and **b**) UTIs in different age groups in 2015. * $P < 0.05$, *** $P < 0.001$

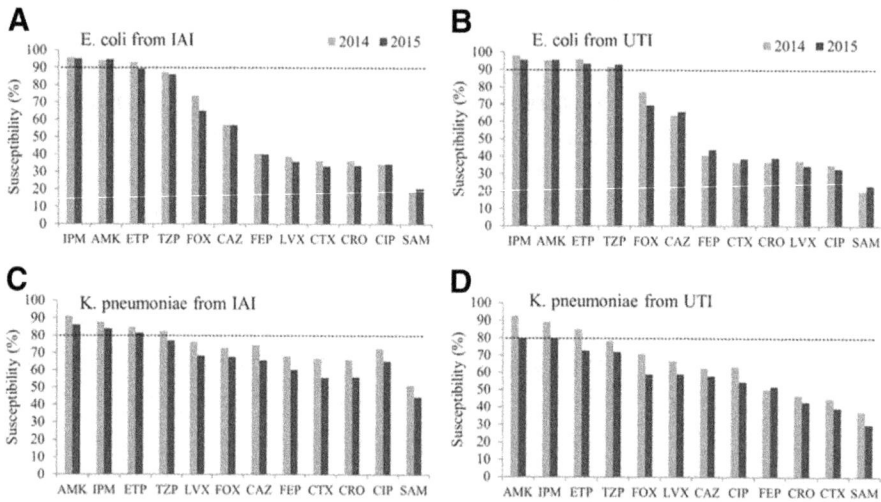

Fig. 3 Comparison of *E. coli* and *K. pneumonia* isolate susceptibilities (IAI and UTI) to 12 common antibiotics between 2014 and 2015. **a** *E. coli* isolated from IAI. **b** *E. coli* isolated from UTI patients. **c** *K. pneumoniae* isolated from IAI patients. **d** *K. pneumoniae* isolated from UTI patients. Dotted lines show the indicated percentages throughout the columns for comparison

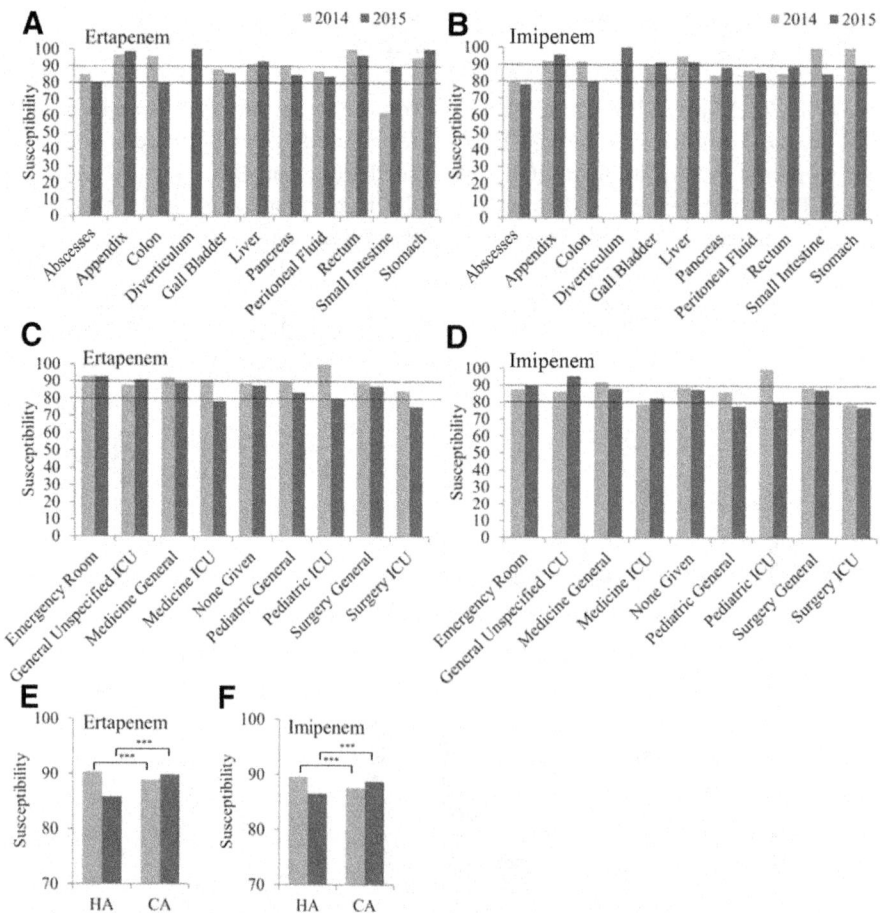

Fig. 4 Susceptibility based on OSWIA in IAI isolates. **a** OSWIA susceptibility of *Enterobacteriaceae* IAI to ETP. **b** OSWIA susceptibility of *Enterobacteriaceae* IAI to IPM. **c** Susceptibilities of *Enterobacteriaceae* UTI and IAI strains to ETP. **d** to IPM. **e** *Enterobacteriaceae* susceptibilities of HA and CA IAI and UTI to ETP. **f** *Enterobacteriaceae* susceptibilities of HA and CA IAI and UTI to IPM. *** $P < 0.001$

Table 2 MIC$_{90}$ values of ETP and IMP for *E. coli* and *K. pneumoniae* in 2014 and 2015

		ETP		IPM	
		2014	2015	2014	2015
E. coli	Abscesses	0.5	2	0.5	1
	Appendix	0.12	0.25	0.25	1
	Colon	0.5	0.25	0.25	≤ 0.5
	Gall Bladder	0.5	1	0.25	1
	Liver	2	0.5	0.5	≤ 0.5
	Pancreas	1	0.5	0.12	≤ 0.5
	Peritoneal Fluid	0.5	0.5	0.5	1
	Rectum	0.25	0.5	2	1
	Small Intestine	1	0.5	0.25	≤ 0.5
	Stomach	≤ 0.03	0.06	0.25	≤ 0.5
	Other	0.5	> 4	0.5	> 32
	Emergency Room	0.12	0.5	0.25	1
	General Unspecified ICU	0.5	1	1	1
	Medicine General	0.5	1	0.25	1
	Medicine ICU	≤ 0.03	4	0.25	> 32
	None Given	0.06	1	0.12	≤ 0.5
	Pediatric General	0.12	≤ 0.03	1	1
	Pediatric ICU	≤ 0.03	≤ 0.03	0.12	1
	Surgery General	0.5	0.5	0.5	1
	Surgery ICU	0.25	2	0.25	1
	HA	0.5	1	0.5	1
	CA	0.5	0.5	0.5	1
K. pneumoniae	Abscesses	> 4	> 4	> 8	> 32
	Appendix	1	0.06	0.5	1
	Colon	≤ 0.03	> 4	0.25	> 32
	Diverticulum		≤ 0.03		≤ 0.5
	Gall Bladder	2	> 4	2	8
	Liver	0.06	≤ 0.03	0.5	1
	Pancreas	0.25	0.25	8	1
	Peritoneal Fluid	> 4	> 4	> 8	> 32
	Rectum	0.12	0.12	0.12	2
	Small Intestine	4		0.12	≤ 0.5
	Stomach	0.25		0.5	1
	Other	> 4	> 4	> 8	> 32
	Emergency Room	1	0.5	2	2
	General Unspecified ICU	> 4	0.25	> 8	1
	Medicine General	0.5	4	1	2
	Medicine ICU	> 4	> 4	> 8	> 32
	None Given	≤ 0.03	0.06	0.12	≤ 0.5
	Pediatric General	≤ 0.03	≤ 0.03	0.25	≤ 0.5
	Pediatric ICU		> 4		> 32
	Surgery General	> 4	> 4	8	32

Table 2 MIC$_{90}$ values of ETP and IMP for *E. coli* and *K. pneumoniae* in 2014 and 2015 *(Continued)*

		ETP		IPM	
		2014	2015	2014	2015
	Surgery ICU	> 4	> 4	> 8	> 32
	HA	1	> 4	1	> 32
	CA	> 4	4	> 8	2

from IAI or UTI, suggesting a high prevalence of ESBL production, which is an extension of the trend shown previously between 2002 and 2011 [1]. A similar but less dramatic pattern has been observed for *K. pneumoniae*, but in contrast to *E. coli*, *K. pneumoniae* showed a decreasing susceptibility to all tested antibiotics from 2014 to 2015 (Fig. 3). Though ESBL-producing *E. coli* and *K. pneumoniae* strains should be susceptible to cefoxitin, both species, whether found in IAI or UTI, were < 80% susceptible to cefoxitin, which suggests that besides ESBL production other resistance mechanisms may be on the rise [13]. In particular *K. pneumoniae* showed a decreasing susceptibility to carbapenems, which was more pronounced in UTI isolates and indicated that carbapenemases or other mechanisms of carbapenem resistance have developed in *K. pneumoniae* strains, which has also been previously noted since carbapenem resistant *K. pneumoniae* strains isolated in Shanghai between July 2014 and May 2015 harbored all or at least one of the ESBL genes plus mainly New Delhi metallo-β-lactamase-1 (NDM-1) and IMP-4 or *Klebsiella pneumoniae* carbapenemase (KPC)-2 [14].

However, data from 2015 showed *K. pneumoniae* IAI isolate susceptibilities between 80 and 90% to IPM and ETP in our study, which was much higher than the 43.24% susceptibility to IPM reported for *K. pneumoniae* IAI isolates from a Chinese tertiary-care hospital between 2012 and 2015 [15], but was in a similar range to Chinese isolates from abdominal trauma-associated IAI collected between 2010 to 2015, with susceptibilities of *K. pneumoniae* strains to IPM and ETP of 87.5–90.6% [16].

The distribution of *Enterobacteriaceae* IAI isolates were similar in peritoneal fluid, abscesses and the colon for HA and CA infections, but HA IAIs manifested more in the gall bladder whereas CA infections occurred to a greater extent in appendicitis IAIs in 2015 (Fig. 1), which is a fair finding since acute appendicitis is a common reason for hospital admissions worldwide [17]. In particular, colon IAI-derived strains showed an increased resistance to carbapenems, decreasing to 80% susceptibility to ertapenem and imipenem in 2015. Similarly, IAI strain susceptibilities from abscesses were about 80% to carbapenems in 2015, but the decrease compared to 2014 was less pronounced (Fig. 3). Apart from general pediatric departments, in 2015 lowered susceptibilities particularly to IPM were most obvious in ICUs, which is in agreement with previous studies, in which it was noted that patients infected with carbapenem-resistant *K. pneumoniae* strains were mainly elderly, possessed multiple co-morbidities, were frequently admitted from and discharged to post-acute care facilities, and experienced prolonged hospital stays [18]. In addition, for carbapenem-resistant Gram-negative pathogen infections, previous administration of carbapenems has been shown to be a major factor, particularly in ICUs [19], and isolation of patients harboring carbapenem-resistant *Enterobacteriaceae* and delayed application of alternative antibiotics has been proposed to lead to a spread of these pathogens in ICUs [20].

A limitation of the present study is the missing data about molecular mechanisms of resistances against the included antibiotics.

Conclusions

Susceptibilities of *E. coli* IAI and UTI strains to IPM and ETP were > 90% in 2014 and 2015, while susceptibilities to IPM and ETP of *K. pneumoniae* IAI strains were > 80% in 2014, but decreased to ≤80% in 2015, particularly for UTI strains. Susceptibilities of all IAI *Enterobacteriaceae* strains to IPM and ETP were lowest in the colon and abscesses and *Enterobacteriaceae* susceptibilities of both UTI and IAI isolates to IPM and ETP were lowest in medical, pediatric and surgery ICUs in 2015.

Susceptibilities rates of *E. coli* and *K. pneumoniae* strains to cephalosporins collected from UTIs ranged from 38.6 to 69.5% and for IAI strains from 33.18 to 67.7% in 2015, which suggests that cephalosporins should not be the first choice for empirical UTI and IAI antibiotic therapy.

Abbreviations

AMK: amikacin; CA: community-associated; CAZ: ceftazidime; CIP: ciprofloxacin; CIs: confidence intervals; CLSI: Clinical and Laboratory Standards Institute; CRO: ceftriaxone; CTX: cefotaxime; *E. coli*: *Escherichia coli*; ETP: ertapenem; FEP: cefepime; FOX: cefoxitin; IAI: intra-abdominal infections; IPM: imipenem; *K. pneumoniae*: *Klebsiella pneumoniae*; LVX: levofloxacin; MIC: Minimum inhibitory concentrations; OSWIA: organ-specific weighted incidence antibiograms; QC: quality control; SAM: ampicillin-sulbactam; SMART: Study for Monitoring Antimicrobial Resistance Trends; TZP: piperacillin-tazobactam; UTI: urinary tract infections

Funding

This research was supported by Outstanding Talents Training Funding Project of Dongcheng District, Beijing (2017), The National Key Research and Development Program of China (SQ2018YFC120102), CAMS Innovation Fund for Medical Sciences (CIFMS) (Grant no. 2016-I2M-1-014) and CAMS Initiative for Innovative Medicine (Grant no. 2016-I2M-3-014). This study was supported by funding from Merck Sharp & Dohme (MSD; Whitehouse Station, NJ, USA).

Authors' contributions

All authors have read and approved the manuscript. The authors were solely responsible for the conception and performance of the study and for writing this manuscript. *Conceptualization:* HZ, YXN, QWY, YCX. *Data collection:* HZ, HSK, YSY, AHW, QD, XFJ, SFZ, ZYS, YXN, WPW, YW, KL, HYL, CXY, WXH, BDG, BS, RB, QWY, YCX. *Data analysis:* HZ, YSY, AHW, QD, SFZ, BDG, WPW, RB, QWY, YCX. *Writing original draft:* HZ, YCX. *Writing review & editing:* HZ, HSK, YSY, AHW, QD, XFJ, SFZ, ZYS, YXN, WPW, YW, KL, HYL, CXY, WXH, BDG, BS, RB, QWY, YCX.

Consent for publication

Not applicable.

Competing interests

Robert Badal received financial support in the form of salaries from International Health Management Associates, who receive funding from MSD to administer the SMART program and for SMART-related travel and consultation expenses.

Author details

[1]Division of Microbiology, Peking Union Medical College Hospital, Peking Union Medical College, Chinese Academy of Medical Sciences, No. 1 Shuaifuyuan, Wangfujing Street, Beijing 100730, China. [2]Department of Microbiology, The First Affiliated Hospital of Zhejiang University, Hangzhou 310003, China. [3]Department of Infectious Diseases, SirRunRun Shaw Hospital, School of Medicine, Zhejiang University, Hangzhou 310016, China. [4]Infection Control Center, Xiangya Hospital, Central South University, Changsha 410008, China. [5]Microbiology Laboratory, Jilin Province People's Hospital, Changchun 130021, China. [6]The Fourth Hospital of Harbin Medical University, No. 37 Yiyuan Road, Nangang District, Harbin, China. [7]Division of Microbiology, Haikou People's Hospital, Haikou 570208, China. [8]Department of Laboratory Medicine, Tongji Hospital, Tongji Medical College, Huazhong University of Science and Technology, Wuhan 430030, China. [9]Division of Microbiology, Ruijin Hospital, School of Medicine, Shanghai Jiaotong University, Shanghai 200025, China. [10]Nanjing General Hospital, No. 305 Zhongshan Dong Road, Nanjing, China. [11]Department of Laboratory Medicine, Shandong Provincial Hospital Affiliated to Shandong University, Jinan 250021, China. [12]Division of Microbiology, The First Affiliated Hospital, Sun Yat-Sen University, Guangzhou 510080, China. [13]Zhongshan Hospital Affiliated to Fudan University, No. 180 Fenglin Road, Shanghai 200032, China. [14]Beijing Chao-yang Hospital, 8 Gongren Tiyuchang Nanlu, Chaoyang District, Beijing 100020, China. [15]Division of Microbiology, The First Affiliated Hospital of Chongqing Medical University, Chongqing 400016, China. [16]Clinical laboratory, The Second Affiliated Hospital of Nanchang University, Nanchang 330006, China. [17]First Affiliated Hospital of Kunming Medical University, No. 295 Xichang Road, Kunming 650032, China. [18]Division of Microbiology, International Health Management Associates, Schaumburg, IL 60173-3817, USA.

References

1. Yang Q, Zhang H, Wang Y, Xu Y, Chen M, Badal RE, Wang H, Ni Y, Yu Y, Hu B, et al. A 10 year surveillance for antimicrobial susceptibility of Escherichia coli and Klebsiella pneumoniae in community- and hospital-associated intra-abdominal infections in China. J Med Microbiol. 2013;62(Pt 9):1343–9.
2. Morrissey I, Hackel M, Badal R, Bouchillon S, Hawser S, Biedenbach D. A review of ten years of the study for monitoring antimicrobial resistance trends (SMART) from 2002 to 2011. Pharmaceuticals (Basel). 2013;6(11):1335–46.
3. Yang Q, Zhang H, Wang Y, Xu Z, Zhang G, Chen X, Xu Y, Cao B, Kong H, Ni Y, et al. Antimicrobial susceptibilities of aerobic and facultative gram-negative bacilli isolated from Chinese patients with urinary tract infections between 2010 and 2014. BMC Infect Dis. 2017;17(1):192.
4. Liao K, Chen Y, Wang M, Guo P, Yang Q, Ni Y, Yu Y, Hu B, Sun Z, Huang W, et al. Molecular characteristics of extended-spectrum beta-lactamase-producing Escherichia coli and Klebsiella pneumoniae causing intra-abdominal infections from 9 tertiary hospitals in China. Diagn Microbiol Infect Dis. 2017;87(1):45–8.
5. Hebert C, Ridgway J, Vekhter B, Brown EC, Weber SG, Robicsek A. Demonstration of the weighted-incidence syndromic combination antibiogram: an empiric prescribing decision aid. Infect Control Hosp Epidemiol. 2012;33(4):381–8.
6. Zhang S, Huang W. Epidemiological study of community- and hospital-acquired intraabdominal infections. Chin J Traumatol. 2015;18(2):84–9.

7. CLSI: Clinical and Laboratory Standards Institute (CLSI) M07-A10. Methods for dilution antimicrobial susceptibility tests for bacteria that grow aerobically; approved standard—tenth edition. Wayne: CLSI; 2015. 2015.

8. CLSI: Clinical and Laboratory Standards Institute (CLSI) M100-S25. Performance standards of antimicrobial susceptibility testing. Twenty-fifth informational supplement. Wyane: CLSI; 2015 2015.

9. Lee S, Han SW, Kim KW, Song DY, Kwon KT. Third-generation cephalosporin resistance of community-onset Escherichia coli and Klebsiella pneumoniae bacteremia in a secondary hospital. Korean J Intern Med. 2014;29(1):49–56.

10. Koksal I, Yilmaz G, Unal S, Zarakolu P, Korten V, Mulazimoglu L, Tabak F, Mete B, Oguz VA, Gulay Z, et al. Epidemiology and susceptibility of pathogens from SMART 2011-12 Turkey: evaluation of hospital-acquired versus community-acquired urinary tract infections and ICU- versus non-ICU-associated intra-abdominal infections. J Antimicrob Chemother. 2017; 72(5):1364–72.

11. Redgrave LS, Sutton SB, Webber MA, Piddock LJ. Fluoroquinolone resistance: mechanisms, impact on bacteria, and role in evolutionary success. Trends Microbiol. 2014;22(8):438–45.

12. Werner NL, Hecker MT, Sethi AK, Donskey CJ. Unnecessary use of fluoroquinolone antibiotics in hospitalized patients. BMC Infect Dis. 2011;11:187.

13. Shi W, Li K, Ji Y, Jiang Q, Wang Y, Shi M, Mi Z. Carbapenem and cefoxitin resistance of Klebsiella pneumoniae strains associated with porin OmpK36 loss and DHA-1 beta-lactamase production. Braz J Microbiol. 2013;44(2):435–42.

14. Zhang X, Chen D, Xu G, Huang W, Wang X. Molecular epidemiology and drug resistant mechanism in carbapenem-resistant Klebsiella pneumoniae isolated from pediatric patients in Shanghai, China. PLoS One. 2018;13(3):e0194000.

15. Liu Q, Ren J, Wu X, Wang G, Wang Z, Wu J, Huang J, Lu T, Li J. Shifting trends in bacteriology and antimicrobial resistance among gastrointestinal fistula patients in China: an eight-year review in a tertiary-care hospital. BMC Infect Dis. 2017;17(1):637.

16. Fan S, Wang J, Li Y, Li J. Bacteriology and antimicrobial susceptibility of ESBLs producers from pus in patients with abdominal trauma associated intra-abdominal infections. Eur J Trauma Emerg Surg. 2017;43(1):65–71.

17. Davies GM, Dasbach EJ, Teutsch S. The burden of appendicitis-related hospitalizations in the United States in 1997. Surg Infect. 2004;5(2):160–5.

18. Perez F, Endimiani A, Ray AJ, Decker BK, Wallace CJ, Hujer KM, Ecker DJ, Adams MD, Toltzis P, Dul MJ, et al. Carbapenem-resistant Acinetobacter baumannii and Klebsiella pneumoniae across a hospital system: impact of post-acute care facilities on dissemination. J Antimicrob Chemother. 2010;65(8):1807–18.

19. Routsi C, Pratikaki M, Platsouka E, Sotiropoulou C, Papas V, Pitsiolis T, Tsakris A, Nanas S, Roussos C. Risk factors for carbapenem-resistant gram-negative bacteremia in intensive care unit patients. Intensive Care Med. 2013;39(7): 1253–61.

20. Zurawski RM. Carbapenem-resistant enterobacteriaceae: occult threat in the intensive care unit. Crit Care Nurse. 2014;34(5):44–52.

Prevalence and antibiotic susceptibility of Uropathogens from cases of urinary tract infections (UTI) in Shashemene referral hospital, Ethiopia

Wubalem Desta Seifu[1]* and Alemayehu Desalegn Gebissa[2]

Abstract

Background: Urinary tract infection (UTI) remains to be one of the most common infectious diseases diagnosed in developing countries. And a widespread use of antibiotics against uropathogens has led to the emergence of antibiotic resistant species. A laboratory based cross-sectional survey was conducted in Shashemene referral hospital to determine the prevalence and antibiotic susceptibility of uropathogens.

Methods: We have collected 384 clean catch mid-stream urine samples from all suspected UTI outpatients using sterile screw capped container. The urine samples were cultured and processed for subsequent uropathogens isolation. The isolated pure cultures were grown on BiOLOG Universal Growth agar (BUG) and identified using GEN III OmniLog® Plus ID System identification protocols. The identified species were then exposed to selected antibiotics to test for their susceptibility.

Results: The overall prevalence of urinary tract infection in the area was 90.1%. Most frequently isolated uropathogen in our study was *Escherichia coli* (39.3%). While, *Staphylococcus* species (20.2%), *Leuconostoc* species (11.4%), *Raoultella terrigena/Klebsiella spp./* (8.4%), *Salmonella typhimurium* (6.3%), *Dermacoccus nishinomiyaensis* (6.3%), *Citerobacter freundii* (5.2%) and *Issatchenkia orientalis/Candida krusei/* (2.7%) were the other isolates. We find that the relationship between uropathogens and some of UTI risk factors was statistically significant ($P < 0.05$). Gentamicin was the most effective drug against most of the isolates followed by chloramphenicol and nitrofurantoin. In contrast, amoxicillin, vancomycin and cephalexin were the antibiotics to which most of the isolates developed resistance.

Conclusion: Urinary tract infection was highly prevalent in the study area and all uropathogens isolated developed a resistance against mostly used antibiotics.

Keywords: Antibiotic sensitivity test, Prevalence, Urinary tract infection

Background

Urinary tract infection remains to be one of the most common infectious diseases diagnosed in outpatients [1]. It is most often caused due to bacteria, but may also include fungal and viral infections [2]. Gram-negative bacteria cause 90% of UTI cases while gram-positive bacteria cause only 10% of the cases. The most frequent isolated uropathogen is *Escherichia coli*, accounting for 65%–90% of urinary tract infections [3, 4]. The relative frequency of uropathogens varies depending upon age, sex, catheterization, hospitalization and previous exposure of antimicrobials [5–7].

The emergence of antibiotic resistance in the management of UTIs is a serious public health issue. Particularly in the developing world where there is high level of poverty, illiteracy and poor hygienic practices, there is also high prevalence of fake and spurious drugs of questionable quality in circulation [4, 8]. The easy availability in the community without prescription and low cost make the drugs subject to abuse [9]. With regards to resistance rates in Ethiopia, a report showed that high

* Correspondence: marry.moj@gmail.com
[1]Department of Biotechnology, Wolkite University, Wolkite, Ethiopia
Full list of author information is available at the end of the article

incidence of resistance to the commonly prescribed antibiotic agents was observed in some regions [6, 10, 11].

Even though, there are few published information concerning the etiology and resistance pattern of UTIs in some hospitals of Ethiopia [6, 10–12], there was no previous study and published information on UTI in the study area. This study was conducted in order to assess the prevalence of bacterial uropathogens and their in vitro susceptibility patterns to commonly used antibiotic agents amongst outpatients with complaints of UTI in Shashemene referral hospital.

Methods

Prior to sample collection, we obtained ethical clearance from Shashemene City Administration Health Affairs Bureau Research Ethics Review Committee (Ref. WEFB-33644/484/04) and informed consent from all research participants. Three hundred and forty eight [13] outpatients volunteered in June–December of 2016. Laboratory and questionnaire-based cross-sectional survey study was used to collect samples from the outpatients. Questionnaire was developed to assess the possible risk factors associated with UTI and register clinical profile of the volunteer. Clean catch mid-stream urine samples were collected from all UTI suspected outpatients attending Shashemene referral hospital using sterile screw capped container. Outpatients with dysuria, frequency, urgency, supra-pubic pain/tenderness and occasional hematuria were considered as possible suspects for UTI. Name, age, sex, clinical history and treatment history of the screened outpatients were recorded and the four age categories considered in this study were children (under 18), young (18–29), adults (30–45) and old (above 45) years (Additional file 1).

Isolation of bacteria from urine samples and preservation

Urine dipstick test was done by using Multisticks of Medi-Test combi 10°SGL leukocyte esterase and nitrite [14]. The urine samples were also examined microscopically for pus cells and then inoculated on MacConkey agar and Blood agar media. Inoculated agar plates were incubated aerobically at 37 °C for 24 to 48 h. The cultured plates were examined for growth and mixed colonies on a plate were re-inoculated further on blood agar and nutrient agar medium for growth of discrete colony. Gram staining was done for all isolates as per the standard procedures and the smears were examined microscopically for their morphology and staining reactions [15].

Isolates were streaked on BUG agar for further identification using standard operation protocols for aerobic bacterial identification in GEN III OmniLog® Plus ID System of BiOLOG [16].

Antibiotic susceptibility tests for Uropathogens

The antibiotic susceptibility test was done by the standard disk diffusion method on Mueller-Hinton agar (MHA) using commercial disks [17]. Turbidity standard protocol was followed in order to have homogenized bacterial inoculum suspension [15]. The following antibiotic discs, manufactured by Oxoid Ltd. Bashingstore Hampaire, UK were used for the disc diffusion tests: amoxicillin (AML, 30 μg), chloramphenicol (C, 30 μg), ciprofloxacin (CIP, 30 μg), gentamicin (GN, 10 μg), nalidixic acid (NA, 30 μg), nitrofurantoin (NTR, 300 μg), trimethprime-sulfamethoxazole (TMP-SMX) (SXT, 25 μg), tetracycline (TTC, 25 μg), vancomycin (VA, 30 μg), cephalexin (Ceph, 30 μg), ceftriaxone (CRO, 30 μg) [17, 18].

Statistical methods

Our data were analyzed using SPSS for Windows, version 16.0 (SPSS, Inc., Chicago, Ill). Pearson Chi-square test was employed to test the existence of association between discrete variables. P-value of <0.05 was considered to indicate statistically significant differences. A binary logistic regression analysis was used to calculate odds ratio (OR); Crude Odds Ratio (COR) and Adjusted Odds Ratio (AOR) to ascertain the degree of association between risk factors and UTI.

Results

Prevalence of urinary tract infection among outpatients in Shashemene referral hospital

We examined a total of 384 (Table 1) outpatients with complaints of urinary tract infection in Shashemene referral hospital and found 90.1% overall prevalence of UTI in the study area (Table 2). The laboratory test results indicate that all samples 384 (100%) were positive for leukocyte esterase, while 88.5% were positive for nitrite and 11.5% were negative (Table 2). On the basis of microscopy of urine, it was found that 90.1% of the samples were positive for both pyuria and bacteriuria (Table 2). Of the total urine samples, 346 (90.1%) were positive and 38 (9.9%) were negative for the growth of different uropathogens on blood agar media (Additional file 2: Fig. S1.1c). On the other hand, 340

Table 1 Number of outpatients enrolled in the study and their corresponding age group

Age group	Gender		
	Female	Male	Total
<18	10 (2.6%)	2 (0.5%)	12 (3.1%)
18–29	92 (24%)	31 (8.1%)	123 (32%)
30–45	68 (17.7%)	36 (9.4%)	104 (27.1%)
>45	96 (25%)	49 (12.8%)	145 (37.1%)
Total	266 (69.3%)	118 (30.7%)	384 (100%)

Table 2 Characteristics of patients at time of presentation with symptoms of cystitis or pyelonephritis and their association with positivity of uropathogens in the study area

Characteristics			The frequency (%) of occurrence of clinical symptoms	The prevalence (%) of UTI		P-value	X^2
Clinical symptoms				Positive	Negative		
	Fever	Yes	165 (43)	155 (44.8)	10 (26.3)	0.002*	9.287
		No	219 (57)	191 (55.2)	28 (73.7)		
	Dysuria	Yes	73 (19)	66 (19.1)	7 (18.4)	0.494	0.468
		No	311 (81)	280 (80.9)	31 (81.6)		
	Urgency	Yes	265 (69)	250 (72.3)	15 (39.5)	0.000*	20.69
		No	119 (31)	96 (27.7)	23 (60.5)		
	Frequency	Yes	231 (60.2)	210 (60.7)	21 (53.3)	0.010*	6.597
		No	153 (39.8)	136 (39.3)	17 (44.7)		
	Flank pain	Yes	220 (57.3)	200 (57.8)	20 (52.6)	0.066	3.385
		No	164 (42.7)	146 (42.2)	18 (47.4)		
	Supra-pubic pain	Yes	266 (69.3)	262 (75.7)	4 (10.5)	0.000*	39.917
		No	118 (30.7)	84 (24.3)	34 (89.5)		
	Age categories (year)		No of positive (%)				
			Female	Male	Total		
Age	<18		9 (2.34)	1 (0.26)	10 (2.6)		
	18–29		86 (22.4)	29 (7.55)	115 (29.94)		
	30–45		58 (15.1)	29 (7.55)	87 (22.65)		
	>45		90 (23.43)	44 (11.45)	134 (34.89)		
	Total		243 (63.3)	103 (26.8)	346 (90.1)		
Urinalysis and urine microscopy			No of positive	No of negative			
	Leucocyte esterase		384 (100)	–			
	Nitrite		340 (88.5)	44 (11.5)			
	Bacteruria		346 (90.1)	38 (9.9)			
	Pyuria		346 (90.1)	38 (9.9)			
	MacConkey Agar		346 (90.1)	38 (9.9)			
	Blood Agar		340 (88.5)	44 (11.5)			

*Statistically significant at P < 0.05

(88.5%) were positive and 44 (11.5%) were negative on MacConkey's agar (Table 2; Additional file 2: Fig. S1.1b).

From the total patients with UTI compliant, 134 (34.89%) were in the old age group while 115 (29.94%) were in the young age group (Table 2).

Clinical symptoms associated with urinary tract infection
Clinical symptoms of UTI are the result of a complex series of host pathogen interactions that could lead to bacterial invasion and persistence and ultimately to disease [19]. In this study, clinical symptoms were used in the diagnosis to determine the course of infections.

Data of clinical symptoms and their associations with UTI of study subjects is shown in Table 2. Of the total outpatients, 155 (44.8%), 66 (19.1%), 250 (72.3%), 210 (60.7), 200 (57.8) and 262 (75.5) of them showed fever, dysuria, urgency, frequency, flank pain and supra-pubic

pain respectively. Statistical analysis revealed that there is significant relation between the majority of clinical symptoms (fever, urgency, frequency, suprapubic pain) and UTI ($P < 0.005$).

The prevalence of Uropathogens from urine samples of UTI positive patients
The relative prevalence of uropathogens isolated from mid-stream urine samples is shown in Table 3. Totally, 429 isolates of ten different kinds of uropathogens were identified from the urine samples. Of these, 417 (97.2%) belonged to bacteria while the rest, 12 (2.8%) were fungi.

The most frequently isolated microbial species was *Escherichia coli* (39.3%). *Staphylococcus* species (20.2%), *Leuconostoc* species (11.4%), *Raoultella terrigena/Klebsiella spp.* (8.4%), *Salmonella typhimurium* (6.3%), *Dermacoccus nishinomiyaensis* (6.3%), *Citerobacter freundii* (5.2%) and

Table 3 Prevalence of uropathogens among positive patients by sex, place of residence and age group

Identified uropathogens	Midstream urine sample								
	Sex		Residence		Age group				
	Female (%)	Male (%)	Urban (%)	Rural (%)	<18 (%)	18–29 (%)	30–45 (%)	>45 (%)	Total (%)
Gram-negative uropathogens									
Escherichia coli	121 (39.3)	48 (39.7)	65 (40.9)	104 (38.5)	3 (37.5)	27 (29.0)	127 (42.5)	12 (41.4)	169 (39.4)
Raoultella terrigena	25 (8.1)	11 (9.1)	17 (10.7)	19 (7.0)	1 (12.5)	11 (11.8)	24 (8.0)	0	36 (8.38)
Salmonella Typhimurium	16 (5.2)	11 (9.1)	11 (6.9)	16 (5.9)	1 (12.5)	5 (5.4)	19 (6.4)	2 (6.9)	27 (6.29)
Citerobacter freundii	17 (5.5)	5 (4.1)	3 (1.9)	19 (7.0)	–	3 (3.2)	17 (5.7)	2 (6.9)	22 (5.12)
Gram-positive uropathogens									
Staphylococcus intermedius	21 (6.8)	14 (11.6)	15 (9.4)	20 (7.4)	–	8 (8.6)	24 (8.0)	3 (10.3)	35 (8.15)
Staphylococcus epidermidis	38 (12.3)	14 (11.6)	18 (11.3)	34 (12.6)	1 (12.5)	18 (19.4)	31 (10.4)	2 (6.9)	52 (12.12)
Leuconostoc citreum	22 (7.1)	6 (4.9)	11 (6.9)	17 (6.3)	1 (12.5)	8 (8.6)	18 (6.0)	1 (3.4)	28 (6.52)
Dermacoccus nishinomiyaensis	22 (7.1)	5 (4.1)	7 (4.4)	20 (7.4)	1 (12.5)	5 (5.4)	20 (6.7)	1 (3.4)	27 (6.29)
Leuconostoc mesenteroides	14 (4.5)	7 (5.8)	7 (4.4)	14 (5.2)	–	4 (4.3)	16 (5.4)	1 (3.4)	21 (4.89)
Fungus									
Issatchenkia orientalis	12 (3.9)	0	5 (3.1)	7 (2.3)	–	4 (4.3)	3 (1.0)	5 (17.2)	12 (2.79)
Total	308 (71.7)	121 (28.3)	159 (37.1)	270 (62.9)	8 (1.86)	93 (21.67)	299 (69.69)	29 (6.75)	429 (100)

Issatchenkia orientalis/Candida krusei/ (2.7%) were the other isolated microbes (Fig. 1).

Prevalence of uropathogens among UTI positive patients by sex

Our result shows, of the total positive patients for uropathogens, while 71.7% were female, 28.3% were male (Table 3). Statistical analysis revealed that there was a significant relationship between sex and the prevalence of uropathogens $P = 0.041$, $X^2 = 4.192$ and AOR = 2.396 (Table 4).

Prevalence of uropathogens among UTI positive patients by place of residence

For all uropathogens isolate, the highest prevalence was observed in patients from the rural area (62.9%) than patients from the urban (37.1%) (Table 3). Statistical analysis revealed that there is significant relation between place of residence and UTI causing microorganisms ($X^2 = 13.089$, $P = 0.000$, COR = 4.648) (Table 5).

Prevalence of uropathogens among UTI positive patients by age group

The highest prevalence of microbial isolates was observed in adult age group (69.69%) followed by the young (21.67%) (Table 3) and it was statistically significant $P = 0.022$, $X^2 = 5.235$ and AOR = 3.404 (Table 4). This might be due to active sexuality of the age group [20, 21]. However, it will require further investigations to validate.

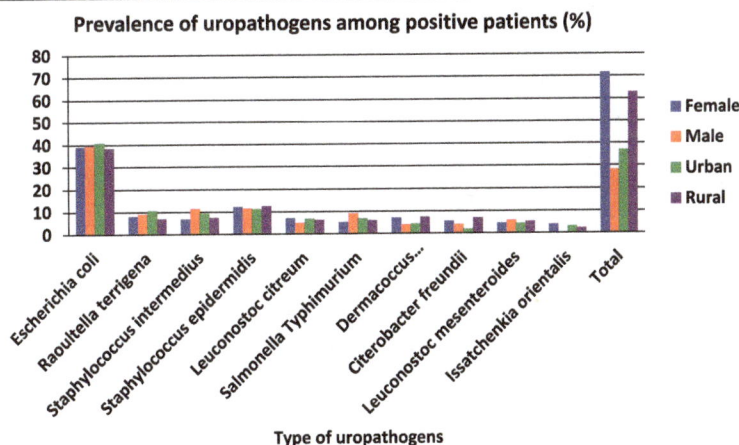

Fig. 1 Sex and place of residence based prevalence of uropathogens

Table 4 Multivariate logistic regression of risk factors for the prevalence of UTI in male and female patients

Association between risk factors and UTI

Risk factors	The frequency (%) of occurrence of risk factors		The prevalence (%) of UTI		P-value	X^2	AOR (95% CI)
			Negative	Positive			
Catheter use	Yes	39(10.2)	3(7.9)	36(10.4)	0.628	0.235	0.738(0.216–2.555)
	No	345(89.8)	35(92.1)	310(89.6)			1
Severe underlying illness	Yes	47(12.2)	2(5.3)	45(13.0)	0.183	1.771	0.372(0.086–1.597)
	No	337(87.8)	36(94.7)	301(87.0)			1
Improper storage	Yes	247(64.3)	10(26.3)	237(68.5)	0.000*	21.882	0.164(0.077–0.350)
	No	137(35.7)	28(73.7)	109(31.5)			1
Place of residence	Rural	223(58.1)	29(76.3)	214(61.8)	0.000*	17.316	5.224(2.398–11.381)
	Urban	161(41.9)	9(23.7)	132(38.2)			1
Age	Child	12(3.1)	1(2.6)	11(3.2)	0.900	0.016	1.158(0.11–11.491)
	Young	123(32)	13(34.2)	110(31.8)	0.302	1.066	1.580(0.663–3.767)
	Adult	104(27.1)	6(15.8)	98(28.3)	0.022*	5.235	3.404(1.192–9.720)
	Old	145(37.8)	18(47.4)	127(36.7)			1
Sex	Female	266(69.3)	23(60.5)	243(70.2)	0.041*	4.192	2.396(1.038–5.531)
	Male	118(30.7)	15(39.5)	103(29.8)			1

N.B.*significant at p < 0.05, Numbers in bracket indicates percentages, *AOR* Adjusted Odds Ratio, *CI* Confidence Interval and 1 = Reference category

Risk factors to urinary tract infection

We have considered various risk factors that might play a role in escalating UTI such as sex, age, spermicide or diaphragm use, catheter use, severe underlying illness, genital hygiene, frequent sex and improper urine storage.

Logistic regression analysis was used to calculate odds ratio (OR) to ascertain the degree of association between these risk factors and UTI. Both urine storage and place of residence had positive and statistically significant relationships with UTI (X^2 = 23.691, P = 0.000 COR = 0.121 and X^2 = 13.089, P = 0.000 COR = 4.648, respectively) (Table 5).

Among risk factors pertinent to females, statistical analysis revealed that there was no significant relationship between use of diaphragm and the prevalence of

Table 5 Univariate logistic regression of risk factors for the prevalence of UTI in male and female patients

Association between risk factors and UTI

Risk factors	The frequency (%) of occurrence of risk factors		The prevalence (%) of UTI		P-value	X^2	COR (95% CI)
			Positive	Negative			
Catheter use	Yes	39(10.2)	3(7.9)	36(10.4)	0.348	0.881	0.507(0.122–2.096)
	No	345(89.8)	35(92.1)	310(89.6)			1
Severe underlying illness	Yes	47(12.2)	2(5.3)	45(13.0)	0.082	3.033	0.240(0.048–1.196)
	No	337(87.8)	36(94.7)	301(87.0)			1
Improper storage	Yes	247(64.3)	10(26.3)	237(68.5)	0.000*	23.691	0.121(0.052–0.284)
	No	137(35.7)	28(73.7)	109(31.5)			1
Place of residence	Rural	223(58.1)	29(76.3)	214(61.8)	0.000*	13.089	4.648(2.022–10.683)
	Urban	161(41.9)	9(23.7)	132(38.2)			1
Age	Child	12(3.1)	11(3.2)	1(2.6)	0.737	0.113	1.436(0.174–11.883)
	Young	123(32)	110(31.8)	13(34.2)	0.716	0.132	1.152(0.537–2.468)
	Adult	104(27.1)	98(28.3)	6(15.8)	0.085	2.97	2.332(0.891–6.106)
	Old	145(37.8)	127(36.7)	18(47.4)			1
Sex	Female	266(69.3)	243(70.2)	23(60.5)	0.206	1.60	1.569(0.781–3.153)
	Male	118(30.7)	103(29.8)	15(39.5)			1

N.B.*significant at p < 0.05, Numbers in bracket indicates percentages, *AOR* Crude Odds Ratio, *CI* Confidence Interval and 1 = Reference category

UTI ($P > 0.05$) (Additional file 3: Table S1a and b). This might be due to the fact that most females were not using diaphragm.

Antibiotic susceptibility test
In-vitro antibiotic susceptibility tests were done on a total of 30 isolates using a standard method of agar disk diffusion technique following the National Committee for Clinical Laboratory Standards. Eleven antibiotic agents were used for the test (Amoxicillin, Chloramphenicol, Ciprofloxacin, Gentamicin, Nalidixic acid, Nitrofurantoin, Trimethprime-Sulfamethoxazole (TMP-SMX), Tetracycline, Vancomycin, and Cephalexin, Ceftriaxone (Additional file 2: Fig. S1.6a–c).

As it can be seen from Additional file 4: Table S2, 93.3%, of the isolates were sensitive to gentamicin. Similarly, 60%, 60%, 56.6%, 46.6%, 40%, 33.3%, of the isolates were sensitive to chloramphenicol, nitrofurantoin, ciprofloxacin, Trimethprime-Sulfamethoxazole (TMP-SMX), ceftriaxone and nalidixic acid, respectively. Moreover, 10–20% of the isolates were sensitive to vancomycin, tetracycline and cephalexin. On the contrary, none of the isolates showed sensitivity to amoxicillin (96.6%) followed by vancomycin (80%) and cephalexin (70%). Likewise, 40–56.6% of the isolates showed resistance to nitrofurantoin, ceftriaxone, nalidixic acid and tetracycline.

Discussion
We have shown that the overall prevalence of UTI was 90.1%. In accordance with [22, 23], the prevalence of UTI is higher in females (63.3%) than males (26.8%) (Table 2). This might be due to the anatomical differences of urogenital organs between the two sexes [24, 25]. Prevalence difference has been also observed among various age groups. This difference suggests that age is one risk factor associated with UTI. The high incidence of UTI amongst the old age group could be due to genito-urinary atrophy and vaginal prolapse after menopause in female which in turn increases the risk of bacteriuria by increasing vaginal pH and decreasing vaginal *Lactobacillus* thereby allowing gram-negative bacteria to grow and act as uropathogens [26]. Moreover, it was indicated in another study [21, 27] that UTI is the most common infection in elderly populations. The high prevalence recorded amongst young age group could be due to increased sexual activity in the age group [26].

Fever, dysuria, urgency, frequency, flank pain and suprapubic pain were the observed clinical symptoms in our study and is comparable with report of [28]. In contrast, dysuria and flank pain were symptoms statistically not significant. Even though statistically not significant, flank pain was the symptom in which positive cases were noted in 200 (57.8%) patients, next to supra-pubic pain and urgency.

Bacterial species were the more prevalent uropathogens compared to other groups of microbes. This result is in accordance with that reported by [2] which indicated that among different microorganisms causing UTIs, bacteria accounts for more than 95% and the rest may also include fungal and viral infections. Among the isolates, gram-negative bacteria, gram-positive bacteria and fungi constituted 59.2%, 38% and 2.7%, respectively. The highest prevalence of gram-negative bacteria in this study is in agreement with that reported by [29, 30].

Moreover, the prevalence of *E. coli* (39.3%) in the current study is comparable with that reported from Nigeria, Zaria by [31], but higher than the reports of [32] from Brazil, [18] from Pakistan, and [33] from Mekele hospital, Ethiopia.

The prevalence of *Staphylococcus epidermidis* 12.1% in our study is also comparable with the study reported by [34] which was 13%. Similarly, the prevalence of other non–*E.coli* aerobic gram-negative rods is comparable with the study reported by [35], which was generally ranging from 5 to 10%.

Dermacoccus nishinomiyaensis (Micrococcus nishinomiyaensis) prevalence is 6.3%. According to the study conducted by [36], it was reported that *Dermacoccus nishinomiyaensis* is prevalent in urinary tract during microbial urethral stent colonization (MUSC). In similar study conducted by [37], urethral stents inserted during urinary tract infection were more frequently colonized (59%) by urophatogens compared to those placed in sterile urine (26%). Female sex and continuous stenting were significant risk factors for MUSC.

In agreement with [38], our study also showed that there was mixed bacterial species infection per a patient. Studies reported that mixed infections (poly-microbial) are more likely to occur in patients with underlying disorders that interfere with free urine flow. Moreover, it is frequent in those with indwelling catheter. The similarities and differences in the type and distribution of uropathogens may result from different environmental conditions and the prevailing practices in each country and region.

Furthermore, we assessed the relationship between various risk factors and UTI. Sex was one of the considered factors and the result indicated that UTI prevalence was higher in females than males for each isolate. Previously, [25, 39, 40] have shown that incidence of UTI was found to be higher in females than in males. This is probably due to multiple factors contributing to the problems among females. The first possible reason would be the anatomical feature of the female urethra, which is much shorter than males' urethra. The Shortness of the urethra, allow the pathogens easy access to the bladder during sexual intercourse. This in turn results in increased bacterial counts in the bladder after intercourse [41, 42].

Statistical analysis showed that patients who were holding urine in their bladder for a long period of time had more probability of having UTI than those who were not holding. In a study done on risk factors of UTI in Pakistan, improper holding of urine in bladder was found to be one of the main causes of urinary tract infection, which produces a favorable environment for the growth of urinary tract pathogens [26, 43].

Among the risk factors of UTI pertinent to females, active sexuality/frequent sex/ has a positive and statistically significant relationship with the prevalence of UTI (Additional file 3: Table S1a). Statistical analysis revealed that there was a significant difference between the prevalence of UTI in patients who were practicing frequent sexual activity and those who were not (Additional file 3: Table S1a and b). This indicates that those patients who were practicing frequent sexual activity would have more probability of having UTI than those who were not. This is consistent with the findings reported by many authors. They showed the incidence of UTI is higher in sexually active females causing 75–90% of bladder infections, [21, 44, 45].

Similarly, keeping genital hygiene has a positive and statistically significant relationship with the prevalence of UTI. Statistical analysis done using both univariate and multivariate logistic regression revealed that there was a significant difference in the prevalence of the UTI between females keeping their genital hygiene and those who were not (Additional file 3: Table S1a and b). This indicates that those patients who were not keeping their genital hygiene had more probability of contracting UTI than those who were keeping their genital hygiene. This could be attributed to multiple factors probably contributing to the increasing problem of infection among these females. One of such factors was most of the female patients were from rural areas, and they have poor hygienic practices. Poor hygienic practice results in direct fecal contamination of urinary tract from the anus in females. Consequently it provides easier access to the pathogens overgrowth and ascent to bladder [41].

The results also revealed that among eleven antibiotics used for susceptibility test, gentamicin was the most effective antibiotics 93.3% followed by chloramphenicol and nitrofurantoin. This might be due to the fact that gentamicin is offered in injection form and its unavailability in tablet form in the community, minimized the chance to abuse (Unpublished data).

We have shown there was multiple antibiotic resistances on many of the identified species. Thus, E. coli, L. cetreum and S. typhimurium were members resistant to more than five antibiotics while the rest of the isolates were resistant to three to five antibiotics. The development of higher resistance against the above-mentioned antimicrobials could be due to repeated use or prolonged exposure of uropathogens to the antibiotics [46]. Repeated use of antibiotics can damage peri-urethral flora, allowing uropathogens to colonize and subsequently infect the urinary tract. Hence, leaving clinicians with very few choices of drugs for the treatment of UTI. Moreover, this condition enables bacteria to exchange their genetic material through horizontal gene transfer resulting in resistant gene that confer resistance to a particular antibiotic [47].

Conclusions

Urinary tract infection is the most common problem throughout the world, particularly in developing countries. In addition, emergence of bacterial strains resistant to commonly used antibiotic agents is widespread phenomenon all over the world. From the results of our study, we concluded that, UTI is prevalent in the study area and the most frequently isolated uropathogen was E. coli followed by Staphylococcus spp. In addition, Leuconostoc species, Raoultella terrigena (Klebsiella spp), Salmonella typhimurium, Dermacoccus nishinomiyaensis, Citerobacter freundii and Issatchenkia orientalis were isolated. Female sex, poor hygienic practice of the rural residents, improper urine storage, frequent sex and lack of genital hygiene, were the major risk factors for the high prevalence of UTI. Gentamycin was the most effective antibiotic for the area followed by chloramphenicol and nitrofurantoin. In contrast, amoxicillin, vancomycin and cephalexin were the drugs to which the isolates developed resistance. Generally, as there was no previous study and published information on UTI in the study area, this study has provided baseline data on the prevalence, drug sensitivity, and some potential risk factors of UTI and is, therefore, of clinical and epidemiological significance.

Additional files

Additional file 1: Questionnaire.

Additional file 2: Figures S1. Different pictures of laboratory processes. The picture indicates the detail of processes followed in the study including outpatients interview, bacterial inoculation and incubation and further analyses.

Additional file 3: Tables S1. Univariate and Multivariate logistic regression of risk factors pertinent to females for the prevalence of UTI. Univariate and multivariate logistic regression were used to correlate risk factors and prevalence of UTI. Except diaphragm use, the rest risk factors have significant association with prevalence of UTI in females.

Additional file 4: Table S2. The proportion of sensitive, intermediate and resistant bacterial isolates to eleven different antibiotics. The table indicates the sensitivity of isolates to various antibiotics used in the study.

Abbreviations
BUG: BiOLOG Universal Growth medium; DM: Diabetes mellitus; MUSC: Microbial Urethral Stent Colonization; TMP-SMX: Trimethprime-Sulfamethoxazole; UTI: Urinary Tract Infection

Acknowledgements
We would also like to express my sincere gratitude to Shashemene Town Health Bureau for their permission to conduct the study in the hospital. We are also highly indebted to Dr. Wuhib G/Hiwot, Medical Director of Shashemene Referral Hospital, Ato Ahimed Adem, Head of the hospital laboratory and all laboratory technicians of the hospital, for providing me laboratory space, reagents and kindly assisting me in all of the technical works during sample collection and interviewing of patients. Our special appreciation also goes to all staff members of Wendogenet College of Forestry and Natural Resources for providing us laboratory space and equipment during bacterial isolation.

Funding
No specific grant was received for this research from funding agencies in the public, commercial, or not-for-profit sectors.

Author's contributions
Both authors contribute equally for this research. Both authors read and approved the final manuscript.

Consent for publication
Not applicable.

Competing interests
The authors declare that they have no competing interests.

Author details
[1]Department of Biotechnology, Wolkite University, Wolkite, Ethiopia.
[2]Department of Biology, Haramaya University, Alemaya, Ethiopia.

References
1. Gales AC, et al. Activity and spectrum of 22 antimicrobial agents tested against urinary tract infection pathogens in hospitalized patients in Latin America: report from the second year of the SENTRY antimicrobial surveillance program (1998). J Antimicrob Chemother. 2000;45(3):295–303.
2. Amdekar S, Singh V, Singh DD. Probiotic therapy: immunomodulating approach toward urinary tract infection. Curr Microbiol. 2011;63(5):484–90.
3. Gupta K, Hooton TM, Stamm WE. INcreasing antimicrobial resistance and the management of uncomplicated community-acquired urinary tract infections. Ann Intern Med. 2001;135(1):41–50.
4. Weekes LM. Antibiotic resistance changing management of urinary tract infections in aged care. Med J Aust. 2015;203(9):352.
5. Haider G, Zehra N, Afroze Munir A. Risk factors of urinary tract infection inpregnancy. J Pak Med Assoc. 2010;60
6. Emiru T, et al. Associated risk factors of urinary tract infection among pregnant women at Felege Hiwot referral hospital, Bahir Dar, north West Ethiopia. BMC Research Notes. 2013;6(1):292.
7. Raz R, et al. Demographic characteristics of patients with community-acquired bacteriuria and susceptibility of urinary pathogens to antimicrobials in northern Israel. Isr Med Assoc J. 2000;2(6):426–9.
8. Fagan M, et al. Antibiotic resistance patterns of bacteria causing urinary tract infections in the elderly living in nursing homes versus the elderly living at home: an observational study. BMC Geriatr. 2015;15(1):98.
9. Manikandan S, et al. Antimicrobial susceptibility pattern of urinary tract infection causing human pathogenic bacteria. Asian Journal of Medical Sciences. 2011;
10. Wolday D, Erge W. Increased incidence of resistance to antimicrobials by urinary pathogens isolated at Tikur Anbessa hospital. Ethiop Med J. 1997;35(2):127–35.
11. Moges F, Mengistu G, Genetu A. Multiple drug resistance in urinary pathogens at Gondar College of Medical Sciences Hospital, Ethiopia. East Afr Med J. 2002;79(8):415–9.
12. Ringertz, S., et al., Antibiotic susceptibility of Escherichia Coli isolates from inpatients with urinary tract infections in hospitals in Addis Ababa and Stockholm. Bull World Health Organ. 1990; 68 (1): p. 61-68.
13. Wiegand H, Kish L. Survey sampling. John Wiley & Sons, inc., New York, London 1965, IX + 643 S., 31 Abb., 56 tab., Preis 83 s. Biom Z. 1968;10(1):88–9.
14. Alper BS, Curry SH. Urinary tract infection in children. Am Fam Physician. 2005;72(12):2483–8.
15. Cheesbrough M. District laboratory practice in tropical countries, part 2, 2nd edition. Cambridge: Cambridge University Press; 2006.
16. BiOLOG: GEN III OmniLog® ID System. [cited 2016 April 20, 2016]; Available from: http://www.biolog.com/products-static/microbial_identification_fully_autometed_systems.php.
17. (NCCLS), N.C.f.C.L.S., Performance standards for antimicrobial discs and dilution susceptibility for bacteria isolated from animals, vol. 22 approved standards, 2nd edition. 2002.
18. Beyene G, Tsegaye W. Bacterial uropathogens in urinary tract infection and antibiotic susceptibility pattern in jimma university specialized hospital, Southwest Ethiopia. Ethiop J Health Sci. 2011;21(2):141–6.
19. Wazait HD, et al. Catheter-associated urinary tract infections: prevalence of uropathogens and pattern of antimicrobial resistance in a UK hospital (1996-2001). BJU Int. 2003;91(9):806–9.
20. Tan CW, Chlebicki MP. Urinary tract infections in adults. Singap Med J. 2016;57(9):485–90.
21. Nicolle LE. Urinary tract infections in the elderly. Clin Geriatr Med. 25(3):423–36.
22. Haque R, Akter ML, Salam MA. Prevalence and susceptibility of uropathogens: a recent report from a teaching hospital in Bangladesh. BMC Research Notes. 2015;8(1):416.
23. Ayoade F, Moro DD, Ebene OL. Prevalence and antimicrobial susceptibility pattern of asymptomatic urinary tract infections of bacterial and parasitic origins among university students in redemption camp, Ogun state, Nigeria. Open Journal of Medical Microbiology. 2013;03(04):8.
24. Flores-Mireles AL, et al. Urinary tract infections: epidemiology, mechanisms of infection and treatment options. Nat Rev Micro. 2015;13(5):269–84.
25. Foxman B. Epidemiology of urinary tract infections: incidence, morbidity, and economic costs. Am J Med. 2002;113(Suppl 1A):5s–13s.
26. Scholes D, et al. Risk factors for recurrent urinary tract infection in young women. J Infect Dis. 2000;182(4):1177–82.
27. Shortliffe LM, McCue JD. Urinary tract infection at the age extremes: pediatrics and geriatrics. Am J Med. 2002;113(Suppl 1A):55s–66s.
28. Bent S, et al. Does this woman have an acute uncomplicated urinary tract infection? JAMA. 2002;287(20):2701–10.
29. Lazarevic G, Petreska D, Pavlovic S. Antibiotic sensitivy of bacteria isolated from the urine of children with urinary tract infections from 1986 to 1995. Srp Arh Celok Lek. 1998;126(11–12):423–9.
30. Mirzarazi M, et al. Antibiotic resistance of isolated gram negative bacteria from urinary tract infections (UTIs) in Isfahan. Jundishapur J Microbiol. 2013;6(8):e6883.
31. Ehinmidu JO. Antibiotics susceptibility patterns of urine bacterial isolates in Zaria, Nigeria. Trop J Pharm Res. 2003;2(2):223–28.
32. Ullah F, Malik S, Ahmed J. Antibiotic susceptibility pattern and ESBL prevalence in nosocomial Escherichia Coli from urinary tract infections in Pakistan. Afr J Biotechnol. 2009;8(16):3921–26.
33. Tesfahunegn Z, et al. Bacteriology of surgical site and catheter related urinary tract infections among patients admitted in Mekelle hospital, Mekelle, Tigray, Ethiopia. Ethiop Med J. 2009;47(2):117–27.
34. Naber KG. Use of Quinolones in urinary tract infections and Prostatitis. Rev Infect Dis. 1989;11(Supplement_5):S1321–37.
35. Hooton TM, Stamm WE. Diagnosis and treatment of uncomplicated urinary tract infection. Infect Dis Clin N Am. 1997;11(3):551–81.
36. Bonkat G, et al. Improved detection of microbial ureteral stent colonisation by sonication. World J Urol. 2011;29(1):133–8.

37. Klis R, et al. Relationship between urinary tract infection and self-retaining double-J catheter colonization. J Endourol. 2009;23(6):1015–9.

38. Siegman-Igra Y, et al. Polymicrobial and monomicrobial bacteraemic urinary tract infection. J Hosp Infect. 1994;28(1):49–56.

39. Moraes D, et al. Prevalence of uropathogens and antimicrobial susceptibility profile in outpatient from Jataí-GO. Jornal Brasileiro de Patologia e Medicina Laboratorial. 2014;50:200–4.

40. Stamm WE. An epidemic of urinary tract infections? N Engl J Med. 2001; 345(14):1055–7.

41. Gupta K, Scholes D, Stamm WE. Increasing prevalence of antimicrobial resistance among uropathogens causing acute uncomplicated cystitis in women. JAMA. 1999;281(8):736–8.

42. Neumann I, Moore P. Pyelonephritis (acute) in non-pregnant women. BMJ Clin Evid. 2014;2014:0807.

43. Remis RS, et al. Risk factors for urinary tract infection. Am J Epidemiol. 1987; 126(4):685–94.

44. Fihn SD. Acute uncomplicated urinary tract infection in women. N Engl J Med. 2003;349(3):259–66.

45. Heffner VA, Gorelick MH. Pediatric urinary tract infection. Clinical Pediatric Emergency Medicine. 2008;9(4):233–7.

46. Hillier S, et al. Prior antibiotics and risk of antibiotic-resistant community-acquired urinary tract infection: a case-control study. J Antimicrob Chemother. 2007;60(1):92–9.

47. Alemu A, et al. Bacterial profile and drug susceptibility pattern of urinary tract infection in pregnant women at University of Gondar Teaching Hospital, Northwest Ethiopia. BMC Res Notes. 2012;5:197.

Distribution of virulence genes and their association with antimicrobial resistance among uropathogenic *Escherichia coli* isolates from Iranian patients

Yalda Malekzadegan[1], Reza Khashei[1]* (iD), Hadi Sedigh Ebrahim-Saraie[1] and Zahra Jahanabadi[2]

Abstract

Background: Urinary tract infections (UTIs) are one of the most frequent diseases encountered by humans worldwide. The presence of multidrug-resistant (MDR) uropathogenic *Escherichia coli* (UPEC) harboring several virulence factors, is a major risk factor for inpatients. We sought to investigate the rate of antibiotic resistance and virulence-associated genes among the UPECs isolated from an Iranian symptomatic population.

Methods: A total of 126 isolates from inpatients with UTI from different wards were identified as UPEC using the conventional microbiological tests. After identification of UPECs, all the isolates were subjected to antimicrobial susceptibility test and polymerase chain reaction (PCR) to identify the presence of 9 putative virulence genes and their association with the clinical outcomes or antimicrobial resistance.

Results: The data showed that the highest and the lowest resistance rates were observed against ampicillin (88.9%), and imipenem (0.8%), respectively. However, the frequency of resistance to ciprofloxacin was found to be 55.6%. High prevalence of MDR (77.8%) and extended-spectrum β-lactamase (ESBL) (54.8%) were substantial. PCR results revealed the frequency of virulence genes ranged from 0 to 99.2%. Among 9 evaluated genes, the frequency of 4 genes (*fimH*, *sfa*, *iutA*, and PAI marker) was > 50% among all the screened isolates. The *iutA*, *pap GII*, and *hlyA* genes were more detected in the urosepsis isolates with significantly different frequencies. The different combinations of virulence genes were characterized as urovirulence patterns. The isolates recovered from pyelonephritis, cystitis, and urosepsis cases revealed 27, 22, and 6 virulence patterns, respectively. A significant difference was determined between ESBL production with *pap GII*, *iutA*, and PAI marker genes.

Conclusions: Our study highlighted the MDR UPEC with high heterogeneity of urovirulence genes. Considering the high rate of ciprofloxacin resistance, alternative drugs and monitoring of the susceptibility profile for UPECs are recommended.

Keywords: *Escherichia coli*, Urinary tract infections, Antimicrobial resistance, Virulence genes

* Correspondence: re.khashei@gmail.com; khasheir@sums.ac.ir
[1]Department of Bacteriology and Virology, School of Medicine, Shiraz University of Medical Sciences, Shiraz, Iran
Full list of author information is available at the end of the article

Background

Urinary tract infections (UTIs) are the most frequent human infections occurring to people of all ages, which cause morbidity and significant mortality globally [1, 2]. UTIs are mostly (70–90%) caused by the uropathogenic *Escherichia coli* (UPEC), one of the extraintestinal pathogenic *E. coli* pathotypes (ExPEC) [1, 3]. UPEC strains account for up to 90% of community-acquired UTIs and 50% of nosocomial UTIs [4]. UPEC strains usually carry a series of virulence markers, including adhesins, toxins and iron uptake systems (siderophores) that enable them to invade, colonize, and survive in the urinary tract, and prevent them from removal during urination [1, 4, 5]. Indeed, it is suggested that UPEC isolates usually harbor the largest number of pathogenicity-associated islands (PAIs) encoding a variety of virulence determinants involved in adhesion, invasion, and bacterial resistance to host defense and consequently influencing the pathogenicity of symptomatic or complicated UTIs [6, 7]. Initially, UPECs colonize the bladder and cause cystitis. Then, in an ascending manner would be able to move to the kidney, causing an acute pyelonephritis or disseminates to the blood leading to urosepsis [4, 6].

On the other hand, increasing antimicrobial resistance among UPEC isolates has been increasing dramatically and has turned out to be a serious health concern. The issue is mainly due to the emergence of multidrug-resistant (MDR) strains which contain genes encoding extended-spectrum β-lactamase (ESBLs) and resistance to sulfamethoxazole-trimethoprim (SXT) and fluoroquinolones [4]. UTIs caused by ESBL-producing UPEC strains are associated with prolonged hospitalization and hygiene cost [8]. The rate of MDR-UPEC strains in developed and developing countries is variable and in Iran as a developing country, has been estimated as 49.4% [9]. Given the increased resistance to the first line antimicrobial agents used in empiric therapy, UTI treatment in clinical practice has become somehow challenging. Indeed, the study of urovirulence genes and antimicrobial resistance can serve as a key element in developing new therapeutic targets. These factors can influence and be utilized as a useful marker to predict the clinical outcomes of UTIs caused by UPECs. There have been limited published epidemiologic studies on virulence genes and antimicrobial resistance among the UPECs isolated from symptomatic patients with UTI in Iran, hence, the present study aimed to evaluate the important characteristics of UPEC isolates, as well as investigate the correlation between the urovirulence genes and the type of clinical disease or antibiotic resistance from Shiraz, Iran.

Methods

Study population and bacterial isolates

A total of 126 non-repetitive *E. coli* isolates (one per patient) were obtained from inpatients who presented with symptomatic UTI at 3 teaching tertiary care hospitals (Nemazee, Faghihi and Dastgheib) in Shiraz, southwest of Iran, over a period ranging from April to August 2016. The study was approved by the Ethics Committee of Shiraz University of Medical Sciences (EC IR.SUMS.REC.1395.S77). The samples were collected as clean-catch midstream urine from the studied participants. UTI was defined as the presence of a positive urine culture (≥ 10^5 colony-forming units [CFU]/mL) and pyuria (≥10^4 leukocyte/mL of urine).

UPEC isolates were divided into three groups: 1) isolates associated with pyelonephritis ($n = 73$, 58%), 2) isolates associated with cystitis ($n = 42$, 33.3%), and 3) isolates related to urosepsis ($n = 11$, 8.7%). Fever, dysuria, urgent voiding, flank pain, nausea and vomiting are the characteristic symptoms of acute pyelonephritis. Cystitis was characterized by urinary frequency, internal dysuria and suprapubic or pelvic pain, whereas urosepsis was identified clinically by fever, tachycardia, tachypnea, and respiratory alkalosis. The isolation and identification *E. coli* strains were performed by standard microbiological and biochemical tests [10]. Confirmed *E. coli* isolates were kept frozen in tryptic soy broth (Merck Co., Germany) containing 20% glycerol (Merck KGaA, Germany) at − 70 °C until further experiments.

Antimicrobial susceptibility testing

Antibiotic susceptibility of all isolates to ampicillin, ceftazidime, cefoxitin, gentamicin, amikacin, ciprofloxacin, sulfamethoxazole-trimethoprim (SXT or Co-trimoxazole), nalidixic acid, nitrofurantoin, and imipenem (Mast Co., UK) was carried out on Muller- Hinton agar (Oxoid Co., UK) using the disk diffusion method, as recommended by the Clinical and Laboratory Standards Institute (CLSI) [11]. *E. coli* ATCC 25922 was used as the quality control strain for antibacterial susceptibility testing. The isolates non-susceptible to ≥1 agent in ≥3 different antimicrobial categories were considered as MDR [12]. Moreover, the MIC (minimum inhibitory concentration) values of ciprofloxacin (as the most common antibiotic prescribed by clinicians in our region) were determined using the Epsilometer test (E-test). The test was performed with E-test strips (Liofilchem s.r.l., Roseto degli Abruzzi, Italy) as described by CLSI [11]. The isolates with MIC values ≤1, and ≥ 4 µg/mL were considered as susceptible, and resistant, respectively. Based on the antibiotic-susceptibility test results, the presence of resistance to both ciprofloxacin and nalidixic acid, indicates the isolates are marked as high-level quinolone-resistant bacteria, whereas nalidixic acid-resistant or intermediate isolates and ciprofloxacin-susceptible isolates are referred to as low level quinolone-resistant bacteria [13].

Phenotypic detection of ESBL

Ceftazidime (as a third-generation cephalosporin) resistant isolates were selected for the ESBL test. ESBL-producing UPEC isolates were detected by the combined disk method using the ceftazidime-clavulanic acid (30/10 μg) disk. According to the CLSI guidelines, an increase of ≥5 mm in the diameter of the inhibition zones around disks containing clavulanic acid as compared to the inhibition zones around disks free of clavulanic acid indicated as ESBL producers [11]. *E. coli* ATCC 25922 and *Klebsiella pneumoniae* ATCC 700603 were used as negative and positive control strains, respectively.

DNA extraction and virulence genotyping

Genomic DNA was extracted from all UPEC isolates using the Cinna-pure kit (CinnaGen Co., Iran) according to manufacturer's instructions and subjected to polymerase chain reaction (PCR) after evaluating determining concentration and quality by measuring absorbance of A_{260} and A_{280} nm using a spectrophotometer and agarose gel electrophoresis, respectively. Isolated DNA was stored in Tris-EDTA buffer at -20 °C until required for assays.

UPEC isolates were investigated for 9 virulence genes. The targeted genes and nucleotide sequences of the oligonucleotide primers used in this study were chosen as described elsewhere [14]. Simplex PCR was used to determine the presence of 9 virulence factors related to adhesion [*pap GI-III* alleles (P-fimbriae or pilus associated with pyelonephritis), *fimH* (type-1 fimbriae), *sfa* (S-fimbriae), *afa* (afimbrial adhesin)], toxins [*hlyA* (hemolysin)], siderophores [*iutA*], and PAI markers. Band sizes of the above-mentioned genes were 461, 190, 258, 508, 240, 559, 1177, 300, and 930 bp, respectively [14].

Amplification of DNA was performed using thermal cycler 5530 (Ependrof master, Germany), in a total volume of 25 μL, containing 3 μL DNA template, 2.5 μL PCR buffer (1X), 1 μL deoxyribonucleotide triphosphates solution (dNTPs, 200 μM), 1.5 μL MgCl₂ (1.5 mM), 0.25 μL Taq DNA polymerase (1 Unit) and 1 μL of each specific primer (1 μM). The cycling conditions were set up as follows: 5 min at 94 °C as initial denaturation, 30 cycles of denaturation at 94 °C for 45 s, annealing (the temperature was depended on the primer sequence), extension at 72 °C for 1 min, and final extension at 72 °C for 10 min. All the reagents were obtained from Ampliqon Co., Denmark. Electrophoresis of amplicons was performed using 1.5% agarose gels, run in 1x Tris-acetate-EDTA buffer for 1 h in a horizontal electrophoresis system at 95 V. Gels were stained with safe

stain load dye (CinnaGen Co., Iran) and visualized through UV transillumination.

DNA sequence analysis

To confirm the accuracy of amplified gene of *afa* (two samples), the amplicons were submitted for sequencing (Bioneer Co., Munpyeongseoro, Daedeok-gu, Daejeon, South Korea) and the sequences were compared using online BLAST software (http://www.ncbi.nlm.nih.gov/BLAST/) (Additional file 1). For the rest of genes, *E. coli* ATCC 25922 was used as control strain.

Data analysis

The Chi-square (χ^2) test was performed to analyze significant differences between the studied virulence genes with clinical outcomes or antimicrobial resistance, using SPSS (ver. 21.0; IBM Co., Armonk, NY, USA) software. The results of demographic and clinical manifestations were presented as descriptive statistics in terms of relative frequency. P value < 0.05 was considered to be significant.

Results
Subject characteristics

The recruited patients in our study were 50 females and 76 males aged from 1 to 100 years old with a mean age of 48.9 ± 28.8 years. There was no statistically significant difference in age and gender of subjects within the three studied disease groups. The recovered UPEC isolates from different wards were as follows: Intensive Care Unit or ICU ($n = 76$, 60.4%), Internal wards ($n = 36$, 28.6%), Surgery ($n = 7$, 5.6%), and Transplantation ($n = 7$, 5.6%). Moreover, the frequencies of cases in different wards were as follows: cystitis (ICU = 23, Internal ward = 12, Surgery = 2, Transplantation = 5), pyelonephritis (ICU = 44, Internal ward = 22, Surgery = 5, Transplantation = 2) and urosepsis (ICU = 9, Internal ward = 2, Surgery = 0, Transplantation = 0).

Distribution of virulence genes

Frequency of the studied virulence genes among clinical groups is depicted in Table 1. Overall, 14.3% (18/126) of the UPEC isolates examined were positive for at least two of virulence markers. No significant difference was observed between virulence genes and isolates from different wards (data not shown). The frequency of only 4 genes (*fimH*, *sfa*, *iutA*, and PAI marker) was $> 50\%$ among all the isolates examined. The majority of virulence genes were determined in different proportions among the three clinical groups (Table 1). Among adhesins, the most prevalent gene in all groups was *fimH* (99.2%), followed by *sfa* (79.4%), and *pap GII* and *afa* were found 46%, equally. Neither *pap GI* nor *GIII* gene was detected among all of the clinical isolates. The *iutA*,

Table 1 Distribution of virulence genes among different clinical diseases

Genes	Cystitis No. (%)	Pyelonephritis No. (%)	Urosepsis No. (%)
fimH	41 (97.6)	73 (100)	11 (100)
PAI	36 (85.7)	61 (83.6)	11 (100)
sfa	33 (78.6)	58 (79.5)	9 (81.8)
iutA[a]	24 (57.1)	52 (71.2)	10 (90.9)
pap GII[b]	15 (35.7)	34 (46.6)	9 (81.8)
afa	19 (45.2)	36 (49.3)	3 (27.3)
hlyA[b]	10 (23.8)	19 (26)	7 (63.6)

[a]The presence of this gene among urosepsis isolates was significantly higher than cystitis isolates (P < 0.05)
[b]The presence of this gene among urosepsis isolates was significantly higher than cystitis and pyelonephritis isolates (P < 0.05)
Abbreviations: fimH = type-1 fimbriae, PAI = pathogenicity-associated island, sfa = S-fimbriae, iutA = iron uptake transfer (ferric aerobactin receptor), pap = pilus associated with pyelonephritis, afa = afimbrial adhesion, hlyA = hemolysin

pap GII, and hlyA genes were found essentially in urosepsis isolates with significantly different (P < 0.05) frequencies (Table 1). As shown in Table 1, among the clinical diseases, UPEC isolates recovered from urosepsis cases had the highest rate of designated genes. As for the distribution of the virulence genes, the isolates exhibited 35 distinct arrangements of virulence patterns, referred to as UPEC followed by an Arabic numeral (Table 2). The isolates recovered from pyelonephritis, cystitis, and urosepsis cases showed 27, 22, and 6 virulence patterns, respectively (Table 2). UPEC 1 was the most frequent pattern (16.7%), with the presence of iutA-fimH-PAI-sfa-afa virulence genes.

Antimicrobial resistance among UPEC isolates

The highest resistance rate was observed against ampicillin (88.9%), followed by nalidixic acid (81%), sulfamethoxazole-trimethoprim (72.2%), ceftazidime (65.1%), ciprofloxacin (55.6%), cefoxitin (20.6%), gentamicin (19.8%), amikacin (7.9%), nitrofurantoin (4.8%), and imipenem (0.8%). The majority of isolates (n = 98, 77.8%) were MDR with predominant patterns for ampicillin, sulfamethoxazole-trimethoprim, nalidixic acid, ceftazidime, ciprofloxacin (15.1%), followed by ampicillin, sulfamethoxazole-trimethoprim, nalidixic acid, and ceftazidime with the frequency of 11.1%. Antibiotic susceptibility patterns were different depending on the place recovery of isolates. The frequencies of MDR isolates from ICU, Internal, Surgery, and Transplantation wards were 81.6, 69.4, 71.4, and 85.7%, respectively. Moreover, the isolates from urosepsis cases were more resistant than those recovered from cystitis and pyelonephiritis cases (81.8% vs. 78.6, and 76.7%, respectively, P > 0.05). Analysis of antibiotic resistance in terms of the gender and age of participants revealed no statistically significant differences among them (P = 0.82).

Relationship between the distribution of virulence genes and resistance to multiple drugs was also investigated. Among the studied genes, 100 and 78.6% of UPEC isolates harboring fimH and sfa were MDR, respectively. On the other hand, 60.7, 53.6, and 60.7% of the isolates carrying iutA, pap GII, and hlyA found to be susceptible to antimicrobial agents, respectively (data not shown). Further analysis revealed that the rate of ESBL-producing isolates was 54.8% (69/126). There was a significant correlation (P < 0.05) between ESBL-producing isolates and antibiotic resistance to all the antibiotics tested, except for amikacin, nitrofurantoin, and imipenem (Table 3). A significant difference was also observed between ESBL production and MDR positive isolates (97.1% ESBL producers vs. 54.4% non-ESBL producers, P < 0.001). Among the seven evaluated genes, a statistically significant difference was determined between ESBL production with pap GII, iutA, and PAI marker genes, and ESBL-negative isolates with afa gene (Table 4).

According to disk diffusion results, 60 (47.6%) isolates were high-level quinolone-resistant bacteria with ciprofloxacin MIC ≥6 µg/mL, while 42 (33.3%) isolates were identified as low level quinolone-resistant bacteria (MIC ≤1). In overall, the MIC range of all 70 ciprofloxacin-resistant isolates was between 6 and > 32 µg/mL, and both MIC_{50} and MIC_{90} were estimated > 32 µg/mL.

Discussion

A better knowledge of the virulence markers of UPEC strains, especially in hospitalized patients allows the physicians to follow up the trend of pathogenicity of strains causing the urinary tract infections. The studied samples in the present investigation were originated from 126 inpatients with pyelonephritis, cystitis and urosepsis, which were evaluated for the presence of nine urovirulence genes and their corresponding antibiotic susceptibility patterns.

Genes encoding adhesins are the most frequently occurring virulence factors in UPECs [15]. Fimbriae are important to establish the UTI and probably in the progression to urosepsis [16]. It is suggested that type 1 and P fimbriae are common among cystitis and pyelonephritis-associated UPEC strains, respectively [5]. As we expected, in our study almost all the isolates (99.2%) carried the fimH gene, encoding of the type 1 fimbriae, consistent with some previous reports [1, 5, 7, 17, 18]. Conversely, in a recent study from Mexico, the prevalence of fimH was reported 61.3% [15], which was in agreement with some other published data [19, 20]. Recently, in an investigation on 183 UPEC isolates [5], the fimH was found to be associated with cystitis cases, but in the current work no correlation was

Table 2 Virulence patterns identified among UPEC isolates

Type No.	Virulence pattern	Total		Pyelonephritis		Cystitis		Urosepsis	
		No.	%	No.	%	No.	%	No.	%
UPEC1	*iutA-fimH-PAI-sfa-afa*	21	16.7	9	12.3	10	23.8	2	18.2
UPEC2	*papGII-iutA-fimH-PAI-hlyA-sfa-afa*	11	8.7	7	9.6	1	2.4	3	27.3
UPEC3	*papGII-iutA-fimH-PAI-hlyA-sfa*	11	8.7	4	5.5	4	9.5	3	27.3
UPEC4	*iutA-fimH-PAI-sfa*	9	7.1	6	8.2	3	7.1	0	0
UPEC5	*papGII-iutA-fimH-PAI-sfa-afa*	9	7.1	6	8.2	3	7.1	0	0
UPEC6	*fimH-sfa*	8	6.3	6	8.2	2	4.8	0	0
UPEC7	*papGII-iutA-fimH-PAI-sfa*	6	4.8	5	6.8	0	0	1	9.1
UPEC8	*fimH-PAI*	4	3.2	1	1.4	3	7.1	0	0
UPEC9	*iutA-fimH-PAI*	4	3.2	4	5.5	0	0	0	0
UPEC10	*fimH-PAI-sfa*	3	2.4	2	2.7	1	2.4	0	0
UPEC11	*papGII-iutA-fimH-PAI*	3	2.4	2	2.7	0	0	1	9.1
UPEC12	*iutA-fimH-PAI-afa*	3	2.4	2	2.7	1	2.4	0	0
UPEC13	*fimH-PAI-hlyA-sfa*	3	2.4	2	2.7	1	2.4	0	0
UPEC14	*papGII-fimH-PAI-sfa-afa*	3	2.4	1	1.4	2	4.8	0	0
UPEC15	*papGII-fimH*	2	1.6	2	2.7	0	0	0	0
UPEC16	*fimH-afa*	2	1.6	1	1.4	1	2.4	0	0
UPEC17	*papGII-fimH-sfa*	2	1.6	1	1.4	1	2.4	0	0
UPEC18	*iutA-fimH-sfa*	2	1.6	1	1.4	1	2.4	0	0
UPEC19	*papGII-fimH-PAI-sfa*	2	1.6	1	1.4	1	2.4	0	0
UPEC20	*papGII-fimH-PAI-hlyA-sfa*	2	1.6	2	2.7	0	0	0	0
UPEC21	*iutA-fimH-PAI-hlyA-sfa*	2	1.6	2	2.7	0	0	0	0
UPEC22	*iutA-fimH*	1	0.8	1	1.4	0	0	0	0
UPEC23	*fimH-hlyA*	1	0.8	0	0	1	2.4	0	0
UPEC24	*papGII-fimH-PAI*	1	0.8	0	0	1	2.4	0	0
UPEC25	*fimH-PAI-afa*	1	0.8	0	0	1	2.4	0	0
UPEC26	PAI-*sfa-afa*	1	0.8	0	0	1	2.4	0	0
UPEC27	*papGII-fimH-PAI-afa*	1	0.8	0	0	1	2.4	0	0
UPEC28	*iutA-fimH-PAI-hlyA*	1	0.8	1	1.4	0	0	0	0
UPEC29	*fimH-PAI-sfa-afa*	1	0.8	1	1.4	0	0	0	0
UPEC30	*papGII-iutA-fimH-PAI-afa*	1	0.8	1	1.4	0	0	0	0
UPEC31	*papGII-iutA-fimH-sfa-afa*	1	0.8	1	1.4	0	0	0	0
UPEC32	*papGII-fimH-PAI-hlyA-afa*	1	0.8	0	0	0	0	1	9.1
UPEC33	*fimH-PAI-hlyA-sfa-afa*	1	0.8	0	0	1	2.4	0	0
UPEC34	*papGII-iutA-fimH-PAI-hlyA-afa*	1	0.8	1	1.4	0	0	0	0
UPEC35	*iutA-fimH-PAI-hlyA-sfa-afa*	1	0.8	0	0	1	2.4	0	0

Abbreviations: *UPEC* = Uropathogenic *Escherichia coli*, *pap* = pilus associated with pyelonephritis, *iutA* = iron uptake transfer (ferric aerobactin receptor), *fimH* = type-1 fimbriae, *PAI* = pathogenicity-associated island, *hlyA* = hemolysin, *sfa* = S-fimbriae, *afa* = afimbrial adhesion

found with clinical manifestations. The *sfa* was the second most prevalent adhesion gene (79.4%) in our isolates, consistent with a study conducted in South Korea with frequency of 100% [1]. On the contrary, in some reports the prevalence of less than 50% [7, 21, 22] or even 0% [23] was cited for this gene. Although the exact role of S-fimbriae is not identified; however, the dissemination of bacterium within the host tissue is suggested for this adhesin [1]. In the present study, the frequency of *pap GII* and *afa* were found to be 46%. It was reported that class II *pap G* allele is related to pyelonephritis cases, while *pap GIII* is primarily associated with UTIs in dogs and cats [18], which is in agreement with our findings. In two studies from South Korea and China [7, 18], no *pap GI* gene

Table 3 Distribution of antibiotic resistant UPEC isolates according to ESBL production

Antibiotic	ESBL-negative Resistant No. (%)	ESBL-positive Resistant No. (%)	P value
Co-trimoxazole	36 (63.2)	55 (79.7)	0.039
Ampicillin	43 (75.4)	69 (100)	< 0.001
Nalidixic acid	35 (61.4)	67 (97.1)	< 0.001
Amikacin	2 (3.5)	8 (11.6)	0.095
Nitrofurantoin	2 (3.5)	4 (5.8)	0.54
Ceftazidime	13 (22.8)	69 (100)	< 0.001
Imipenem	0	1 (1.4)	0.36
Gentamicin	5 (8.8)	20 (29)	0.005
Ciprofloxacin	25 (43.9)	45 (65.2)	0.016
Cefoxitin	17 (29.8)	9 (13)	0.021

Abbreviations: *UPEC* = Uropathogenic *Escherichia coli*, *ESBL* = extended-spectrum β- lactamase

was identified in their isolates, similar to our findings, either. Indeed, it has been suggested that there is a possibility of mutation at the level of a specific gene, resulting in the absence of the corresponding gene in PCR method [19]. The role of *afa* afimbrial adhesin is mentioned in the development of chronic nephritis [19]. Our findings revealed that 49.3% of isolates from pyelonephritis cases were *afa* PCR-positive which is higher than those reported by other investigators [1, 15, 17–19, 22–24]. This discrepancy could be due to differences in type disease (symptomatic or asymptomatic bacteriuria) or geographic region.

The second most common gene in this study was found to be PAI marker (85.7%). The determinants such as toxins, siderophores, and protectins are encoded on UPEC PAIs [15]. This frequency was higher than those previously reported for UPEC

Table 4 Distribution of virulence genes among UPEC isolates according to ESBL production

Gene	ESBL-negative Positive No. (%)	ESBL-positive	P value
pap GII	20 (35.1)	38 (55.1)	0.03
iutA	31 (54.4)	55 (79.7)	0.004
fimH	56 (98.2)	69 (100)	0.45
PAI	42 (73.7)	66 (95.7)	0.001
hlyA	15 (26.3)	21 (30.4)	0.69
sfa	42 (73.7)	58 (84.1)	0.19
afa	35 (61.4)	23 (33.3)	0.002

Abbreviations: *UPEC* = Uropathogenic *Escherichia coli*, *ESBL* = extended-spectrum β- lactamase, *pap* = pilus associated with pyelonephritis, *iutA* = iron uptake transfer (ferric aerobactin receptor), *fimH* = type-1 fimbriae, *PAI* = pathogenicity-associated island, *hlyA* = hemolysin, *sfa* = S-fimbriae, *afa* = afimbrial adhesin)

isolates [15, 23, 24], but lower than that reported in other studies from Iran [25–27].

The *iutA* as a siderophore marker donates the potency of resistance against serum killing to the UPEC strains, thereby enabling them to persist in body fluids such as the blood [24]. The attributed characteristic is important for the pathogenesis of isolates causing urosepsis. As indicated by present findings, 90.9% of UPEC were carrying the *iutA* gene, suggesting the isolates are invasive and a significant association between this gene and clinical groups. According to the obtained data, the frequency in the current study was higher than those previously reported [7, 15], indicating the genes codifying siderophore vary depending on geographic areas and hosts [15]. However, of the three clinical complications, isolates recovered from urosepsis cases had the highest frequency among the studied genes.

The *hlyA* toxin is involved in tissue damage and impairment of local immune responses [19]. There was a significant association between *hlyA* gene and urosepsis isolates, which is consistent with invasive nature of UPECs isolated from urosepsis cases. Our results (28.6%) are in agreement with those found by other studies [7, 19, 28].

On the other hand, in the present investigation, 35 patterns of combinations of the urovirulence markers were characterized. The UPEC 1 pattern with *iutA--fimH*-PAI-*sfa*-*afa* template was the most frequently present. According to different geographic regions and disease status, different patterns of combinations of the virulence genes and antimicrobial resistance phenotypes have been reported in previous studies [7, 15, 23].

According to our data, all UPECs contained at least two virulence genes. This is in contrast to Oliveira et al. [24], who reported 90% UPECs showed at least one of the eight virulence genes. It was shown in a study [19], that UPECs isolated from hospitalized patients offered a great diversity of gene associations, in agreement with our data, indicating heterogeneity in the distribution of virulence genes among UPEC strains in different regions [24].

Increased antibiotic resistance, particularly for third-generation cephalosporins and fluoroquinolones among UPEC isolates has created challenges in clinical practice [29]. Majority of our isolates were remarkably resistant to the most of the tested antibiotics, with 77.8% of strains showing multi-drug resistance, making them the causative agent of an important health problem in our area, in agreement with previous works from different regions [15, 20, 25, 30]. As empirical antimicrobial therapy is usually the first conventional treatment for UTIs, awareness of the local epidemiological data for an efficient therapy is necessary and useful [31]. According to our investigation, 88.9, 81, 72.2, and 55.6%

isolates were resistant to ampicillin, nalidixic acid, sulfamethoxazole-trimethoprim, and ciprofloxacin, respectively, the therapeutic agents used as the first-line empirical treatments for UTIs [24, 32]. Ciprofloxacin is the most common fluroquinolone used to treat UTIs. However, due to its overuse in the last decade, the resistance rate of UPECs to that antibiotic has markedly increased [33]. In comparison to other studies from different countries [18, 20, 24, 28], our rate (55.6%) is high, but it is consistent with another investigation from Iran with frequency of 61.3% [30]. Our findings regarding the MIC study of ciprofloxacin showed that the MIC_{50} and MIC_{90} ranges are higher than their corresponding maximum values in the E-test strip (32 μg/mL). The MIC values of clinical isolates vary based on geographic area and time. In a study from Algeria [28], ciprofloxacin MIC range was mentioned between 0.5 to >128 μg/mL. It seems that in a clinical setting, we cannot surmount this level of resistance even by using the manifold dosages of MIC_{50} and MIC_{90} values. One explanation for our observed high rate in our region could be the wide use of antibiotics for bacterial infections, for example prescription of ciprofloxacin by clinicians in the first visit of patients with uncomplicated UTIs.

Similar to the other studies from Iran and other countries [1, 18, 20, 34, 35], the majority of isolates in the present study were susceptible to imipenem (99.2%) and nitrofurantoin (95.2%). Because of the emergence of antibiotic resistance in Gram-negative rods, imipenem is not preferably included in the first line therapy of UTIs and is recommended as a choice agent for only ESBL-producers [28, 32]. Additionally, in spite of good activity of nitrofurantoin against UPEC isolates, but due to numerous side effects, its application is limited. Nevertheless, because of increasing resistance rate of UPEC strains to sulfamethoxazole-trimethoprim and quinolones, rational use of nitrofurantoin has been recommended again for the re-infection prophylaxis of recurrent non complicated UTIs [36, 37].

Appropriate diagnosis and treatment of UTIs caused by ESBL-producing phenotypes is important for the prevention of long-term clinical outcomes [8]. One of our major concerns is about the observed high rates of MDR among UPEC ESBL-producers (97.1%). The data from a multi-centric study revealed that the rates of UPEC ESBL-producers among Iranian isolates were 42, and 44% of isolates which were MDR [38]. In the present study, the rate of ESBL-positive isolates was 54.8%, which was similar to some other studies [18, 34]. In contrary, in three studies from Iran a range of 22.3–35.7% was observed for UPEC ESBL-producers [20, 39, 40]. Such discrepancies might be due to the differences in epidemiology of isolates or sample size of studies.

Conclusion

In summary, our data point out the battery of multi-drug resistance and genetic heterogeneity among UPEC isolates from southwest of Iran. Moreover, it can be suggested that antibiotic resistance is associated with the isolates harboring certain urovirulence genes, such as *sfa* or the presence of *iutA, pap GII* and PAI marker in ESBL-producers. Taking into account the results, it seems that ciprofloxacin could not be used in empiric antibiotic treatment and the alternative drugs such as cefoxitin and for cystitis cases, nitrofurantoin might be choice options. Taken together, our findings support the importance of some urovirulence genes (e.g., *iutA, pap GII* and *hlyA*) as a marker for developing of symptomatic UTIs. To our knowledge, the present work is the first study in Iran that characterizes the several urovirulence genes in different disease groups and warrants further intensive studies.

Abbreviations
afa: Afimbrial adhesion; ATCC: American type culture collection; CFU: Colony-forming units; CLSI: Clinical and laboratory standards institute; ESBL: Extended-spectrum β-lactamase; E-test: Epsilometer test; ExPEC: Extraintestinal pathogenic *E. coli*; *hlyA*: Hemolysin; MDR: Multidrug resistant; MIC: Minimum inhibitory concentration; PAIs: Pathogenicity-associated islands; *pap*: P-fimbriae or pilus associated with pyelonephritis; PCR: Polymerase chain reaction; *sfa*: S-fimbriae; SXT: Sulfamethoxazole-trimethoprim; UPEC: Uropathogenic *Escherichia coli*; UTI: Urinary tract infection

Acknowledgements
This work is extracted from M.Sc thesis of Mrs. Malekzadegan in partial fulfillment of the requirements for the Medical Microbiology Master's degree.

Funding
This study was supported by Shiraz University of Medical Sciences grant No. 94–9327.

Authors' contributions
YM and RK: conceived the study. YM, ZJ: participated in the acquisition of data and sampling. YM, RK, ZJ, and HS: participated in the design of the study and performed the statistical analysis. YM and HS: interpreted the data. YM and RK: obtained ethical clearance and permission for study. RK and ZJ: Supervised data collectors. RK, YM, and HS: Drafting the article or revisiting it critically for important intellectual content. RK and YM were project leaders and primary investigators of the study. All authors read and approved the final manuscript.

Consent for publication
Not applicable.

Competing interests
The authors declare that they have no competing interests.

Author details
[1]Department of Bacteriology and Virology, School of Medicine, Shiraz University of Medical Sciences, Shiraz, Iran. [2]Department of Urology, School of Medicine, Shiraz University of Medical Sciences, Shiraz, Iran.

References

1. Lee JH, Subhadra B, Son YJ, Kim DH, Park HS, Kim JM, et al. Phylogenetic group distributions, virulence factors and antimicrobial resistance properties of uropathogenic *Escherichia coli* strains isolated from patients with urinary tract infections in South Korea. Lett Appl Microbiol. 2016;62:84–90. https://doi.org/10.1111/lam.12517.

2. Lai YM, Zaw MT, Shamsudin SB, Lin Z. Evaluation of PAIusp subtyping to characterize uropathogenic *E. coli* isolates. J Infect Dev Ctries. 2016;10:1053–8. https://doi.org/10.3855/jidc.6944.

3. Morales-Espinosa R, Hernandez-Castro R, Delgado G, Mendez JL, Navarro A, Manjarrez A, et al. UPEC strain characterization isolated from Mexican patients with recurrenturinary infections. J Infect Dev Ctries. 2016;10:317–28. https://doi.org/10.3855/jidc.6652.

4. Singh SK, Seema K, Gupta M. Detection of AmpC b-lactamase and adherence factors in uropathogenic *Escherichia coli* isolated from aged patients. Microb Pathog. 2016;100:293–8. https://doi.org/10.1016/j.micpath.2016.10.010.

5. Gao Q, Zhang D, Ye Z, Zhu X, Yang W, Dong L, et al. Virulence traits and pathogenicity of uropathogenic *Escherichia coli* isolates with common and uncommon O serotypes. Microb Pathog. 2017;104:217–24. https://doi.org/10.1016/j.micpath.2017.01.027.

6. Alteri CJ, Mobley HL. Metabolism and fitness of urinary tract pathogens. Microbiol Spectr. 2015;3(3). https://doi.org/10.1128/microbiolspec.

7. Yun KW, Kim HY, Park HK, Kim W, Lim IS. Virulence factors of uropathogenic *Escherichia coli* of urinary tract infections and asymptomatic bacteriuria in children. J Microbiol Immunol Infect. 2014;47:455–61. https://doi.org/10.1016/j.jmii.2013.07.010.

8. Flokas ME, Detsis M, Ml A, Mylonakis E. Prevalence of ESBL-producing Enterobacteriaceae in paediatric urinary tract infections: a systematic review and meta-analysis. J Inf Secur. 2016;73:547–57. https://doi.org/10.1016/j.jinf.2016.07.014.

9. Hadifar S, Moghoofei M, Nematollahi S, Ramazanzadeh R, Sedighi M, Salehi-Abargouei A, et al. Epidemiology of multidrug resistant uropathogenic *Escherichia coli* in Iran: a systematic review and meta-analysis. Jpn J Infect Dis. 2017;70:19–25. https://doi.org/10.7883/yoken.JJID.2015.652.

10. Walker KE, Mahon CR, Lehman D, Manuselis G. Enterobacteriaceae. In: Mahon CR, Lehman D, Manuselis G, editors. Textbook of diagnostic microbiology. 5th ed. New York: W. B. Saunders Company; 2015. p. 420–54.

11. Wayne PA. Clinical and Laboratory Standards Institute (CLSI). Performance Standards for Antimicrobial Susceptibility Testing 2015; 25th informational supplement. M100-S25.

12. Magiorakos AP, Srinivasan A, Carey RB, Carmeli Y, Falagas ME, Giske CG, et al. Multidrug-resistant, extensively drug-resistant and pandrug-resistant bacteria: an international expert proposal for interim standard definitions for acquired resistance. Clin Microbiol Infect. 2012;18:268–81. https://doi.org/10.1111/j.1469-0691.2011.03570.x.

13. Oktem IM, Gulay Z, Bicmen M, Gur D. HITIT project study group. *qnrA* prevalence in extended-spectrum beta-lactamase-positive Enterobacteriaceae isolates from Turkey. Jpn J Infect Dis. 2008;61:13–7.

14. Chapman TA, Wu XY, Barchia I, Bettelheim KA, Driesen S, Trott D, et al. Comparison of virulence gene profiles of *Escherichia coli* strains isolated from healthy and diarrheic swine. Appl Environ Microbiol. 2006;72:4782–95.

15. Paniagua-Contreras GL, Monroy-Pérez E, Rodríguez-Moctezuma JR, Domínguez-Trejo P, Vaca-Paniagua F, Vaca S. Virulence factors, antibiotic resistance phenotypes and O-serogroups of *Escherichia coli* strains isolated from community-acquired urinary tract infection patients in Mexico. J Microbiol Immunol Infect. 2017;50:478–85. https://doi.org/10.1016/j.jmii.2015.08.005.

16. Narciso A, Nunes F, Amores T, Lito L, Melo-Cristino J, Duarte A. Persistence of uropathogenic *Escherichia coli* strains in the host for long periods of time: relationship between phylogenetic groups and virulence factors. Eur J Clin Microbiol Infect Dis. 2012;31:1211–7. https://doi.org/10.1007/s10096-011-1431-7.

17. Rahdar M, Rashki A, Miri HR, Rashki Ghalehnoo M. Detection of *pap, sfa, afa, foc*, and *fim* adhesin-encoding operons in uropathogenic *Escherichia coli* isolates collected from patients with urinary tract infection. Jundishapur J Microbiol. 2015;8:e22647. https://doi.org/10.5812/jjm.22647.

18. Qin X, Hu F, Wu S, Ye X, Zhu D, Zhang Y, et al. Comparison of adhesin genes and antimicrobial susceptibilities between uropathogenic and intestinal commensal *Escherichia coli* strains. PLoS One. 2013;8:e61169. https://doi.org/10.1371/journal.pone.0061169.

19. Tarchouna M, Ferjani A, Ben-Selma W, Boukadida J. Distribution of uropathogenic virulence genes in *Escherichia coli* isolated from patients with urinary tract infection. Int J Infect Dis. 2013;17:e450–3. https://doi.org/10.1016/j.ijid.2013.01.025.

20. Tabasi M, Asadi Karam MR, Habibi M, Yekaninejad MS, Bouzari S. Phenotypic assays to determine virulence factors of uropathogenic *Escherichia coli* (UPEC) isolates and their correlation with antibiotic resistance pattern. Osong Public Health Res Perspect. 2015;6:261–8. https://doi.org/10.1016/j.phrp.2015.08.002.

21. Mohajeri P, Khademi H, Ebrahimi R, Farahani A, Rezaei M. Frequency distribution of virulence factors in uropathogenic *Escherichia coli* isolated from Kermanshah in 2011-2012. Int J Appl Basic Med Res. 2014;4:111–6. https://doi.org/10.4103/2229-516X.136794.

22. Santo E, Macedo C, Marin JM. Virulence factors of uropathogenic *Escherichia coli* from a university hospital in Ribeirão Preto, São Paulo, Brazil. Rev Inst Med Trop Sao Paulo. 2006;48:185–8.

23. Firoozeh F, Saffari M, Neamati F, Zibaei M. Detection of virulence genes in *Escherichia coli* isolated from patients with cystitis and pyelonephritis. Int J Infect Dis. 2014;29:219–22. https://doi.org/10.1016/j.ijid.2014.03.1393.

24. Oliveira FA, Paludo KS, Arend LN, Farah SM, Pedrosa FO, Souza EM, et al. Virulence characteristics and antimicrobial susceptibility of uropathogenic *Escherichia coli* strains. Genet Mol Res. 2011;10:4114–25. https://doi.org/10.4238/2011.

25. Samei A, Haghi F, Zeighami H. Distribution of pathogenicity island markers in commensal and uropathogenic *Escherichia coli* isolates. Folia Microbiol (Praha). 2016;61:261–8. https://doi.org/10.1007/s12223-015-0433-8.

26. Firoozeh F, Soleimani-Moorchekhorti L, Zibaei M. Evaluation of pathogenicity islands in uropathogenic *Escherichia coli* isolated from patients with urinary catheters. J Infect Dev Ctries. 2017;11:557–62. https://doi.org/10.3855/jidc.8660.

27. Navidinia M, Najar Peerayeh S, Fallah F, Bakhshi B. Phylogenetic groups and pathogenicity island markers in *Escherichia coli* isolated from children. Jundishapur J Microbiol. 2013;6:e8362. https://doi.org/10.5812/jjm.8362.

28. Yahiaoui M, Robin F, Bakour R, Hamidi M, Bonnet R, Messai Y. Antibiotic resistance, virulence, and genetic background of community-acquired uropathogenic *Escherichia coli* from Algeria. Microb Drug Resist. 2015;21:516–26. https://doi.org/10.1089/mdr.2015.0045.

29. Chiu CC, Lin TC, Wu RX, Yang YS, Hsiao PJ, Lee Y, et al. Etiologies of community-onset urinary tract infections requiring hospitalization and antimicrobial susceptibilities of causative microorganisms. J Microbiol Immunol Infect. 2017;50:879–85. https://doi.org/10.1016/j.jmii.2016.08.008.

30. Neamati F, Firoozeh F, Saffari M, Zibaei M. Virulence genes and antimicrobial resistance pattern in uropathogenic *Escherichia coli* isolated from hospitalized patients in Kashan, Iran. Jundishapur J Microbiol. 2015;8:e17514. https://doi.org/10.5812/jjm.17514.

31. Tandogdu Z, Wagenlehner FM. Global epidemiology of urinary tract infections. Curr Opin Infect Dis. 2016;29:73–9. https://doi.org/10.1097/QCO.0000000000000228.

32. Stultz JS, Doern CD, Godbout E. Antibiotic resistance in pediatric urinary tract infections. Curr Infect Dis Rep. 2016;18:40.

33. Fasugba O, Gardner A, Mitchell BG, Mnatzaganian G. Ciprofloxacin resistance in community- and hospital-acquired *Escherichia coli* urinary tract infections: a systematic review and meta-analysis of observational studies. BMC Infect Dis. 2015;15:545. https://doi.org/10.1186/s12879-015-1282-4.

34. Haghighatpanah M, Mozaffari Nejad AS, Mojtahedi A, Amirmozafari N, Zeighami H. Detection of extended-spectrum β-lactamase (ESBL) and plasmid-borne *bla*CTX-M and *bla*TEM genes among clinical strains of *Escherichia coli* isolated from patients in the north of Iran. J Glob Antimicrob Resist. 2016;7:110–3. https://doi.org/10.1016/j.jgar.2016.08.005.

35. Farshad S, Japoni A, Hosseini M. Low distribution of integrons among multidrug resistant *E. coli* strains isolated from children with community-acquired urinary tract infections in shiraz, Iran. Pol J Microbiol. 2008;57:193–8.

36. Stock I. Nitrofurantoin--clinical relevance in uncomplicated urinary tract infections. Med Monatsschr Pharm. 2014;37:242–8.

37. El Sakka N, Gould IM. Role of old antimicrobial agents in the management of urinary tract infection. Expert Rev Clin Pharmacol. 2016;9:1047–56. https://doi.org/10.1080/17512433.2016.1189325.

38. Ramos NL, Dzung DT, Stopsack K, Jankó V, Pourshafie MR, Katouli M, et al. Characterisation of uropathogenic *Escherichia coli* from children with urinary tract infection in different countries. Eur J Clin Microbiol Infect Dis. 2011;30:1587–93. https://doi.org/10.1007/s10096-011-1264-4.

39. Asgharzadeh Kangachar S, Mojtahedi A. The presence of extended-spectrum β-lactamase as a risk factor for MDR in clinical isolation of *Escherichia coli*. Trop Biomed. 2017;34:1–12.

40. Ghadiri H, Vaez H, Razavi-Azarkhiavi K, Rezaee R, Haji-Noormohammadi M, Rahimi AA, et al. Prevalence and antibiotic susceptibility patterns of extended-spectrum ß-lactamase and metallo-ß-lactamase-producing uropathogenic *Escherichia coli* isolates. Lab Med. 2014;45:291–6. https://doi.org/10.1309/LMHEP4VQHEY2POOK.

Prevalence of antimicrobial resistant *Escherichia coli* from patients with suspected urinary tract infection in primary care, Denmark

Gloria Córdoba[1]* , Anne Holm[1], Frank Hansen[2], Anette M. Hammerum[2] and Lars Bjerrum[1]

Abstract

Background: *Escherichia coli* is the most common pathogen causing Urinary Tract Infections (UTI). Data from the current National Surveillance program in Denmark (DANMAP) may not accurately represent the prevalence of resistant *E. coli* in primary care, because only urine samples from complicated cases may be forwarded to the microbiological departments at hospitals for diagnostic examination. The aim of this study was to assess the prevalence of resistant *E. coli* to the most commonly used antimicrobial agents in primary care in a consecutive sample of patients from general practice.

Methods: Observational study carried out from December 2014 to December 2015. Thirty-nine general practices from The Capital Region of Denmark included adult patients with urinary tract symptoms and suspected UTI. All urine samples were sent to the central laboratory Statens Serum Institut (SSI). Significant bacteriuria was interpreted according to the European Urinalysis Standards. Susceptibility testing was performed and interpreted according to the European Committee on Antimicrobial Susceptibility Testing (EUCAST) standards.

Results: From the 39 general practices 505 patients were recruited. Completed data were obtained from 485 (96%) patients. According to the European Urinalysis Standards, 261 (54%) patients had positive bacteriuria. The most common uropathogen in patients with uncomplicated (uUTI) and complicated (cUTI) urinary tract infection was *E. coli* 105 (69%) and 76 (70%), respectively. Eighty-two (45%) of 181 *E. coli* isolates were resistant to at least one of the tested antibiotics and 50 out of 82 isolates were resistant to two or more antimicrobial agents. The highest resistance-rate was found against ampicillin 34% (95% CI 24;42) in uUTI and 36% (24;46) in cUTI. There were no differences in the distribution of resistance between uncomplicated and complicated cases. The prevalence of resistance was similar to the one reported in DANMAP 2014.

Conclusion: In *E. coli* from uUTI there is high resistance rates to antimicrobial agents commonly used in primary care. There was no difference in the distribution of resistant *E. coli* in suspected uUTI vs cUTI. In Denmark, data from the National Surveillance program DANMAP can guide the decision for choice of antibiotic in patients with suspected UTI seeking care in primary care.

Keywords: *E. coli*, Antibiotic resistance, Urinary tract infections

* Correspondence: gloriac@sund.ku.dk
[1]The Research Unit for General Practice and Section of General Practice, Department of Public Health, University of Copenhagen; Øster Farimagsgade 5, 1014 Copenhagen, Denmark
Full list of author information is available at the end of the article

Background

Antimicrobial resistance is one of the most important threats to human health [1]. Multiple surveillance programs have been launched worldwide to monitor the spread of resistant strains in community acquired and nosocomial infections [2, 3].

Urinary tract infection (UTI) is the second most common bacterial infection managed in primary care [4, 5] and *Escherichia coli* is the most common pathogen causing UTI [6, 7]. *E. coli* resistant to antibiotics is on the rise, with great variation across regions [8, 9].

Experts recommend [10, 11] that choice of antibiotics in patients with suspected complicated UTI should be based on the results of a urine culture and susceptibility test, while the choice of antibiotics in patients with suspected uncomplicated UTI should be based on up-to-date surveillance data of patients from primary care. Thus, prospective surveillance of resistant patterns of uropathogens isolated from all patients attending primary care is crucial for guiding first and second line antibiotic selection.

Previous studies have suggested a systematic bias in surveillance data because uncomplicated UTIs (uUTI) are underrepresented, leading to an overestimation of resistance rates in primary care [12, 13]. This is problematic because general practitioners (GPs) need an accurate knowledge of the prevalence of resistance to the most commonly used antibiotics in primary care in order to make an appropriate treatment decision (i.e. choosing the right antibiotic).

In Denmark, the DANMAP programme is used for surveillance of antimicrobial consumption and antimicrobial resistance in bacteria from animals, food and humans [2]. DANMAP reports the prevalence of resistance for bacteria from clinical samples analyzed at the departments of clinical microbiology in Denmark. Part of the urine samples analyzed at the microbiology departments come from general practice.

The inferred prevalence of resistant strains in primary care may suffer from selection bias as GPs may predominantly send urine samples to culture in patients with complicated UTI or treatment failure.

In this paper, we report the results of a study aiming to assess the prevalence of resistant *E. coli* to the most commonly used antimicrobial agents in Denmark in patients with suspected (both complicated and uncomplicated) UTI seeking care at primary care level.

Methods

Study design

Prospective observational study carried out from December 2014 to December 2015.

Participants

Five-hundred practices from The Capital Region of Denmark were randomly invited to participate. Thirty-nine practices accepted to consecutively recruit patients with the following characteristics: i.) inclusion criteria: Adult patients (i.e. > 18 years of age) seeking care in general practice during office hours with dysuria and/or urinary frequency as the main reason for consultation, and in which GPs suspected a UTI; ii.) exclusion criteria: a) Currently taking antibiotics, b) Inability to provide a urine sample, c) Inability to sign an informed consent, d) Previous participation in this study.

Data collection

The day of the index consultation, all patients provided 10 mL of urine, which was sent to Statens Serum Institut (SSI). The urine sample was preserved in boric acid and sent by certified post the same day of the consultation.

Culture and susceptibility testing at the reference laboratory

At SSI, the culture was analyzed by a medical laboratory scientist, who had no information about the clinical history of the patient. A positive culture was defined as growth of $\geq 10^3$ Colony Forming Unit per milliliter (CFU/mL) for *E. coli* according to the European Urinalysis Standards [14].

Aerobic urine culture was carried out with 1 μL on Blood agar plate and "Blue" agar plate (SSI Diagnostics; Hillerød, Denmark) and 100 μL on ESBL chromogenic culture media (Brilliance ESBL AGAR; Oxoid, UK).

ESBL plates were examined after one day of incubation and read according to the colour chart provided by the manufacturer. Phenotypic confirmation of ESBL production was performed by the Total ESBL Confirm Kit 98,014 (Rosco Diagnostics, Taastrup, Denmark).

Susceptibility testing was performed and interpreted according to EUCAST standards [15] on Mueller-Hinton agar plates using Neo-Sensitabs (Sulfamethoxazole, trimethoprim, ampicillin, amoxicillin-clavulanic acid, cefpodoxime, ciprofloxacin, nitrofurantoin and mecillinam (Rosco Diagnostics).

Data analysis

We considered UTI as uncomplicated if the patient was a non-pregnant woman, under 65-year old without reported co-morbidity and assessed by the nurse or GP as not having an acute complicated cystitis or suspected pyelonephritis. In contrast, we considered UTI as complicated if the patient was a man, a pregnant woman, a woman 65-year or older or with a reported co-morbidity or assessed by the nurse or GP to have complicated cystitis or pyelonephritis.

The proportions of susceptible and resistant *E. coli* isolates were compared between uncomplicated and complicated UTI. Proportion of resistant *E. coli* isolates in our study was compared to the proportion of resistant *E. coli* isolates from primary healthcare from the National surveillance program

DANMAP 2014. Significance of the differences between the independent samples were performed by using the Pearson's Chi-Square test (alpha 5%; CI 95%) and Fisher exact test when appropriate. Descriptive analyses were performed using SAS software, Version 9.3 of the SAS System for Windows 7.

Results
Baseline characteristics
From the 39 practices, 505 patients were recruited. There was completed information for 485 (96%) of the patients, from which 261 (54%) had positive bacteriuria. Of the 261 cases, 152 (58%) were classified as uncomplicated UTI and 109 as complicated UTI. The most common uropathogen in uncomplicated and complicated cases was *E. coli* 105 (69%) and 76 (70%), respectively - Fig. 1.

Antimicrobial resistance for *E. coli* isolates
Eighty-two (45%) of the 181 *E. coli* isolates were resistant to at least one of the tested antimicrobial agents. Fifty (28%) of the 181 *E. coli* isolates were resistant to more than one antimicrobial agent. The distribution of resistance for the tested antimicrobial agents was not significantly different for the uncomplicated and complicated cases - Fig. 2 and Additional file 1: Table S1.

The highest resistance rates were found for ampicillin: 34% (95% CI 24;42) of the *E. coli* from uncomplicated cases and 36% (95% CI 24;46) of the *E. coli* from complicated cases. It was followed by sulfamethoxazole: 31%, (95% CI 21;39) of the *E. coli* from uncomplicated cases and 24% (95% CI 14;33) of the *E. coli* from complicated cases. Resistance to pivmecillinam (first line antibiotic in Denmark) was 1% (95% CI 0;5) in *E. coli* from uUTI and 9% (95% CI 2;15)

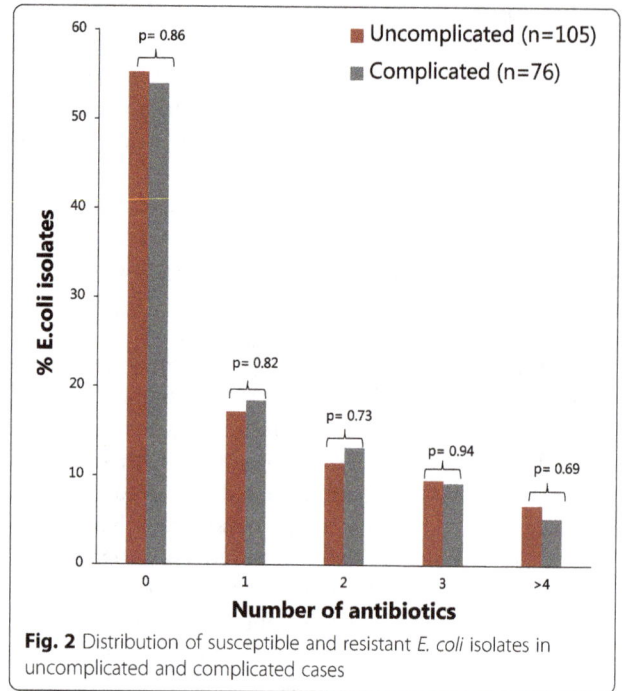

Fig. 2 Distribution of susceptible and resistant *E. coli* isolates in uncomplicated and complicated cases

from *E. coli* from cUTI. Resistance to third generation cephalosporins and clavulanate (i.e. ESBL-resistance test) was found in 6% (95% CI 1;10) of *E. coli* from uUTI and 3% (95% CI 0;9) of *E.coli* from cUTI. None of the tested *E. coli* isolates were resistant to nitrofurantoin – Table 1 and Additional file 1: Table S2.

The differences between the resistance rates of *E. coli* isolates from the study population and DANMAP 2014 were lower than 10% across all antibiotics, for which comparison was available. No single difference was statistically significant. – Table 2 and Additional file 1: Table S2.

Discussion
Summary of main finding
This study shows that in uncomplicated cases there was high resistance to antibiotics commonly used in primary

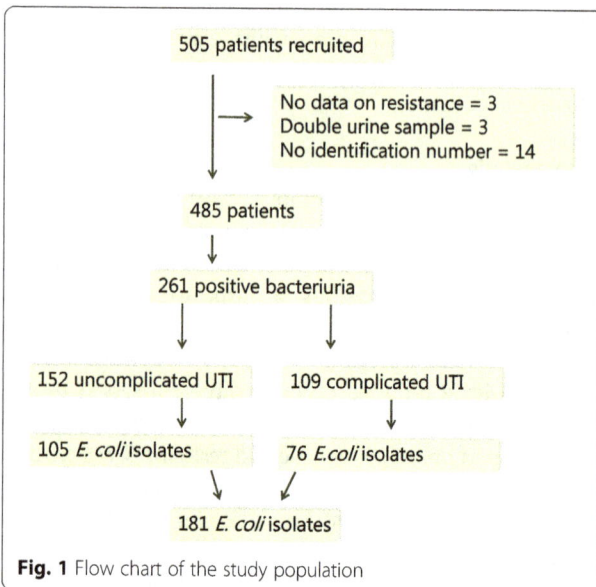

Fig. 1 Flow chart of the study population

Table 1 Resistance rates among *E. coli* isolates from patients seeking care in primary care

	Uncomplicated	Complicated
	n = 105	n = 76
Ampicillin	34% (24;42)	36% (24;46)
Sulfamethoxazole	31% (21;39)	24% (14;33)
Trimethoprim	23% (14;30)	17% (8;25)
Pivmecillinam	1% (0;5)	9% (2;15)
Ciprofloxacin	8% (2;12)	8%(1;14)
Nitrofurantoin	0	0
3rd gen. Cephalosporins + clavulanate[a]	6% (1;10)	3% (0;9)

[a]ESBL status tested with combinations of the third generation cephalosporins (Cefotaxime, Ceftazidime) and clavulanate

Table 2 Comparison of resistance rates for *E. coli* between the National Surveillance program DANMAP and our study

	DANMAP 2014	Our study[a]	*p*-value
Ampicillin	39%	34%	0.19
Sulfamethoxazole	32%	28%	0.2
Trimethoprim	N/A	20%	N/A
Pivmecillinam	5%	4%	0.74
Ciprofloxacin	9%	8%	0.5
Nitrofurantoin	N/A	0	N/A
3rd gen. Cephalosporins + clavulanate[b]	4%	4%	0.96

N/A no data from the National Surveillance program DANMAP 2014
[a]Uncomplicated and complicated cases
[b]ESBL- resistant *E. coli*

care in Denmark. There was no statistically and clinically significant difference in the distribution of resistant *E. coli*, in suspected uncomplicated vs complicated cases. Data from the National Surveillance program (DANMAP 2014) can be used to guide the selection of first and second line antibiotics to treat UTI in primary care in Denmark.

Strengths and limitations

The pragmatic design of the study enabled the inclusion of a wide variety of patients seeking care in primary care due to urinary tract symptoms, thus uncomplicated and complicated cases were equally likely to be included in the study. It maximized generalizability to the patient population seeking care in primary care settings in Denmark.

Furthermore, all patients had a urine culture interpreted at the same reference laboratory. The laboratory technician had no access to clinical data. It minimized the risk for review bias and inter-observer variability.

The main limitation of our study is the small sample size resulting in lack of power to counteract the type II error (i.e. accepting the null hypothesis of lack of difference, when there is a difference between the groups). Nonetheless, the results of this study should be interpreted considering clinically relevant differences rather than statistically significant differences.

For example, in DANMAP 2014 the resistance rate of *E. coli* isolates to Sulfamethoxazole was 32%, while in our study it was 28%. The difference between estimates was not statistically significant and is not clinically relevant too. The Infectious Disease Society of America (IDSA) recommends that resistance rates above 20% is the threshold at which sulfamethoxazole is no longer recommended for empirical treatment [10].

Another example is the lower percentage of *E.coli* isolates from the uUTI group resistant to pivmecillinam in comparison to the cUTI group. Due to the small sample size, we cannot rule out that the difference in the point estimate was caused by chance.

Another limitation was that we relied on GPs judgment as part of the operationalization of the uncomplicated versus complicated variable. Thus, we cannot rule out that some patients may have been miss-classified as having uncomplicated UTI by their GP. Currently, there is no agreement about the criteria of classifying a patient as a uUTI or cUTI [16]. We chose to take into consideration the GPs' assessment because it reflects more accurately the challenges for classifying patients as uUTI and cUTI during everyday practice.

Comparison with other studies

The distribution of resistant *E. coli* in uncomplicated cases is similar to the distribution reported in other studies from Greece, Germany, Austria, Sweden, Portugal and the United Kingdom, in which ampicillin has the highest resistance and nitrofurantoin the lowest resistance rate [13, 17–20]. It confirms that *E. coli* resistant to antibiotics commonly used in primary care is an increasing problem, even in low prevalence settings such as the Danish context.

ESBL-producing *E. coli* was found in both uncomplicated and complicated cases seeking care at primary care level. Previous studies have already pointed out that ESBL-producing *E. coli* strains have the potential for spread beyond the hospital environment [21, 22]. Studies carried out in China [23] and Spain [24] have shown the constant increase of healthy carriers colonized with ESBL-producing *E. coli*. Thus, treating community-acquired urinary tract infections caused by ESBL-producing *E. coli* is a growing problem to be dealt with at primary care level as the therapeutic options are limited [25].

Relevance

In Denmark, there are different guidelines made by different health authorities [26–28]. All guidelines agree on recommending pivmecillinam and sulfametizol as the first line options in patients with suspected uncomplicated UTI. All agree on pivmecillinam as first line options in patients with suspected complicated UTI, while only two suggest trimethroprim as an option too.

IDSA recommends that the selection of empirical antibiotics takes into consideration that resistance rates should not exceed 10% for fluoroquinolones and 20% for trimethoprim-sulfamethoxazole [10].

Based on the results of our study pivmecillinam is a good first option, while the routine use of sulfamethizol needs to be re-considered. In other countries, nitrofurantoin has started to gain importance as part of the first line antibiotics for the management of UTIs in primary care [10, 11]. A recent systematic reviews [29] about the efficacy and toxicity of short-term use (i.e. <14 days) of nitrofurantoin reported no differences in the rates for adverse events when compared to other antimicrobial agents and did not report cases of pulmonary fibrosis and hepatotoxicity.

Another alternative is Fosfomycin [30]. It gives good bacterial coverage with low toxicity and limited effect in fecal flora, although it has low efficacy against *Staphylococcus saprophyticus*. A systematic review reported fewer adverse effect of fosfomycin in pregnant women in comparison to other antibiotics used in primary care [31]. However, fosfomycin is not licensed for use in Denmark; hence, it was not included for assessment in this study.

Conclusion

Antimicrobial resistance is a rising problem that do not belong exclusively to patients attended in secondary care or complicated cases seen in primary care. In uncomplicated cases, there were high resistance rates to antibiotics commonly used in primary care. In Denmark, the National Surveillance program DANMAP can guide the decision for choice of antimicrobial agents in patients with suspected UTI seeking care in primary care.

Abbreviations
cUTI: Complicated Urinary Tract Infection; DANMAP: Danish Programme for surveillance of antimicrobial consumption and resistance in bacteria from animals, food and humans; EUCAST: European Committee on Antimicrobial susceptibility testing; GPs: General Practitioners; IDSA: Infectious Diseases Society of America; SSI: Statens Serum Institute; UTI: Urinary Tract Infection; uUTI: Uncomplicated Urinary Tract Infection

Acknowledgements
We would like to acknowledge the General Practitioners and patients that contributed with data for the study. We would like to thank as well Nadia Xenia Olsen for her excellent technical assistance.

Funding
This study was in part supported by The Danish Ministry of Health as part of the Danish Integrated Antimicrobial Resistance Monitoring and Research Programme (DANMAP), 2016 fund (grant from the University of Copenhagen to promote interdisciplinary research), b) KAP-H (agency for quality in primary care at the capital region), c) læge Sofus Carl Emil Friis og Hustru Olga Doris Friis' legat.

Authors' contributions
GC AH FH AMH LB designed the study and participated in data collection. GC wrote the first draft and all authors critically revised the manuscript and approved the final version.

Consent for publication
not applicable.

Competing interests
The authors declare that they have no competing interests.

Author details
[1]The Research Unit for General Practice and Section of General Practice, Department of Public Health, University of Copenhagen; Øster Farimagsgade 5, 1014 Copenhagen, Denmark. [2]Department for Bacteria, Parasites and Fungi, Statens Serum Institut, Copenhagen, Denmark.

References
1. World Economic Forum. Global Risks 2013. Geneva. 2013. http://www3.weforum.org/docs/WEF_GlobalRisks_Report_2013.pdf. Accessed 8 June 2017.
2. Statens Serum Institut. DANMAP 2014-use of antimicrobial agents and occurrence of antimicrobial resistance in bacteria from food animals, food and humans in Denmark. 2014. http://www.danmap.org/~/media/projekt%20sites/danmap/danmap%20reports/danmap%202014/danmap_2014.ashx. Accessed 8 June 2017.
3. Swedres– Svarm 2014.Consumption of antibiotics and occurrence of antibiotic resistance in Sweden. 2014. http://www.sva.se/globalassets/redesign2011/pdf/om_sva/publikationer/swedres_svarm2014.pdf. Accessed 8 June 2017.
4. O'Brien K, Bellis TW, Kelson M, Hood K, Butler CC, Edwards A. Clinical predictors of antibiotic prescribing for acutely ill children in primary care: an observational study. Br J Gen Pract. 2015;65:e585–92.
5. Pace WD, Dickinson LM, Staton EW. Seasonal variation in diagnoses and visits to family physicians. Ann Fam Med. 2004;2:411–7.
6. Etienne M, Lefebvre E, Frebourg N, Hamel H, Pestel-Caron M, Caron F. Antibiotic treatment of acute uncomplicated cystitis based on rapid urine test and local epidemiology: lessons from a primary care series. BMC Infect Dis. 2014;14:1–8.
7. Schito GC, Naber KG, Botto H, Palou J, Mazzei T, Gualco L, et al. The ARESC study: an international survey on the antimicrobial resistance of pathogens involved in uncomplicated urinary tract infections. Int J Antimicrob Agents. 2009;34:407–13.
8. Allocati N, Masulli M, Alexeyev MF, Di Ilio C. Escherichia coli in Europe: an overview. Int J environ res. Public Health. 2013;10(12):6235–54.
9. The European Antimicrobial Resistance Surveillance Network (EARS-Net). http://www.ecdc.europa.eu/en/activities/surveillance/EARS-Net/Pages/index.aspx. Accessed 8 June 2017.
10. Gupta K, Hooton TM, Naber KG, Wullt B, Colgan R, Miller LG, et al. International clinical practice guidelines for the treatment of acute uncomplicated cystitis and pyelonephritis in women: a 2010 update by the Infectious Diseases Society of America and the European Society for Microbiology and Infectious Diseases. Clin Infect Dis. 2011;52:e103–20.
11. Scotish Intercollegiate Guidelines Network. Management of suspected bacterial urinary tract infection in adults: a national clinical guideline. 2015. http://www.sign.ac.uk/guidelines/fulltext/88/. Accessed 8 June 2017.
12. Hillier S, Bell J, Heginbothom M, Roberts Z, Dunstan F, Howard A, et al. When do general practitioners request urine specimens for microbiology analysis? The applicability of antibiotic resistance surveillance based on routinely collected data. J Antimicrob Chemother. 2006;58:1303–6.
13. Kamenski G, Wagner G, Zehetmayer S, Fink W, Spiegel W, Hoffmann K. Antibacterial resistances in uncomplicated urinary tract infections in women: ECO·SENS II data from primary health care in Austria. BMC Infect Dis. 2012;12:1–8.
14. European Confederation of Laboratory Medicine. European urinanalysis guidelines. Scand J Clin Lab Invest Suppl. 2000;231:1–86.
15. European Committee on Antimicrobial susceptibility testing. www.eucast.org. Accessed 8 June 2017.
16. Johansen TE, Botto H, Cek M, Grabe M, Tenke P, Wagenlehner FM, et al. Critical review of current definitions of urinary tract infections and proposal of an EAU/ESIU classification system. Int J Antimicrob Agents. 2011;38:64–70.
17. Schmiemann G, Gágyor I, Hummers-Pradier E, Bleidorn J. Resistance profiles of urinary tract infections in general practice - an observational study. BMC Urol. 2012;12:1–5.
18. Falagas ME, Polemis M, Alexiou VG, Marini-Mastrogiannaki A, Kremastinou J, Vatopoulos AC. Antimicrobial resistance of Esherichia coli urinary isolates from primary care patients in Greece. Med Sci Monit. 2008;14:Cr75–9.
19. Kahlmeter G, Poulsen HO. Antimicrobial susceptibility of *Escherichia coli* from community-acquired urinary tract infections in Europe: the ECO.SENS study revisited. Int J Antimicrob Agents. 2012;39(1):45–51.
20. Shaifali I, Gupta U, Mahmood SE, Ahmed J. Antibiotic susceptibility patterns of urinary pathogens in female outpatients. N Am J Med Sci. 2012;4:163–9.
21. Pitout JD, Laupland KB. Extended-spectrum β-lactamase-producing Enterobacteriaceae: an emerging public-health concern. Lancet Infect Dis. 2008;8:159–66.
22. Hertz FB, Nielsen JB, Schønning K, Littauer P, Knudsen JD, Løbner-Olesen A, et al. Population structure of drug-susceptible, –resistant and ESBL-producing *Escherichia coli* from community-acquired urinary tract infections. BMC Microbiol. 2016;16:1–6.
23. Tian SF, Chen BY, Chu YZ, Wang S. Prevalence of rectal carriage of extended-spectrum β-lactamase-producing *Escherichia coli* among elderly

Prevalence of antimicrobial resistant Escherichia coli from patients with suspected urinary tract infection...

205

people in community settings in China. Can J Microbiol. 2008;54:781–5.

24. Vinue L, Saenz Y, Martinez S, Somalo S, Moreno MA, Torres C, et al. Prevalence and diversity of extended-spectrum beta-lactamases in faecal *Escherichia coli* isolates from healthy humans in Spain. Clin Microbiol Infect. 2009;15:954–7.

25. Prakash V, Lewis JS, Herrera ML, Wickes BL, Jorgensen JH. Oral and parenteral therapeutic options for outpatient urinary infections caused by Enterobacteriaceae producing CTX-M extended-Spectrum β-Lactamases. Antimicrob Agents Chemother. 2009;53:1278–80.

26. Institute for rational pharmacotherapy. Systemic antibiotics. 2016. http://www. irf.dk/dk/rekommandationsliste/baggrundsnotater/infektionssygdomme/ antibiotika_systemisk_brug.htm. Accessed 8 June 2017.

27. Arendrup K, Arpi M, Lindhardt B, Carlsen C, Unkerskov J, Møller N, Jakobsen H. Guidelines for antibiotic use in General practice - Capital region. 2016. https://www.regionh.dk/til-fagfolk/Sundhed/Sundhedsfaglige-raad- ogkomiteer/klinisk-mikrobiologi/Documents/24-juni-antibiotikavejledning- 20160614.pdf. Accessed 8 June 2017.

28. Region Sjælland. Guideline for use of antibiotics in General Practice - North Region. 2016. http://kap-s.dk/wp-content/uploads/2016/04/infektioner-pjece. pdf. Accessed 8 June 2017.

29. Huttner A, Verhaegh EM, Harbarth S, Muller AE, Theuretzbacher U, Mouton JW. Nitrofurantoin revisited: a systematic review and meta-analysis of controlled trials. J Antimicrob Chemother. 2015;70:2456–64.

30. Sastry S, Doi Y. Fosfomycin: resurgence of an old companion. J Infect Chemother. 2016;22(5):273–80.

31. Falagas ME, Vouloumanou EK, Togias AG, Karadima M, Kapaskelis AM, Rafailidis PI, et al. Fosfomycin versus other antibiotics for the treatment of cystitis: a meta-analysis of randomized controlled trials. J Antimicrob Chemother. 2010;65:1862–77.

Permissions

All chapters in this book were first published in ID, by BioMed Central; hereby published with permission under the Creative Commons Attribution License or equivalent. Every chapter published in this book has been scrutinized by our experts. Their significance has been extensively debated. The topics covered herein carry significant findings which will fuel the growth of the discipline. They may even be implemented as practical applications or may be referred to as a beginning point for another development.

The contributors of this book come from diverse backgrounds, making this book a truly international effort. This book will bring forth new frontiers with its revolutionizing research information and detailed analysis of the nascent developments around the world.

We would like to thank all the contributing authors for lending their expertise to make the book truly unique. They have played a crucial role in the development of this book. Without their invaluable contributions this book wouldn't have been possible. They have made vital efforts to compile up to date information on the varied aspects of this subject to make this book a valuable addition to the collection of many professionals and students.

This book was conceptualized with the vision of imparting up-to-date information and advanced data in this field. To ensure the same, a matchless editorial board was set up. Every individual on the board went through rigorous rounds of assessment to prove their worth. After which they invested a large part of their time researching and compiling the most relevant data for our readers.

The editorial board has been involved in producing this book since its inception. They have spent rigorous hours researching and exploring the diverse topics which have resulted in the successful publishing of this book. They have passed on their knowledge of decades through this book. To expedite this challenging task, the publisher supported the team at every step. A small team of assistant editors was also appointed to further simplify the editing procedure and attain best results for the readers.

Apart from the editorial board, the designing team has also invested a significant amount of their time in understanding the subject and creating the most relevant covers. They scrutinized every image to scout for the most suitable representation of the subject and create an appropriate cover for the book.

The publishing team has been an ardent support to the editorial, designing and production team. Their endless efforts to recruit the best for this project, has resulted in the accomplishment of this book. They are a veteran in the field of academics and their pool of knowledge is as vast as their experience in printing. Their expertise and guidance has proved useful at every step. Their uncompromising quality standards have made this book an exceptional effort. Their encouragement from time to time has been an inspiration for everyone.

The publisher and the editorial board hope that this book will prove to be a valuable piece of knowledge for researchers, students, practitioners and scholars across the globe.

List of Contributors

Ramandeep Singh, Frederike J. Bemelman and Ineke J. M. ten Berge
Department of Internal Medicine, Renal transplant Unit, Division of Nephrology, Academic Medical Center – University of Amsterdam, The Netherlands

Caspar J. Hodiamont
Department of Medical Microbiology, Academic Medical Center – University of Amsterdam, The Netherlands

Mirza M. Idu
Department of Surgery, Division of Vascular Surgery, Academic Medical Center – University of Amsterdam, The Netherlands

Suzanne E. Geerlings
Department of Internal Medicine, Division of Infectious Diseases, Academic Medical Center- University of Amsterdam, The Netherlands

Marya D. Zilberberg
EviMed Research Group, LLC, Goshen, MA 01032, USA

Brian H. Nathanson
OptiStatim, LLC, Longmeadow, MA 01116, USA

Kate Sulham and Weihong Fan
The Medicines Company, 8 Sylvan Way, Parsippany, NJ 07054, USA

Andrew F. Shorr
Washington Hospital Center, 110 Irving St. NW, Washington, DC 20010, USA

Catherine Zatorski and Gillian Brooks
Department of Emergency Medicine, The George Washington University, 2120 L Street, NW Suite 4-450, Washington, DC 20037, USA

Mark Zocchi
Center for Healthcare Innovation & Policy Research, The George Washington University, 2100 Pennsylvania Avenue Suite 300, Washington, DC 20037, USA

Sara E. Cosgrove
Department of Medicine, Division of Infectious Diseases, Johns Hopkins Medical Institutions, Osler 425, 600 N. Wolfe St., Baltimore, MD 21287, USA

Cynthia Rand
Division of Pulmonary and Critical Care Medicine, The Johns Hopkins Institutions, 5501 Hopkins Bayview Circle, Baltimore, MD 21224, USA

Larissa May
Department of Emergency Medicine, UC Davis Medical Center, 4150 V Street, Suite 2100, Sacramento, CA 95817, USA

M. M. P. S. C. Fernando, J. K. N. D. Miththinda, R. D. S. S. Wickramasinghe, B. S. Sebastiampillai, M. P. M. L. Gunathilake and F. H. D. S. Silva
Professorial Medical Unit, North Colombo Teaching Hospital, Ragama, Sri Lanka

W. A. N. V. Luke
Department of Clinical Pharmacology, Faculty of Medicine, University of Kelaniya, Kelaniya, Sri Lanka

R. Premaratna
Department of Medicine, Faculty of Medicine, University of Kelaniya, Kelaniya, Sri Lanka

Monique R. Bidell and Thomas P. Lodise
Albany College of Pharmacy and Health Sciences, 106 New Scotland Avenue, Albany 12208-3492, NY, USA

Melissa Palchak Opraseuth, Min Yoon and John Mohr
Merck & Co., Inc., Kenilworth, NJ, USA

Dean Ironmonger and Obaghe Edeghere
Field Epidemiology Service, Public Health England, 5 St Philips Place, Birmingham, UK

Savita Gossain
Public Health Laboratory, Public Health England, Heart of England NHS Foundation Trust, Birmingham, UK

Peter M. Hawkey
Public Health Laboratory, Public Health England, Heart of England NHS Foundation Trust, Birmingham, UK
Institute of Microbiology and Infection, Biosciences, University of Birmingham, Birmingham, UK

Joel Manyahi and Sabrina J. Moyo
Department of Clinical Science, University of Bergen, Bergen, Norway
Department of Microbiology and Immunology, Muhimbili University of Health and Allied Sciences, Dar es Salaam, Tanzania

Bjørn Blomberg and Nina Langeland
epartment of Clinical Science, University of Bergen, Bergen, Norway
National Centre for Tropical Infectious Diseases, Department of Medicine, Haukeland University Hospital, Bergen, Norway

Faustine Ndugulile and Willy Urassa
Department of Microbiology and Immunology, Muhimbili University of Health and Allied Sciences, Dar es Salaam, Tanzania

Marit Gjerde Tellevik
National Centre for Tropical Infectious Diseases, Department of Medicine, Haukeland University Hospital, Bergen, Norway

Matifan Dereje
Department of medicine, Collages of medicine and health sciences, Ambo University, Ambo, Ethiopia

Yimtubezinesh Woldeamanuel and Daneil Asrat
Department of Microbiology, Immunology & Parasitology, School of Medicine, Addis Ababa University, Addis Ababa, Ethiopia

Fekade Ayenachew
Addis Ababa Hamlin Fistula Hospital, Addis Ababa, Ethiopia

Teresa L Kauf
Shire International GmbH, Zug, Switzerland

Rebekah H. Borse and Shuvayu S. Sen
Merck & Co., Inc., Kenilworth, NJ, USA

Goran Medic and Jennifer Gaultney
MAPI Group, Houten, The Netherlands

Benjamin Miller
Shire, Lexington, MA, USA

Anirban Basu
University of Washington, Seattle, WA, USA

Vimalanand S. Prabhu
Merck & Co., Inc., Kenilworth, NJ, USA
Merck & Co., Inc., 2000 Galloping Hill Rd., Kenilworth, NJ 07033, USA

Eliana S. Armstrong, Janelle A. Mikulca, Daniel J. Cloutier, Caleb A. Bliss and Judith N. Steenbergen
Merck & Co., Inc., 2000 Galloping Hill Road, Kenilworth, NJ 07033, USA

Aurélien Dinh, Constance Blanc, Alexis Descatha and Jérôme Salomon
Infectious Disease Unit, Garches PIFO University Hospital, AP-HP, Versailles Saint Quentin University, Garches, France

Adnène Toumi
Infectious Diseases Unit, University Hospital, Monastir, Tunisia

Frédérique Bouchand
Pharmacy, University Hospital, AP-HP, Versailles Saint Quentin University, Garches, France

Thomas Hanslik
Internal Medicine Unit, University Hospital, AP-HP, Versailles Saint Quentin University, Boulogne-Billancourt, France

Benjamin Bernuz and Pierre Denys
Physical Medicine and Rehabilitation Department, University Hospital, AP-HP, Versailles Saint Quentin University, Garches, France

Louis Bernard
Infectious Disease Unit, Bretonneau University Hospital, Tours, France

Sebastiaan Hermanus Johannes Zegers and Jeanne Dieleman
Máxima Medical Center, Veldhoven, The Netherlands

Tjomme van der Bruggen
University Medical Center, Utrecht, The Netherlands

Jan Kimpen and Catharine de Jong-de Vos van Steenwijk
Wilhelmina Children's Hospital, University Medical Center, Utrecht, The Netherlands

Siobhan Kavanagh and Jérôme P. Fennell
Department of Clinical Microbiology, AMNCH, Tallaght Hospital, Dublin 24, Ireland

Fardod O'Kelly, Rustom Manecksha and John Thornhill
Department of Urological Surgery, AMNCH, Tallaght Hospital, Dublin 24, Ireland

Qiwen Yang, Hui Zhang, Yao Wang, Zhipeng Xu, Ge Zhang, Xinxin Chen and Yingchun Xu
Department of Clinical Laboratory, Peking Union Medical College Hospital, Peking Union Medical College, Chinese Academy of Medical Sciences, Beijing 100730, China

Bin Cao
Department of Respiratory and Critical Care Medicine, Clinical Microbiology and Infectious Disease Lab., China-Japan Friendship Hospital, Beijing 100029, China

Haishen Kong
Department of Microbiology, The First Affiliated Hospital of Zhejiang University, Hangzhou 310003, China

Yuxing Ni
Division of Microbiology, Ruijin Hospital, School of Medicine, Shanghai Jiaotong University, Shanghai 200025, China

Yunsong Yu
Department of Infectious Diseases, SirRunRun Shaw Hospital, School of Medicine, Zhejiang University, Hangzhou 310016, China

Ziyong Sun
Department of Laboratory Medicine, Tongji Hospital, Tongji Medical College, Huazhong University of Science and Technology, Wuhan 430030, China

Qiong Duan
Microbiology Lab, Jilin Province People's Hospital, Changchun 130021, China

Shufang Zhang
Division of Microbiology, Haikou People's Hospital, Haikou 570208, China

Haifeng Shao
Division of Microbiology, General Hospital of Nanjing Military Command, Nanjing 210002, China

Robert E. Badal
Division of Microbiology, International Health Management Associates, Schaumburg, IL 60173-3817, USA

Lucinda K. Barrett, Stephanie Warren, Matthew Scarborough and Nicola Jones
Department of Infectious Diseases and Microbiology, Oxford University Hospitals NHS Foundation Trust, John Radcliffe Hospital, Headley Way, Headington, Oxford OX3 9DU, UK

Philippa C. Matthews and Nicole Stoesser
Department of Infectious Diseases and Microbiology, Oxford University Hospitals NHS Foundation Trust, John Radcliffe Hospital, Headley Way, Headington, Oxford OX3 9DU, UK
Nuffield Department of Medicine, University of Oxford, Peter Medawar Building for Pathogen Research, South Parks Road, Oxford OX1 3SY, UK

Mel Snelling
Pharmacy Department, Oxford University Hospitals NHS Foundation Trust, John Radcliffe Hospital, Headley Way, Headington, Oxford OX3 9DU, UK

Yu Bin Seo and Jacob Lee
Division of Infectious Diseases, Department of Internal Medicine, Kangnam Sacred Heart Hospital, Hallym University College of Medicine, Seoul, Republic of Korea

Young Keun Kim and Hyo Youl Kim
Department of Internal Medicine, Yonsei University Wonju College of Medicine, Wonju, Republic of Korea

Seung Soon Lee and Jeong-a Lee
Division of Infectious Diseases, Department of Internal Medicine, Hallym University Sacred Heart Hospital, Hallym University College of Medicine, Seoul, Republic of Korea

Young Uh
Department of Laboratory Medicine, Yonsei University Wonju College of Medicine, Wonju, Republic of Korea

Han-Sung Kim
Department of Laboratory Medicine, Hallym University Sacred Heart Hospital, Hallym University College of Medicine, Seoul, Republic of Korea

Wonkeun Song
Department of Laboratory Medicine, Kangnam Sacred Heart Hospital, Hallym University College of Medicine, 1 Shingil-ro, Youngdeungpo-gu, Seoul 150-950, Korea

Kedar Diwakar Mandakhalikar and Paul A. Tambyah
Department of Medicine, Yong Loo Lin School of Medicine, National University of Singapore, 1E, Kent Ridge Road, NUHS Tower Block, Level 10, Singapore 119228, Singapore

Rong Wang
ACI Medical Pte Ltd, Singapore 069534, Singapore

Juwita N. Rahmat and Edmund Chiong
Department of Surgery, Yong Loo Lin School of Medicine, National University of Singapore, Singapore 119228, Singapore

Koon Gee Neoh
Department of Chemical and Biomolecular Engineering, National University of Singapore, Singapore 117585, Singapore

Adane Bitew
Department of Medical Laboratory Sciences, College of Health Sciences, Addis Ababa University, Addis Ababa, Ethiopia

Tamirat Molalign
Department of Medical Laboratory, St. Peter Tuberculosis Specialized Hospital, Addis Ababa, Ethiopia

Meseret Chanie
Arsho Advanced Medical Laboratory Private Limited Company, Addis Ababa, Ethiopia

Ibrahim H. Babikir
College of Medical Laboratory Sciences, Microbiology Department, University of Khartoum, Khartoum, Sudan
College of Medicine, Qassim University, Buraydah, Qassim, Kingdom of Saudi Arabia

Elsir A. Abugroun
Faculty of Medical Laboratory Sciences, University of Science and Technology, Omdurman, Sudan

Naser Eldin Bilal
Khartoum University Central Research Laboratory, University of Khartoum, Khartoum, Sudan

Abdullah Ali Alghasham, Elmuataz Elmansi Abdalla and Ishag Adam
College of Medicine, Qassim University, Buraydah, Qassim, Kingdom of Saudi Arabia

Sebastian Bischoff, Matthias Ebert and Roger Vogelmann
Second Department of Internal Medicine, University Medical Center Mannheim, Medical Faculty Mannheim, Heidelberg University, Theodor-Kutzer Ufer 1-3, D-68167 Mannheim, Germany

Thomas Walter
Emergency Department, University Medical Center Mannheim, Medical Faculty Mannheim, Heidelberg University, Theodor-Kutzer Ufer 1-3, D-68167 Mannheim, Germany

Marlis Gerigk
Department of Microbiology, University Medical Center Mannheim, Medical Faculty Mannheim, Heidelberg University, Theodor-Kutzer Ufer 1-3, D-68167 Mannheim, Germany

Janneke E. Stalenhoef, Willize E. van der Starre and Albert M. Vollaard
Department of Infectious Diseases, Leiden University Medical Center, C5-P, the Netherlands

Ewout W. Steyerberg
Department of Public Health, Erasmus MC - University Medical Center Rotterdam, Rotterdam, The Netherlands

Nathalie M. Delfos
Dept of Internal Medicine, Alrijne Hospital, Leiderdorp, The Netherlands

Eliane M.S. Leyten, Jan W. van't Wout and Jaap T. van Dissel
Dept of Internal Medicine, MCH-Bronovo, The Hague, The Netherlands

Ted Koster
Dept of Internal Medicine, Groene Hart Hospital, Gouda, The Netherlands

Hans C. Ablij
Dept of Internal Medicine, Alrijne Hospital, Leiden, The Netherlands

Cees van Nieuwkoop
Dept of Internal Medicine, Haga Hospital, The Hague, The Netherlands

Hui Zhang, Qiwen Yang and Yingchun Xu
Division of Microbiology, Peking Union Medical College Hospital, Peking Union Medical College, Chinese Academy of Medical Sciences, No. 1 Shuaifuyuan, Wangfujing Street, Beijing 100730, China

Haishen Kong
Department of Microbiology, The First Affiliated Hospital of Zhejiang University, Hangzhou 310003, China

Yunsong Yu
Department of Infectious Diseases, SirRunRun Shaw Hospital, School of Medicine, Zhejiang University, Hangzhou 310016, China

Anhua Wu
Infection Control Center, Xiangya Hospital, Central South University, Changsha 410008, China

Qiong Duan
Microbiology Laboratory, Jilin Province People's Hospital, Changchun 130021, China

Xiaofeng Jiang
The Fourth Hospital of Harbin Medical University, No. 37 Yiyuan Road, Nangang District, Harbin, China

Shufang Zhang
Division of Microbiology, Haikou People's Hospital, Haikou 570208, China

Ziyong Sun
Department of Laboratory Medicine, Tongji Hospital, Tongji Medical College, Huazhong University of Science and Technology, Wuhan 430030, China

Yuxing Ni
Division of Microbiology, Ruijin Hospital, School of Medicine, Shanghai Jiaotong University, Shanghai 200025, China

Weiping Wang
Nanjing General Hospital, No. 305 Zhongshan Dong Road, Nanjing, China

Yong Wang
Department of Laboratory Medicine, Shandong Provincial Hospital Affiliated to Shandong University, Jinan 250021, China

Kang Liao
Division of Microbiology, The First Affiliated Hospital, Sun Yat-Sen University, Guangzhou 510080, China

Chunxia Yang
Beijing Chao-yang Hospital, 8 Gongren Tiyuchang Nanlu, Chaoyang District, Beijing 100020, China

Wenxiang Huang
Division of Microbiology, The First Affiliated Hospital of Chongqing Medical University, Chongqing 400016, China

Bingdong Gui
Clinical laboratory, The Second Affiliated Hospital of Nanchang University, Nanchang 330006, China

Bin Shan
First Affiliated Hospital of Kunming Medical University, No. 295 Xichang Road, Kunming 650032, China

Robert Badal
Division of Microbiology, International Health Management Associates, Schaumburg, IL 60173-3817, USA

Wubalem Desta Seifu
Department of Biotechnology, Wolkite University, Wolkite, Ethiopia

Alemayehu Desalegn Gebissa
Department of Biology, Haramaya University, Alemaya, Ethiopia

Yalda Malekzadegan, Reza Khashei and Hadi Sedigh Ebrahim-Saraie
Department of Bacteriology and Virology, School of Medicine, Shiraz University of Medical Sciences, Shiraz, Iran

Zahra Jahanabadi
Department of Urology, School of Medicine, Shiraz University of Medical Sciences, Shiraz, Iran

Gloria Córdoba, Anne Holm and Lars Bjerrum
The Research Unit for General Practice and Section of General Practice, Department of Public Health, University of Copenhagen; Øster Farimagsgade 5, 1014 Copenhagen, Denmark

Frank Hansen and Anette M. Hammerum
Department for Bacteria, Parasites and Fungi, Statens Serum Institut, Copenhagen, Denmark

Index

A

Allograft Pyelonephritis, 1-2, 4, 9

Amikacin, 33, 35-36, 40, 92-94, 104-107, 111, 125, 131, 175, 180, 192, 194, 196

Aminoglycosides, 15-16, 19, 34, 36-37, 52-53, 84-86, 93-95, 98, 125

Amoxicillin-clavulanic Acid, 3, 5, 9, 55, 58, 61, 63-64, 201

Anti-encrustation Silver Nanoparticle, 133

Antibiotic Prophylaxis, 10, 88, 91-96

Antimicrobial Resistance, 1-3, 5, 8-11, 20, 22-23, 25, 31, 38-39, 44-46, 51, 55-57, 63, 72, 74, 80, 96, 102, 105, 107, 112, 121-123, 146, 158, 164, 174, 181, 189-194, 196, 198, 202, 204

Asymptomatic Bacteriuria, 1-2, 4, 9-10, 63-64, 85-86, 121, 196, 198

Aztreonam, 16, 19, 69-70, 115, 125

B

Bacterial Biofilms, 133, 137, 141

C

C-reactive Protein, 83, 119, 159-160, 173

Carbapenem Resistance, 11-12, 20, 33-34, 37, 40, 112, 179

Cathelicidin, 150-151, 154-156

Cefazolin, 40, 92-93, 144, 146

Cefotaxime, 40, 53, 55-56, 98, 105-108, 111, 115, 125, 175, 180, 202

Cephalosporins, 16, 19, 23, 34-36, 40, 43, 52-53, 85, 92, 98, 105-106, 108, 111, 115, 125, 130, 132, 145, 158, 161-163, 174-175, 177, 180, 196, 202-203

Charlson Comorbidity Index, 15, 124-129

Citrobacter Freundii, 13, 55, 91, 93, 106, 131, 143, 177

Clean Intermittent Bladder Catheterization, 88

Co-amoxiclav, 97, 99-100, 102, 115

Cystitis, 1-5, 7-8, 24-32, 38, 45, 80, 86, 102, 105, 109, 112, 134, 140, 142, 148, 154, 173, 184, 190-195, 197-198, 201, 204-205

Cytomegalovirus, 2, 4, 9-10

D

Dermacoccus Nishinomiyaensis, 182, 184-185, 187-188

E

Enterobacter Cloacae, 13, 54, 91, 93, 106-108, 112, 131, 143, 153, 175, 177

Enterobacteriaceae, 11-13, 15, 17, 20-21, 23, 36, 39-40, 43, 52-54, 56-57, 67, 75-79, 86, 91, 97-99, 101-102, 104-109, 111-112, 114, 117-118, 120-123, 131-132, 164, 174-181, 198, 205

Enterococcus Faecalis, 153, 155

Enzyme-linked Immunosorbent Assay, 155

Ertapenem, 13, 36, 38, 40, 72, 75, 104-109, 111-112, 118, 124-129, 174-175, 179-180

Escherichia Coli, 5, 8-10, 13, 23, 28, 31, 40, 43, 45, 51, 54, 57, 65, 71, 81, 88, 90, 97, 100, 104, 106, 109, 113, 117, 125, 132, 140, 148, 153, 157, 160, 164, 170, 177, 182, 184, 189, 192, 201, 204-205

Extended Spectrum Beta Lactamase, 33, 37-38, 102

F

Facultative Gram-negative Bacilli, 104-105

Febrile Urinary Tract Infection, 82, 84-85, 164-166, 171-173

Fluoroquinolones, 25, 31, 34-36, 39-40, 42, 53, 57, 76-77, 80-81, 84-85, 92, 95, 98, 103, 105-106, 108-109, 111, 122, 158-159, 162-163, 174-175, 177, 192, 196, 203

G

Gentamicin, 38, 40, 52-56, 58-59, 61, 63-64, 92-94, 125, 144-147, 158-163, 182-183, 187-188, 192, 194, 196

Glomerular Filtration Rate, 114, 118-119, 122, 159-160, 163

Gram-negative Pathogens, 11, 39-40, 42, 52, 57, 66-67, 69, 71, 96, 111, 122-123, 164, 174

I

Imipenem, 13, 21, 33, 35-36, 40, 53-55, 69-70, 78, 104-109, 111, 125, 159-162, 174-175, 179-180, 191-192, 194, 196-197

Inappropriate Empiric Therapy, 11-12, 17, 20-22

Initial Appropriate Antibiotic Therapy, 66, 70, 74

Intra-abdominal Infections, 74, 105, 112, 174, 180-181

K

Klebsiella Oxytoca, 13, 57, 91, 93, 105-106, 143, 153, 174

Klebsiella Pneumonia, 143

L

Leuconostoc Species, 182, 184, 188

Leukocyte Count, 83-84

Levofloxacin, 35-36, 40, 69-70, 72, 75-81, 92, 94, 104-105, 107, 109, 111, 144, 146, 173, 175, 180

Linezolid, 144-147

M

Mecillinam, 97-103, 201

Meropenem, 13, 33, 35-37, 40, 68-71, 92-93, 118, 122

Minimum Inhibitory Concentration, 44, 76-77, 79-80, 105, 115, 122, 192, 197

Morganella Morganii, 13, 118, 153, 155

Multi-drug Resistance, 159, 196-197

N

Neurogenic Bladder, 82-86, 96

Nitrofurantoin, 3, 5, 9, 25-28, 33, 35, 53-56, 61, 63-64, 90, 92, 94-96, 103, 108, 114-115, 117, 119-121, 123, 131, 144-147, 182-183, 187-188, 192, 194, 196-197, 199, 201-203, 205

O

Obstetric Fistula, 58-59, 61-62, 64-65

Oral Fosfomycin, 113-114, 116-118, 121-122

P

Piperacillin, 37-38, 40, 42-43, 66-75, 92-93, 104-107, 111, 115, 124-125, 127-132, 142, 144-147, 158-161, 163-164, 175, 180

Pivmecillinam, 97-99, 101-103, 114-115, 120, 123, 202-203

Pneumocystis Jiroveci Pneumonia, 1-2, 9

Pneumonia Severity Index, 165-166, 170, 172-173

Polydopamine, 133-134, 140

Porcine Model, 133-137, 140

Proteus Mirabilis, 13, 21, 71, 90-91, 93, 98, 104, 106, 108-109, 112, 134, 141, 143, 153, 156, 160, 174, 177

Pyelonephritis, 1-2, 4, 7, 9-10, 24-32, 34-35, 45, 75-78, 80-82, 86-87, 105, 109, 112, 114, 131, 142, 154, 156, 159-160, 164, 171-173, 184, 190-198, 201, 204

Q

Quinolones, 34, 52, 98, 189, 197

R

Recto-vaginal Fistula, 58-59

S

Salmonella Typhimurium, 182, 184-185, 188

Sepsis, 11-13, 15-17, 19-23, 34, 36, 38, 82, 86-87, 114, 142, 166, 172

Serratia Odorifera, 175

Spina Bifida, 88-92, 94-96

Staphylococcus Species, 182, 184

Sulfamethoxazole, 1-2, 4, 9-10, 25, 31, 40, 43, 45, 52-56, 74, 87, 92, 94-95, 108, 125, 142, 144-147, 183, 187, 192, 194, 197, 201-203

Sulphydryl Variable, 98

T

Tazobactam, 37-38, 40, 42-43, 66-78, 80, 92-93, 104-107, 111, 124-125, 127-132, 142, 144-147, 158-161, 163-164, 175, 180

Temoneira, 98, 102

Trimethoprim-sulfamethoxazole, 1-2, 4, 9-10, 25, 31, 45, 52-56, 74, 87, 108, 125, 203

U

Urinary Catheter, 83, 133, 158-163, 169

Uropathogens, 24-25, 38, 56, 64, 81, 90-93, 95-96, 98, 108-109, 111, 113, 115, 122, 134, 142-143, 147-149, 154-155, 182-185, 187-190, 201

Urosepsis, 113, 118, 159, 172, 191-196

V

Vancomycin, 102, 142, 144, 146-147, 182-183, 187-188

Vesico-ureteral Reflux, 89

Virulence Genes, 191-194, 196, 198

Vitek-2 Compact System, 152, 156

www.ingramcontent.com/pod-product-compliance
Lightning Source LLC
Chambersburg PA
CBHW082039190326
41458CB00010B/3411